IF WE CAN LOVE

The Mennonite Mental Health Story

Vernon H. Neufeld, Editor

Library of Congress Number 82-083885
International Standard Book Number 0-87303-074-5
Printing in the United States of America
Copyright © 1983 by Faith and Life Press, 718 Main Street, Newton, Kansas 67114

Design by John Hiebert
Printed by Mennonite Press, Inc.

"If we can love: this is the touchstone. This is the key to all the therapeutic program of the modern psychiatric hospital; it dominates the behavior of its staff from director down to gardener. To our patient who cannot love, we must say by our actions that we do love him. 'You can be angry here if you must be; we know you have been wronged. We know too, that your anger will arouse our anger and that you will be wronged again and disappointed again and rejected again and driven mad once more. But we are not angry—and you won't be either, after a while. We are your friends; those about you are all friends; you can relax your defenses and your tensions. As you—and we—come to understand your life better, the warmth of love will begin to replace your present anguish and you will find yourself getting well.' "

—Karl A. Menninger, M.D.

Foreword

The Mennonite Mental Health Story is an exciting story. How much has happened in so short a span of time!

I recall how little we knew about mental illness during our younger years and up to the mid-1930s. We did not know how to deal with persons afflicted with mental disorders except to commit them to state mental hospitals. We did not understand moods of depression, melancholy or despondency. We tended to ignore persons so afflicted or else treat them with a patronizing, judgmental condescension: Why didn't they use willpower to control their "moods" or compensate for their inadequacies?

My own boyhood experience made me sensitively aware of the tragic plight of the mentally ill. The family circles of two of my young friends had to go through the agony of seeing the father in one instance and the mother in another taken from the home and committed to the state *insane asylum* as it was called. I learned something then of the heartbreak and the helpless hopelessness that this involved.

During the years 1936 to 39 my assignment as field secretary of the General Conference Mennonite Church caused me to travel extensively among Russian Mennonite refugees in Canada, Brazil, and Paraguay, victims of horrendous violence during the Russian Revolution. These refugees in conversation often referred to "Bethania," their small mental hospital in Russia. They always spoke of it with pride and gratitude for the service it had rendered mentally ill, epileptic, and retarded persons. What they apparently appreciated most of all was its spirit of caring which surrounded every patient with love and hopefulness and a sense of dignity as a human being.

This made me increasingly sensitive to the fact that in the United States and Canada we also had real mental health problems but as churches we were providing very little care for the mentally ill. I sometimes wondered why. Were we afraid to tackle the problem? Or did we fail to see the problem?

Then the pressures and the disorders of World War II were upon us. Suddenly Mennonite conscientious objectors by the hundreds were working in government mental hospitals in the United States and Canada. How did we get there? We certainly had not planned for it. Actually we landed in the mental hospital program by way of a detour, very similar to the way in which the Apostle Paul landed in Troas. In his mission he had set his sights on Ephesus and Bithynia, but in each instance his plans were thwarted. He landed in Troas, a dirty, dreary old harbor town. He did not want to go to Troas. He had great plans for Ephesus and Bithynia. But it was in Troas that he heard a call, clear and strong, "Come over here. We need you." And Troas turned out to be the gateway to the most significant ministry of his whole life.

During the war we also had our plans. Men in the Civilian Public Service wanted meaningful service, to witness in centers of tension and suffering, but strange circumstances arose to frustrate our brave purposes and plans. One of the most disheartening blows to strike down our high hopes came when the Starnes Amendment forbade all use of conscientious objectors in foreign service. Detouring around frustrating government imposed regulations we finally landed in Staunton, Virginia, August 1942. In a way that was our Troas, because the situation in that mental hospital was so frustrating it almost made us sick. But work in mental hospitals became for us the gateway to a service of profound significance and one which more than any other single experience sparked the Mennonite Central Committee mental health program.

It was surprising and exhilarating to discover young men and young women "seeing visions," Mennonites being inspired to sponsor a mental health service in line with the best of our Mennonite heritage. But there is more. In this same strategic time we hear of "old men" (and women), leaders among their people, "dreaming dreams" (cf. Joel 2:28), that God in his providence appeared to be calling Mennonites to such a mental health venture. And the young and the old learned about each other. What a combination! Young people with vision, drive and creative spirit, and older people with experience, dreams, and a sense of mission, contributing support, counsel, and cash to a venture of faith. Somehow we found one another and our thoughts and efforts were united in this new venture of faith which became the Mennonite mental health story. Clearly, the MMHS venture was "an idea whose time had come." Thank God for the work of his providence in all this undertaking.

Henry A. Fast

Preface

Although I served in Civilian Public Service units during World War II, I didn't understand the impact of Mennonite leadership in the national and international arena of mental health until I served on the MMHS board.

Now, after nine years of direct involvement and close observation, I am deeply moved by how caring and sensitive administrators and staff, motivated by Christian concern, have modeled new therapeutic communities across our continent in response to a crying need of modern society.

MMHS board members felt the urgent need to record this history before the early founders and leaders are gone. The administrators accepted the challenge. *If We Can Love* is the story of a modern miracle—the miracle of love combined with high professional standards in a healing ministry.

—Wesley Prieb[1]

Late in 1979, at the urging of board members like Wesley Prieb, Mennonite Mental Health Services (MMHS) appointed an Editorial Committee composed of Prieb, A. J. Klassen, and Vernon Neufeld to develop a proposal for the MMHS History Project. The next spring MMHS approved a three-fold project: (1) to prepare a comprehensive bibliography of materials related to Mennonites and mental health, (2) to publish a book on the Mennonite mental health experience, and (3) to cooperate with the editor of *Mennonite Quarterly Review* (MQR) in publishing scholarly papers relating to mental health.

The first and third tasks were completed with the January 1982 issue of MQR.[2] This issue presented nine papers on a variety of subjects—historical, theoretical, and practical. Perhaps most significant,certainly for the future, the issue included the most comprehensive bibliography ever compiled of published and unpublished materials related to Mennonite mental health (pp. 116-44). MMHS is indebted to John Oyer, editor, and the staff of MQR for their cooperation and help in the project.

The other task, to record the Mennonite mental health experience, has been completed with the publication of the present book, *If We Can Love.*

In planning and preparing the manuscript, the Editorial Committee agreed to aim for a general readership rather than a more specialized one. Two needs were apparent. One was to inform the church constituency, particularly the younger generation, about what happened in one aspect of the church's mission. The other was to provide information and an historical perspective for the board and staff members of the MMHS centers, especially for use in the orientation of new members. And beyond these potential readers, of course, the committee hoped many who work or are interested in mental health would find the book interesting and informative.

The plan of the book, indicated by the four major sections, is to accomplish four objectives: (1) To provide an adequate background and context for the mental health story in the section called, "How We Started." (2) To tell the story of each of the eight centers or hospitals, under the heading, "How Our Centers Developed." (3) To evaluate the Mennonite mental health experience, using five different themes in the section called, "What We Learned." And finally (4) to have four persons, from different backgrounds and experiences who are not directly connected with MMHS, share their views under the title, "What Others Say."

From the broad, diversified and detailed experiences potentially a part of the Mennonite mental health story, the committee needed to set limits. It was agreed that this account in essence would be the story of MMHS — its origin in the Mennonite Central Committee (MCC), the story of the MCC centers and those independent institutions which joined MMHS. There are other Mennonite programs which might come under this title, but this history follows the MCC-MMHS line of development. The story is also limited to Canada and the United States; it does not include, for example, Paraguay, where an entirely new mental health experience is unfolding, with some ties to MMHS. Moreover, there are Mennonite programs and institutions, some even under MCC or with relationships to MMHS, which work with mentally retarded and other developmentally disabled persons, but the book is limited to efforts in the mental health area. And then, what was most difficult, limits needed to be set on the space allocated to each chapter. What might be volumes needed to be reduced to chapters. The task of condensing so rich and vast an experience was not easy.

The project of publishing the Mennonite mental health story required the effort and cooperation of many people, too many to name individually. Besides the authors named with each chapter, numerous persons at each center helped with research, preparing and reviewing the manuscript. Special recognition is due the members of the Editorial Committee: Wesley Prieb, Larry Yoder, and A. J. Klassen, who was replaced midway through the project by Elmer

Ediger. Their help in planning the book and in reading and rereading the manuscript was indispensable. The role of the editor at times infringed upon the writer's task, and he became more involved than might usually be expected. This was due to a variety of reasons—meeting deadlines, providing additional information, assisting with the writing task.

Finally, and certainly not least important, we express the gratitude of MMHS for those who made this project possible financially. The Mennonite Mutual Aid Fraternal Activities Program provided a significant grant in support of the project. The Mennonite Central Committee, in supporting the outreach efforts of MMHS, also financially underwrote the publication of the book. And the MMHS centers, by allocating hours of staff time and/or funds, cooperated fully and helped make possible the completion of the history project.

Vernon H. Neufeld, Editor

Table of Contents

What We Learned

What Others Say

How We Started

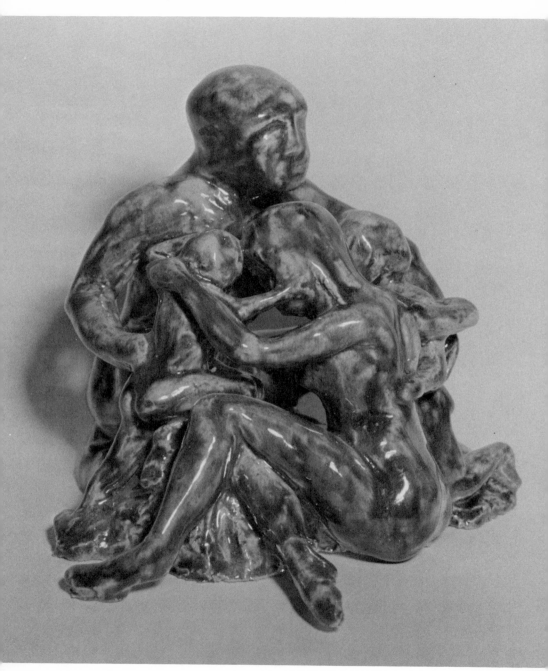

"If we can love," a work of art by a patient at Prairie View.

CHAPTER 1

Roots of the Mennonite Mental Health Story
Elmer M. Ediger*

With only a few church-related psychiatric hospitals in the United States and Canada, it is significant that more than half are Mennonite-related. Who then are the Mennonites and how did they become involved in mental health services?

Scattered around the world, Mennonites have a membership of approximately 500,000 persons. Historically, the heaviest concentrations have been in Switzerland, the Netherlands, Germany, Russia, United States, Canada, Paraguay, and Mexico. As a result of mission activities during the last hundred years, about half of the total membership is located in Africa, Asia, and Latin America.

The Mennonite church began in central Europe in the early 1500s. Originally, they were known as *Anabaptists* because they rebaptized persons as adults who had previously been baptized as infants. Luther, Calvin, and Zwingli, the early Reformation leaders, separated from the Catholic church, preaching salvation by grace through personal faith. However, they continued seeking the power of the church over a given geographical area and a mandatory type of church membership. The early Anabaptist leaders believed the Reformers had not gone far enough in their reforms; consequently, they withdrew from the mainline movements in order to realize their vision of what it meant to be adult followers of Christ and a church of believers. They particularly emphasized the principles of religious freedom of conscience for themselves and others, the separation of church and state, and volunteerism in religion.

The Anabaptists spread rapidly through central Europe. Because of their potential threat to the church and governmental structures of the day, they suffered severe persecution, particularly

*Elmer M. Ediger is Executive Director of Prairie View, Newton, Kansas. Paul W. Pruyser, Ph.D., psychologist, author and theologian of the Menninger Foundation, served as a special resource in the preparation of this historical survey.

3

from 1527 to 1560. A governmental decree in 1529 ordered that "every Anabaptist and rebaptized person of either sex should be put to death by fire, sword, or some other way."[1]

Harold S. Bender in his classic statement, "The Anabaptist Vision," makes the bold declaration that for the Anabaptist the essence of Christianity was discipleship, a way of life seeking to apply love in all human conduct and thus the Christianization of all human relationships. The great word of Anabaptists was not *faith* as it was for the Reformers, but *following Christ*.[2] The church was to be a sharing type of brotherhood in order to provide the support needed to live the life of love. Such an Anabaptist vision renewed by Bender and others during World War II served as the seedbed for a variety of new Mennonite efforts including the worldwide programs of relief and the cause of mental health.

Because of their emphasis upon Christian pacifism and the refusal to go to war, Mennonites are known as a *peace church* along with the Friends and the Church of the Brethren. During World War II at least half of the Mennonite young men registered as conscientious objectors and worked in Civilian Public Service as an alternative to the military. Beginning with World War I, and particularly since World War II, Mennonites have given expression to their belief in love and the way of peace through an extensive worldwide relief service, using the motto, *In the name of Christ*. Today there are more than a thousand volunteers serving one to three years in some type of relief, rehabilitation, and development work. It is within this frame of reference that the modern Mennonite mental health story evolved.

Early Treatment of the Mentally Ill

It is important to get some perspective on how baffling the problem of mental illness has been over the centuries, how deeply rooted its stigma, and how slowly society has gained understanding. The church has been involved in some of the worst treatment of the mentally ill, as well as in pioneering the better ways. The mentally ill have been like a football kicked back and forth in the larger power struggles within society involving scientific, antiscientific, legal, economic, religious, and political forces. The progress has been slow and the art and science of psychiatry are still very young.

Prior to Hippocrates, who lived 300 years before Christ at the time of Socrates, medicine was largely in the realm of the primitive and mystical religions, the temples of healing, and the seeking of advice from oracles along with some use of herbs. The mentally ill were feared, hated, and sometimes incorporated into a religious ceremony to help others. In this prescientific era little thought was given to finding the natural reason for illness.

Hippocrates was the first known physician to be thoroughly committed to clinical observation in the search of "fixed measures" in the physical and natural realm. He boldly introduced psychiatric problems into his study and practice; in fact, he even presented a classification for mental illness which continues in some sense to this day.[3] He described in some detail cases recognizable today (for example, postpartum psychosis). His *Sacred Diseases*, in which he is clinical but also somewhat emotional in the way he responds to religious critics who attributed epilepsy to supernatural forces, is a classic. "It thus does appear to me to be in no way more divine, nor more sacred than other disease, but has a natural cause from which it originates..." Referring to his critics as charlatans, he says, "Such persons thus...use the divinity as a pretext and a screen for their own inability to afford any assistance." He then refers to his clinical observations in cutting open the head and the evidence he found of the disease.[4]

The gains made by Hippocrates have been characterized as "classical medicine." Unfortunately, these gains were not incorporated into the practice of medicine in the centuries that followed. However, the monks preserved a great deal of the knowledge of classical medicine, as well as other learning, in the monasteries during the darkest years of the Middle Ages. During these years mental illness, to the degree that it was treated at all, was largely outside the influence of medicine and became once more dominated by beliefs regarding demon possession.

The mentally ill had their darkest hour at the hands of the Christian church during the Inquisition of the thirteenth century. With growing fears in society and an increasing sense of instability in the world of their day, the Catholic hierarchy sought to consolidate the powers of the church and the state through the Inquisition.[5] Literally hundreds of thousands of mentally ill lost their lives in central Europe in a vigorous effort to exterminate those possessed of the devil. Prime movers of this severe application of the Inquisition were two Dominican brothers, authors of *The Witches' Hammer*(1489). Their goal was to guide exorcists and priestly heresy hunters to do their task efficiently.

Foucault in his *Madness and Civilization* sees madness as having fulfilled a real need for society. He holds that in the ancient and early medieval world the insane gradually took the place of the lepers as the scapegoats of society. Insanity was a part of a subterranean world of evil spirits, and madmen were isolated but somewhat respectfully treated. In the fifteenth century they were even put on sailing boats, "the ship of fools," to keep them away from their homeland until they died.[6] There is a whole literature of moral fables and a long series of "follies" including Erasmus's *In Praise of Follies*. In Erasmus, madness is no longer associated with subterranean forces, it is within man, "in the attachment he bears for himself and by the illusions he entertains."[7]

Then in the sixteenth century madmen were moved to the center of the theatrical stage where as guardians of the truth they said what society might not accept from anyone else. Don Quixote is immortalized only by his insanity and from that perspective brings wisdom with regard to the world. Macbeth represents another type of madness, a desperate, passionate delirium from which flow some nuggets of truth about life and society.[8]

With madness liberated from the supernatural by the new role of reason in society, the fool was no longer seen as a tragic reality with a possible message to society. Madness must now be tamed and confined. By the late eighteenth century there was a new ethic of work and idleness in a society now beset with problems of poverty and unemployment growing out of the industrial revolution. One out of every one hundred persons in Paris—the poor, the unemployed, the prisoners, and the insane—were confined under the law to the same place, The Hospital General. This new institution of confinement was given all authority by the church and government over such "poor," possessed as it were, with the problem of idleness. Society, in a somewhat rational way, was seeking to cope with a social nuisance through confinement, but seeking to make as much use of such confined labor as possible through in-house factories.

Foucault maintains that civilization, liberated by the era of enlightenment, was no longer able to think of the insane as solely the devil-possessed, no longer able to accept the wisdom of madness through the theater, and no longer able to tolerate the wandering people whether insane, poor, or unemployed. As a result, madhouses developed from a fear that society would be overrun with bothersome people.

A Thread of Humane Care

Despite an overwhelming picture of superstition and gross mistreatment, there is also a small thread of Christian, humane programs running through ancient and medieval history. W. Earle Biddle and Gregory Zilboorg, both psychiatrists with church interests, have made helpful surveys providing illustrations of such institutions through the centuries.

The monasteries of Saint Basil (A.D. 329-80) in Caesarea gave mental patients humane care. A similar monastery was founded by Saint Jerome (A.D. 343-420) at Bethlehem. Here the monks were required to make arrangements for the isolation and proper treatment of the mentally ill. The rule of Saint Jerome required that mentally ill persons be given the same care as the physically ill and that every means be used to secure appropriate treatment and speedy recovery.[9]

At Monte Cassino, begun by Saint Benedict (A.D. 480-543), occupational therapy was promoted. The hospice, a forerunner of the modern hospital, was set up to give shelter to wanderers and to provide rehabilitative activity for the mentally ill. In such places as the Hospice of Mont Canis (A.D. 825) and the Hospice of Great Saint Bernard (A.D. 962) the mentally ill could also find refuge.[10] Pinel, to whom we will refer later, commended the care given the mentally ill in Spain, particularly at their first asylum established at Valencia in 1409 by a monk.

One institution, whose facilities were even extravagant and luxurious, with 150 employees to care for twenty patients, was an Arabian asylum at Suleimanie (1560). But, as Biddle adds, "It may be a shock to Christian pride to learn that this institution was conducted by Mohammedans."[11]

Pilgrimages were frequently made to religious shrines during the Middle Ages; and, if a sick person improved, rumors of miraculous cures soon spread. One of the well-known shrines of this type was established in Gheel, Belgium. Because some of its services continue to this day, it has served as an inspiration for community psychiatry in some Mennonite centers and is worthy of description in a little more detail.

According to tradition, Dympna, the daughter of an Irish king, was converted to Christianity and fled with a priest. The father of Dympna, angered over her conversion and elopement, pursued her. After finding Dympna and being unable to dissuade her from Christianity, he beheaded both her and the priest. The legend is that several mentally ill persons who saw the cruel act thus regained their mental health. This was accepted as a miracle and thereafter she became a patron saint for mad persons, Saint Dympna.

Rumors spread about the healing powers at her tomb and this brought many mentally ill pilgrims to Gheel. By the year 1200 a church was erected to help receive many of these pilgrims into the church and community while they were waiting for the cures. Various routines and ceremonies to facilitate the healing also developed in connection with the shrine.

Perhaps the real miracle was the custom that developed for the community to open up its homes to accept these pilgrims while they were waiting to be cured. The Gheel community care pattern has continued even to this day so that one out of every seven homes in the community of 30,000 cares for a mentally ill person, while only a few are in a central hospital.[12]

In later years as the Mennonites were preparing to launch their own mental hospital program, it was not uncommon to hear psychiatrists refer to Gheel, Belgium, as a model for the Mennonites to follow. In the post-World War II era, H. A. Fast, one of the early Mennonite mental health leaders, visited Gheel.

First Revolution of Psychiatry: Moral Treatment Hospitals

The evolution of the modern psychiatric approach to mental illness has been grouped into three major revolutionary developments. The first is focused on the work of Pinel and the Tukes, who began the so-called moral treatment era and advocated the use of the hospital for treatment rather than mere segregation purposes.

Increasing awareness of the deplorable conditions in the hospitals of France and England prepared the way for a reformation in the late eighteenth century. Philippe Pinel (1745-1826) came to Paris as a young doctor eleven years before the French Revolution. He served as physician and chief of the Bicetre where his revolution with the mentally ill began. Pinel had a high respect for rational and scientific writings, including those of Hippocrates. The fact that he was close to those high in government made possible the reformation he undertook. Pinel put into practice his convictions that the principles of the French political revolution should include humane treatment of the mentally ill. What he did had ripple effects in other parts of the world.

After careful observation of many cases at the Bicetre, Pinel made an appeal to the government to allow, in effect, a "bold new approach." Within a few days he liberated over fifty patients from chains and dungeons, and within two years inhuman restraint and confinement were replaced by promenades and workshops.[13]

Pinel was quite aware of the Tukes of England and perhaps even somewhat competitive. He mentioned examining closely the writings of the "English physicians" since they "give themselves credit for a great superiority of skill in moral treatment." He singled out the York Retreat for its "pure and elevated principles of philanthropy...applied...to the moral treatment of insanity."[14]

In writing about the "moral treatment of insanity," Pinel condemned the old system and urged a minimum of coercion, "...use mildness...or firmness as occasion may require, the bland arts of conciliation, or the tone of irresistible authority pronouncing an irreversible mandate." He observed a direct relationship between how patients are treated and how they behave.[15]

Early Quakers

Abuse and neglect of the mentally ill in England at the end of the eighteenth century are also well documented. For many years one of the attractions of London was a visit to Bedlam where the attendants displayed patients like animals at a sideshow. In fact, visitors had to buy admission tickets!

In the midst of such abuses, the Quakers of England became aroused by the mysterious death of a Quaker woman in the York Asylum. This incident was the immediate cause of a proposal by William Tuke to the Society of Friends in 1792 that they erect their own institution where a "milder and more appropriate system of treatment than that usually practiced might be adopted." The York Retreat, opened four years later, marked the beginning of a new era of moral treatment in England and later America. "Restraint and abuse were replaced by kindness and tolerance, by working in the garden and gentle exercise on the surrounding grounds, by light recreations and amusements."[16]

The term *moral* was not used in the ethical sense, but rather stood in oppostion to the physical-medical approach to the mentally ill. It meant roughly psychological and conveyed a sense of the moral rights to decency of the Enlightenment era. It provided respect and esteem to the patient and carried an expectation of reasonable behavior. The approach was not based on scientific theories but on common sense and, for some, on Christian values. It was a treatment program emphasizing the milieu therapy and therapeutic community approaches which were to follow more than a century later.[17]

William Tuke, his son Henry, and grandson Samuel promoted the York Retreat as a model and took many visitors on inspection tours. Included in one such visit was an American educator, Thomas Scattergood. After his visit in 1811, Scattergood proposed to the Philadelphia Yearly Meeting of the Friends that an asylum be established, "for such of our members as may be deprived the use of their reason."[18]

The Friends Asylum in Philadelphia opened in 1817 under the leadership of a farmer named Isaac Bonsall who had no previous experience in the care of the mentally ill. Except for the general principles of moral treatment, Bonsall had little to guide him except his strong sense of human dignity and a passionate belief in order. Bonsall found himself in conflict with the resident physician who wanted to follow generally accepted medical practices of the eigh-

teenth century which included blistering in which burns were in-
flicted on a patient's shaved head. The massive blisters caused by
this treatment were then expected to draw the madness from out of
the patient's body. Other medical treatments included "bleeding,"
using leeches or a barber's razor; chemicals to induce either vomit-
ing or diarrhea; hot and cold showers; and even a form of treatment
using the newly discovered force of electricity. Isaac Bonsall, firmly
committed to the idea of moral treatment, helped develop techniques which would eventually eliminate most of the treatment
methods in use at that time.[19]

The first principle of moral treatment as advocated by William
Tuke of the York Retreat was that no person was ever completely
insane. Regardless of how "mad"a person might seem, there was
always some rationality still present and it was the job of the Asylum
staff to expose and strengthen that healthy portion of the patient's
mind; to "cherish every ray of returning reason." Doing this would
allow the patient himself to then gain some measure of control over
his disorder.[20]

The second principle was that all mentally ill were to be accepted as "brethren and men." The York Retreat community expected each person to become a stable and productive member of
the community. The patients and staff worked together, ate meals
communally, and were housed in the same building.[21]

The third principle was that of patient responsibility, the counterpart of being accepted as "brethren and men." The patient who
became violent would temporarily be removed from the rest of the
patients and placed in a room by himself. When composed again he
would be allowed to rejoin the group. Every patient was also expected to make an attempt at some form of occupation, usually
related to housework or farming.

As moral treatment was undertaken almost simultaneously by
Pinel and Tuke in the last part of the eighteenth century, there were
also parallel efforts by a few reformers in other countries. It is quite
clear that the writings of Enlightenment physician-philosopher
John Locke about inalienable rights influenced men such as Pinel
and Tuke.

Rise of Modern Psychiatric Hospitals

The Quaker effort of 1817 in Philadelphia became the inspiration for establishing other privately endowed mental hospitals in
America—McLean, Bloomingdale, and the Hartford Retreat. Within
thirty years at least eighteen private hospitals were built for the
moral treatment of the mentally ill in this country. From these
private models developed state hospitals also premised on moral

treatment—Lexington, Kentucky; Staunton, Virginia; Columbia, South Carolina; Manhattan State in New York; and the Worcester State Hospital in Massachusetts.[22]

The Worcester State Hospital played an unusual role in the history of moral treatment because of the careful records and reports it issued annually. Though contested by some psychiatrists since that time, the reports from 1833 to 1852 indicate a recovery rate of 61.3 percent to 74.6 percent of all patients discharged. A study in the late 1800s indicated that 48 percent of those discharged as recovered in the 1830s had remained well throughout their lives, or up to the survey about fifteen years after their treatment.[23] Even if some of the figures could be contested, it does seem clear that results of the moral treatment era far exceeded that of the eras both before and soon after that time.

Unfortunately the rapid rise of moral treatment in state hospitals was followed by a similarly rapid decline. This was caused by a variety of factors. The increase of poorly equipped immigrants who became paupers required expansion of state institutions. This in turn greatly changed the complexion of the patient population and what was possible by way of an intimate patient-staff hospital community. Leaders of the moral treatment approach failed to train successors and to conduct adequate research. Treatment by depletion (purges, leeching, bloodletting) as well as phrenology were part of American medical practice at the time. As these became discredited, moral treatment seemed to decline with them. Part of this decline can also be attributed to the rapid rise of scientific, laboratory-based training in the second half of the nineteenth century, and especially the prestige that neurology gained. Mental disorder was increasingly interpreted as brain disease.

Dorothea Dix

In 1841, while moral treatment was still flourishing in the better private and state institutions, Dorothea Lynde Dix, a retired schoolteacher, began a moral crusade against abuse in the care of the indigent insane. She began visiting jails and county hospitals where the mentally ill and mentally retarded were kept. Dix believed that the horrible conditions surrounding the insane were due to an antiquated, ignorant, and callous system of public policy based upon theories and practices which must be revolutionized out of respect to Christianity and advancing civilization.[24]

In 1848 she submitted a "memorial" to the Congress of the United States indicating that she had seen "more than 9,000 idiots, epileptics and insane in the United States, destitute of appropriate care and protection...bound with galling chains, bowed beneath fetters and heavy iron balls attached to drag-chains, lacerated with ropes, scourged with rods and terrified beneath storms of execration and cruel blows; now subject to jibes and scorn and torturing tricks; now abandoned to the most outrageous violations."[25] As a result of her work more than thirty state institutions were either founded or enlarged.

Thus came the rapid rise of the large and highly impersonal state hospital, buildings that greeted conscientious objectors in World War II and are still being used in many states. Although some writers list Dorothea Dix with the pioneering of Pinel and the Tukes, Bockoven points out that in effect Dix operated on the erroneous assumption "that elimination of abuse in *itself* would result in the recovery of the curable." In fact he believed that her rigid opinions introduced an attitude of censorship and faultfinding into hospital psychiatry.[26]

Second Revolution:
Freud, Modern Psychiatry

The second major revolution in mental health centered around Sigmund Freud (1856-1939) and his development of a set of assumptions and methodologies known as *psychoanalysis*. As one writer put it, "All that Freud did stems from one simple discovery...that beneath the surface manifestations of human life there are deeper motives and feelings and purposes which the individual conceals not only from others but even from himself."[27] While the established psychiatry previously had been only descriptive, it was now possible with Freud's presuppositions to develop a body of knowledge and skills with which to treat mental illness. This became the basis for modern psychotherapy and its more optimistic outlook.

Freud began as a neurologist working in the scientific laboratory and then moved to the direct study of people. His discoveries began when he noted the power of suggestion of the physician over patients. Then through hypnosis he noted the emotional release experienced when they were able to talk about deeply disturbing experiences. Later he discovered that people could experience the same emotional release without hypnosis through the use of what he called free association.

Although professionals and lay people disagree with various aspects of Freud's theories and methods, there is, nevertheless, a rather general acceptance of his postulation of the unconscious as a storehouse of experiences of the individual. The more deeply repressed materials of the unconscious may influence attitudes and actions that are not easily changed and may produce behavior which does not seem reasonable on the surface.[28]

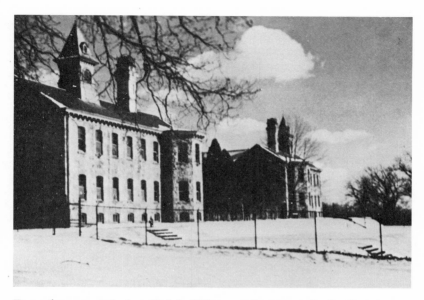

Two of many state hospital buildings at Greystone Park, New Jersey, housing more than 5,000 patients with a thousand employees, including 100 in CPS Unit #77 during World War II.

Freud's use of free association led to the development of psychotherapy, which covers a much broader range of helping technologies than psychoanalysis. Used to relieve symptoms of psychic origin, psychotherapy includes methods such as suggestion, persuasion, exhortation, hypnosis, dynamic psychotherapy, and group therapy, as well as psychoanalysis proper. Most modern psychiatric hospitals use a number of these methods, chosen to be appropriate to the patient's needs.

Psychiatry and Religion

Many Christians have tended to react against anything Freudian because of what they have perceived as Freud's critical attitude toward religion. Freud's views about religion were, however, quite complex. He was obviously much fascinated by religion and paid much attention to it in his writings.[29]

Some other outstanding psychiatrists have given special attention to the role of religion though not necessarily in ways pleasing to all believers. Carl G. Jung (1875-1961), a one-time colleague of Freud, went on to develop his own school of thought stressing the importance of the ego and the spiritual aspect of the individual. Out of the German death camps of World War II came Viktor Frankl,

Viennese psychiatrist, who placed a strong emphasis upon the need to understand man's search for meaning and the significance of the spiritual dimension of life. His method is called *logotherapy*. Karl Menninger's supportive stance toward religion and his personal views have become well known through his book, *Whatever Became of Sin?*.

As in any other profession, there are individuals in psychiatry who are nonreligious or even antireligious. However, in 1951 a supportive statement released at the International Congress on Mental Health said, "Religion can contribute to the mental health of an individual by providing security, self-respect, goodwill, unselfishness and companionship with God, and it provides a philosophy of the real meaning of life... True religion and true psychology are mutually enriching and having nothing to fear from each other."[30]

Psychiatry's Continuing Search

The history of psychiatry is marked by an unending search for somatic causes and physical methods of treatment. Adolph Meyer (1866-1950), who was biologically as well as psychologically oriented, did much to promote the belief that mental disorder could be understood as stress reactions and in effect reversed through treatment. His treatment methods included the somatic (physical) such as electroconvulsive therapy.

Leaders in emphasizing interpersonal relationships, namely that other people are involved both in the origin and healing of mental illness, were Karen Horney (1885-1952) and Harry Stack Sullivan (1892-1949). This emphasis on the "here and now" and the "interpersonal" has greatly influenced the Mennonite mental health centers.

Two methods were discovered in the 1930s to relieve symptoms of schizophrenia and manic-depressive psychosis. One of these was insulin shock therapy and the other electroconvulsive therapy. In the 1940s psychosurgery was also common. In recent years chemotherapy has been added. Great changes have been made possible in hospital and other treatment by the discovery of antipsychotic medications and antidepressant drugs. The earlier antipsychotic medications derived from the plant Rauwolfia Serpentina have almost entirely replaced deep insulin treatment and psychosurgery. Later the antidepressants greatly reduced but not totally replaced electroconvulsive treatments for depression.

Third Revolution:
Community Mental Health

The first revolution in mental health care was a move from

primitive forms of confinement to care in hospitals which sought a humane approach that would lead to recovery. The second revolution was a breakthrough in thinking about mental illness in such a way that explanatory knowledge could be accumulated and skills developed for treatment. The third revolution sought to bring many forms of treatment and support to the local community where they would be accessible to everyone, where early treatment could take place, and illness might even be prevented.

There are many antecedents of community mental health including features in the first two revolutions.

Citizen awareness. The plight of the mentally ill and citizen demand for better resources were basic to the community health movement. Clifford Beers, released from a state hospital, published *A Mind That Found Itself* in 1908 and devoted himself to the promotion of a local and national mental hygiene movement that was to become worldwide by 1930. Following World War I this movement concerned itself with the "shell shock" victims of World War I, out of which emerged what are known today as *mental health associations*.

Geographical decentralization. As early as 1906 Adolph Meyers was talking about aftercare and envisioning the creation of community mental hygiene districts to coordinate services of schools, playgrounds, churches, law enforcement agencies, and others in an effort to prevent mental illness.[31] Later, state hospitals placed patients in wards according to their area of residence prior to hospitalization. This geographical pattern began as a device for following up discharged patients and soon became a means of establishing working relationships between the hospitals and the communities. These developments took place largely after World War II, following the effort of many states to reform their state hospital programs whose poor conditions had been exposed by the conscientious objectors and various psychiatric leaders during World War II.

Therapeutic community. The introduction of the therapeutic community concept by Maxwell Jones of England in about 1953 was a tremendous step forward in transforming hospitals into healing communities. Jones indicates that the concept of the therapeutic community was in a sense a recovery of the values of the moral treatment era.[32] It was based on the premise that therapeutic potential resided in the patients as well as the staff. Community psychiatry, guided by assumptions of the therapeutic community idea, was a leap from within the walls of the hospital out into the larger community. The basic assumption is that communities have resources that can be mobilized to prevent disorders, as well as provide care for persons in need of special support and understanding.

Pharmacology. A summary has already been given of gains

made during the 1950s through new drugs. Not only did these drugs enable more effective realization of the therapeutic community idea in the hospital, but they also made possible the treatment of more patients at home, thereby forestalling hospitalization.

Crisis Intervention. The basic assumption of crisis intervention is that service provided during a period of crisis can usually be effective in staving off the development of mental disorders. The military applied this particularly in the Korean War. Community mental health centers have capitalized on this approach in working with police who intervene in times of family conflict, providing special services during disasters, and helping individuals cope with transitional stress periods.[33]

Prevention. The concept of prevention of disease has been adapted from public health, focusing on controlling factors that are detrimental to mental health. Terms and concepts borrowed from public health include: health promotion (primary prevention), early recognition and prompt treatment of incipient cases (secondary prevention), and rehabilitation of the ill (tertiary prevention).

All of these emerging ideas and action patterns are components that contributed to the third revolution—the community mental health movement. The large number of psychiatric casualties in World War II gave added impetus, leading eventually to the community mental health legislation enacted by the United States government during the 1960s.

National Legislation for Mental Health

After the National Institute of Mental Health was initiated in 1948, the Joint Commission for Mental Health and Illness was appointed by Congress in 1955 to devise an overall strategy. *Action for Mental Health*, the findings of this Joint Commission, was published in 1961. It recommended to the American public that mental hospitals be reformed as mental health centers; that is, as part of an integrated community service, the centers were to include outpatient and aftercare facilities as well as inpatient services.[34]

The Community Mental Health Centers Act of 1963 which became law under President John F. Kennedy, represented a bold new approach to the problems of mental illness and mental health. This law defined the essential functions of a comprehensive mental health center as: 1) inpatient services, 2) outpatient services, 3) partial hospitalization—at least day-care service, 4) emergency services provided twenty-four hours per day and available within at least one of the first three services listed above, and 5) consultation and educational services to community agencies and professional personnel.

In addition to these required services, centers were urged to include five others: 6) diagnostic services, 7) vocational and educational programs, 8) precare and aftercare services in the community (foster home placement, home visiting, and halfway houses), 9) training, and 10) research and program evaluation. These ten services constituted the blueprint for which the federal government planned to provide both construction and staffing grant money to help start centers for every population area of 200,000 persons in the United States. It was this legislation which was to implement the third revolution in a massive and dramatic way, a movement in which Mennonite mental health centers were to be used as a model and in which they were to make a significant contribution.

Church Mental Health Programs in the Modern Era

Although special church-sponsored mental health facilities stand out in modern history by their scarcity, the fostering of mental health is actually an integral and common element of the church's pastoral ministry. From this pastoral concern developed the Clinical Pastoral Education movement which in turn has had a major impact on the pastoral ministry to people suffering from spiritual and psychological problems. From the broad perspective of the church's concern for the psyche (or soul), it seems strange that the church has been involved so little in providing special programs for the mentally ill.

Since World War II psychiatric wards have become relatively common in general hospitals sponsored by both Catholic and Protestant churches. These, however, have not involved the church as deeply as the church-sponsored psychiatric hospital where the church takes primary responsibility for the professional treatment as well as the hospital care.

The Roman Catholic Church

The Roman Catholic church has had a long history of relating to the needs of mentally ill. Previous sections of this chapter have illustrated this in terms of the early monastic hospices and through the church's struggle with the problem of demon possession.

After an earlier period of resisting modern psychiatry, the Catholic church in 1953 under Pope Pius XII looked "...with satisfaction at the new paths opened by psychiatry... It knows that the recovery of a spirit from insanity, whether by prevention or by cure, is like the first step toward gaining him for Christ." Pope Pius XII made other papal pronouncements which sought to accept but also to set limits on the role of psychiatry for Christians. Though recognizing the power of dynamic drives in people, he stressed the need of personal responsibility in directing them. The pope warned against exempting abnormal people from moral responsibility and urged moral limits on exploring the psyche through free association. Another papal pronouncement was against unlimited disclosure of confessional secrets. The pope also held that a purely psychotherapeutic treatment could not eliminate genuine guilt[35] These statements illustrate the new attitude and the new role of the Catholic church in seeking to cooperate with and yet set limits to the modern psychiatric disciplines.

Protestant Efforts

Protestant facilities for treating the mentally ill have been provided largely through the work of the Quakers, the Christian Reformed Church, the Seventh-Day Adventists, and the Mennonites.

As Kin Van Atta points out, for the *Quakers*, it was very necessary to find a cure for the mentally ill due to one of the central tenets of that Society..."that in every man there is a 'divine principle'..."[36] This helps to account for the Friends' sense of divine mission regarding this cause.

In addition to the Quaker role in the York Retreat of England and the Friends Hospital of Philadelphia, individual members of the Society of Friends have been unusually influential in the history of American psychiatry. They include Thomas Kirkbride, a physician of the Friends Hospital, who provided the primary leadership in establishing the American Psychiatric Association, and Phiny Earle, a psychiatric leader in the moral treatment era. Erich Lindemann, author of a landmark paper on crisis intervention in bereavement, was a Quaker. The well-known Sheppard and Enoch Pratt Hospital at Baltimore, though not formally a Quaker institution, has for a long time had a majority of Quakers on its board of directors.[37]

Modern Friends of Jungian persuasion seek to nurture their Christian and professional role in *Inward Light*, a publication sponsored by the Friends Conference on Religion and Psychology. The editor states that this magazine is a "special blend of experiential religion and what we have termed mystical psychology."[38]

The Christian Reformed Church in America is a Protestant group whose concern for the mentally ill goes back to Europe, in the Netherlands. This group, whose membership is approximately the size of the Mennonite constituency in the United States, has founded three psychiatric hospitals. The one in Wyckoff, New Jersey, has twenty-five beds for acute and seventy-five beds for long-term patients. Bethesda Hospital located in Denver, Colorado, combines a hospital and a community mental health center. The Christian Psychopathic Hospital and Pine Rest Sanitarium in Grand Rapids, Michigan, began in the early 1900s and is the largest of the three, with approximately 200 beds for patients of all ages. Most of the patients in these hospitals come from their supporting constituency which has assumed a heavy financial responsibility to subsidize the care and treatment of their mentally ill.

In the *Seventh-Day Adventist Church*, the mental health interest is fostered by members as a part of their commitment to health based on the spiritual vision of Ellen White (1863). This broad emphasis has led to education on such practices as temperance, diets, and vegetarianism, and the launching of their own medical school at Loma Linda University in California. Harrison Evans, chairman of the psychiatric department, writes, "Psychology as such has been viewed with some skepticism by the church ...although it is well accepted here at Loma Linda University."[39]

The Harding Hospital, in Worthington, Ohio, founded in 1916, has developed a strong program of treatment, education, and clinical research largely through the efforts of several generations of the Harding family, who are staunch members of this denomination.

The Mennonites in Mental Health

Bethania Hospital in southern Russia was the first psychiatric hospital of the Mennonites. Though it operated for only a relatively

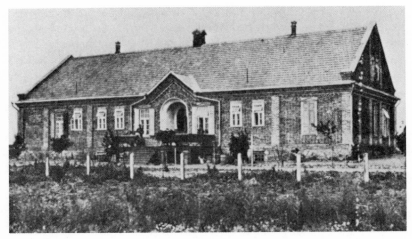

Men's building of the Mennonite psychiatric hospital in Russia known as Bethania.

short period of time (1910-1927), it was destined to have considerable impact upon Mennonites in other parts of the world. Bethania was established in the Chortitza Settlement, Russia, and was patterned after Bodelschwingh's Bethel-in-Bielefeld, Germany. It had a capacity for 76 patients and statistics indicate that of the 204 patients in 1925, 101 were Russian, 87 German, and 16 Jewish. After the revolution, Bethania was taken over by the province and in 1925 by the federal government. Bethania came to an end in 1927 when its buildings came under the backwaters of the Dneprostroy power dam.[40]

The second Mennonite mental hospital, Bethesda, was located in Vineland, Ontario. It was started in 1932 by Henry P. Wiebe, who had spent three years on the staff of Bethania in Russia. A Mennonite minister who had experienced a nervous breakdown was threatened with deportation. He was brought to Wiebe who took care of the patient in his home until he was able to return to his family. In 1937 Wiebe and his family purchased a farm near Vineland, Ontario, and immediately began taking in other patients.[41] In 1945 the Ontario Conference of the Mennonite Brethren churches officially took over the work of operating Bethesda as a small home-hospital for the mentally ill and the deficient.[42] Still later the home was converted to care more exclusively for the mentally deficient and was financed by the government.

Bertram D. Smucker, making a visit to Bethesda Hospital in March, 1946, on behalf of the Mental Health Study Committee appointed by the Mennonite Central Committee, had this general comment, "The whole spirit of this hospital is in the tradition of a genuine, warm Christian family in contrast to the harshness of a huge state mental institution. The patients carry on quite a normal life, not living under lock and key, daily working on the farm, eating and worshipping together... It is this type of custom which builds a real sense of security more valuable than most highly developed scientific therapy."[43]

The second institution to grow directly out of the Bethania experience in Russia was Hoffnungsheim in the Chaco of Paraguay. This hospital was established by Mennonite immigrants in 1945 carved out of the jungle on the edge of Filadelfia. It began as a seven-room house, although a series of cottages were later added. A psychiatrist from Germany gave leadership to the program soon after its beginning. Although set up to serve primarily the mentally ill, it also included some mentally deficient.

The Hoffnungsheim program is now in the process of being absorbed into a larger three-colony program known as *Servicios Menonitas de Salud Mental*. Under the leadership of Heinz Ratzlaff, a psychologist, the new program planned for the mentally ill and the mentally retarded is strongly oriented toward community education and support services. Ratzlaff has been assisted by Mennonite Mental Health Services of the United States and Canada, and his program efforts also reflect the influence of MMHS centers of North America.[44]

In the United States, a relatively unknown effort that did not result in the establishment of an institution for the mentally ill occurred in 1937 when the General Conference Mennonites considered the possibility of a facility presumably to be located in Kansas. "Repeated inquiries have come to the Bethel Hospital in Newton, Kansas, as to whether this institution could care for demented, feeble-minded, or epileptic individuals,"[45] wrote C. E. Krehbiel in his annual report of 1937. However, a subsequent survey of all General Conference Mennonite churches in the United States indicated inadequate support to proceed further. Thirty-nine (of a possible 139) congregations reported a total of sixty-three cases; twenty-nine were for the establishment of some central institution, ten were against or doubtful, and three had no opinion. Those in favor indicated such reasons as "crying need," "Christian duty," "Christian influence." Those opposed listed "expense," "distance," "help," "location," "state duty," "state more effective," and "danger of violence and tragedy."[46] Although the interest of the Kansas Mennonites cannot be traced directly to Bethania, a considerable awareness of it among leaders of that time was evident.

Conscientious Objectors in State Mental Hospitals

The alternative-service experiences of conscientious objectors in state mental hospitals (1942-1946) had a major impact on the establishment of Mennonite mental health services in the United States. Not as well known is the impact of these conscientious objectors on the history of public mental hospitals throughout the United States. In many ways their impact was comparable to that of Dorothea Dix in helping to create a turning point in the quality of care for the mentally ill. Ironically it was these same large, inhuman institutions developed out of the efforts of Dorothea Dix that had become the "snake pits" to which the conscientious objectors were assigned beginning in 1942.

The United States Selective Service and Training Act of 1940 provided an alternative to military service for conscientious objectors during World War II, known as Civilian Public Service (CPS). The men of draft age came from about 100 different church denominations, although the majority were Mennonites, Brethren, Friends, and Methodists. These men, working without pay, were assigned by the United States government to large work projects such as Soil Conservation, the Forest Service, and the National Park Service.

Such tasks did not fully satisfy the need of those conscientious objectors who wanted to do "meaningful work" by rendering a more direct human service. Many would have preferred to do relief work in war-torn countries, but national policy did not permit such work overseas by conscientious objectors. By 1942 an earnest search by the United States government and the churches led to the assignment in the state mental hospitals and the training schools for the mentally retarded. The Mennonites who volunteered for their work were distributed over twenty-six hospital or training units in twenty-two states in groups of fifteen to one hundred sixty men. Greystone Park in New Jersey, for example, had 5,000 patients, 1,000 employees, and 100 CPS men, 94 of whom served as attendants.

Eventually, the more than 3,000 conscientious objectors who worked for two to four years in the hospitals of twenty-two states shared their observations with the public to help effect some reforms. Frank Wright, author of *Out of Sight Out of Mind*, claims that conscientious objectors amassed the greatest wealth of factual material about conditions in mental hospitals that had ever been gathered in one place.

The conditions in the state hospitals were far from satisfactory before the war and they became desperate during the war. Because of wartime demands for manpower, parts of hospitals were being closed, patients were being denied admission, and the situation was deemed dangerous for lack of help.[47] For example, the Philadelphia State Hospital, with a capacity of 2,500 patients had 6,000 who were served by only 200 attendants![48] This desperate situation prevailed in state after state.

Based on the documentary evidence gathered over four years by CPS men, the May 6, 1946, issue of *Life* magazine exposed the deplorable state of affairs in an article entitled, "Bedlam 1946, Most U.S. Mental Hospitals Are a Shame and Disgrace." "Through public neglect and legislative penny-pinching, state after state has allowed its institutions for the care and cure of the mentally sick to degenerate into little more than concentration camps on the Belsen pattern."[49]

The *Life* article goes on to say dramatically:

> Yet beatings and murders are hardly the most significant of the indignities we have heaped upon most of the 400,000 guiltless patient-prisoners of over 180 state mental institutions.
>
> We jam-pack men, women and sometimes even children into hundred-year-old firetraps in wards so crowded that the floors cannot be seen between the rickety cots, while thousands more sleep on

ticks, on blankets or on the bare floors. We give them little and shoddy clothing at best. Hundreds—of my own knowledge and sight—spend 24 hours a day in stark and filthy nakedness. Those who are well enough to work slave away in many institutions for 12 hours a day, often without a day's rest for years on end...

Thousands spend their days—often for weeks at a stretch—locked in devices euphemistically called "restraints": thick leather handcuffs, great canvas camisoles, "muffs," "mitts," wristlets, locks and straps and restraining sheets. Hundreds are confined in "lodges"—bare, bedless rooms reeking with filth and feces...[50]

The *Life* article concludes, "...their reports leave no shadow of doubt as to the need for major reforms in the mental-hospital systems of almost every state."[51]

Conditions were particularly bad in the Cleveland State Hospital. Although the administration was resistant to facing the facts, outside community leadership used data from the conscientious objector study to get publicity and force investigations. As a result the Friends CPS unit at Cleveland was closed down. Later under a new superintendent, a Mennonite unit took up the service again, and conditions were greatly improved both at Cleveland and statewide as a result of these CPS efforts. A similar story could be told about the units in Virginia where, for example, a member of the Mennonite unit at Staunton worked seven months before he had a day off duty![52]

Another illustration of how CPS men influenced practices in state hospitals came from a Lima, Ohio, institution for the criminally insane.

All the inmates had criminal records. It had been the practice for all attendants to carry black-jacks for protection, but when the unit of CPS men came, they asked to go on the wards without these clubs. Permission was granted with the warning that it was a dangerous action. It worked out so well, however, that the practice of carrying black-jacks was abandoned for all employees and a new and different patient and attendant attitude was created.[53]

Actually, the typical Mennonite CPS unit in a state hospital was less focused on reform than some of these vignettes may suggest. What stood out was the honest day's work done by a generally wholesome, rural-type of person who had genuine interest in the patient. The *Anniversary Review* of the Harrisburg CPS No. 93 gives an excellent crosssection of such an approach. Gordon Engle writes, "Many expect the 'way of life' in everyday living to produce drastic changes immediately. The CPS attendants have discovered this to be merely an illusion... Are we willing and patient enough to bide our time in seeking results?"[54] The CPS units did produce some results. Among other things, they made life a little more pleasant, provided some turning points toward wellness, and gave support to progressive state hospital leaders.

Long Range Reform Efforts

By 1944 CPS men from various units banded together to become better prepared for the hospital work they were doing and to take steps toward a longer-range reform. A special Mental Hygiene Program was thus initiated at Philadelphia through leadership from the Friends unit of that location.

Their first project was beginning a monthly magazine known as *The Attendant* which later became *The Psychiatric Aide*. The circulation of this informative periodical expanded rapidly in the state hospitals with CPS units, and it eventually became national and even international in its coverage. By 1946 the Mental Hygiene Program became the National Mental Health Foundation, with its own board of substantial citizens and its own sources of funding. Included in the Board of Directors were such persons as Anton Boison, the father of the Clinical Pastoral Training movement; Owen J. Roberts,

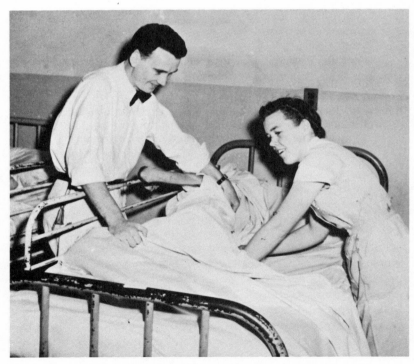

CPS Unit #63 at Marlboro State Hospital, Marlboro, New Jersey.

member of the United States Supreme Court; and various prominent psychiatrists. In the professional advisory group were persons
such as R. H. Felix, M.D., General Chief of the Mental Hygiene
Division of the United States Public Health Service; and Karl Menninger, M.D., of Topeka. The Foundation launched a national program. In addition to the publications already listed, the Foundation
published an impressive list of pamphlets on mental illness and
mental deficiency: *Toward Mental Health* (Public Affairs Pamphlet
#120); *Forgotten Children; From Folly...to Fetters...to Freedom; What to
Look for in a Mental Hospital; Where Does Your State Stand;* and many
others.

A series of eight radio dramatizations were transcribed for
United States and Canadian use. The legal division of the Foundation prepared briefs on existing mental hygiene laws of forty-eight
states and produced a model law for consideration by states. The
education division worked with summer and year-round college
and church volunteer service units in mental hospitals. The executive director wrote in April 1947, "Now, we believe, the substance,
power and vision are all at hand to keep a wave of understanding
and reform rolling..."[55]

Eventually the National Mental Health Foundation merged
with the National Committee for Mental Hygiene in a new organization which continues to function today, The National Committee for
Mental Health, Incorporated. Richard Hunter, a CPS man from one
of the Mennonite hospital units, continues to this day serving as an
executive for this association.

All these efforts were greatly aided by the determination of
leaders such as William C. Menninger of the Veterans Administration. As a latter-day Dorothea Dix, he raised the consciousness of
legislators and persuaded the governments of many states to allo-
cate substantial funds for mental health programs.

Movement Toward Mennonite Mental Hospitals

Parallel to the above developments were discussions by the
young men in Mennonite CPS hospital units which eventually led to
the establishment of the Mennonite mental hospitals in the United
States. An excellent collection of such discussions was brought
together by Robert Kreider, the educational secretary of the Mennonite Central Committee CPS units, in "A Symposium, Should the
Churches Establish and Maintain Hospitals for the Mentally Ill?"
This collection from nine contributors was released in February
1945, near the end of the war.

In this symposium William J. Ellis, the state mental health
commissioner of New Jersey, recognized the modern hospital as the

outgrowth of Quaker efforts in England and urged that the church think of continuing this work today. Such a hospital, he maintained, "...under church auspices should be small enough to serve as a demonstration center and would do well to align itself with one of the medical schools or other teaching institutions."[56]

Paul Goering a CPS hospital leader, who also referred to the precedence of the Quakers, cited the advantages of such a hospital in terms of "spirit of love," "removing corruption," and "higher caliber of attendant help." Eugene Weed, a non-Mennonite CPS man, viewed Mennonites with their heritage of wholesome living as being able to provide the basics for good care but also to offer "something central around which to reorganize life."[57] Loris Habegger, another CPS leader, urged consideration of psychiatric wings in general hospitals.

Arthur Jost, a CPS unit leader and later director of one of the Mennonite hospitals, urged the establishment of mental hospitals as a way of creating interest in prevention of mental illness, implementing the ideals of love and nonviolence, making it easier for people to come for treatment, and using the larger reserve of qualified attendants produced by CPS.

P. C. Hiebert, chairman of the Mennonite Central Committee, favored church mental hospitals as an expression of Christian ideals, in line with the Mennonite demonstration in Russia. D. D. Eitzen, a Mennonite pastoral counseling professor, was affirmative but called for professional adequacy.[58]

Some raised questions. For example, O. R. Yoder, the superintendent of Ypsilanti State Hospital in Michigan, questioned whether conservative, traditional, religionists had the objectivity to deal with problems of mental illness.[59] On the whole, however, the responses were predominantly favorable toward the establishment of a church mental hospital and reflect a degree of self-confidence based on the wartime experiences, the potential of the Mennonite church groups, and the precedence of the Quakers and the Russian Mennonites.

Mental Health, a Mennonite Cause

By the end of World War II mental health work was becoming a sizable undertaking largely dependent upon professionals. In addition to the special fears some church people had of "Freudianism," psychiatry continued to be mystifying and overwhelming to the general public. Why then did Mennonites enter the mental health field?[60]

No other church group had ever had such a concentrated experience with mental illness as the American Mennonites during

World War II. During a four-year period 1,500 Mennonites had a "hands on" involvement with mental illness which they shared freely with their home congregations. They developed a vision of what might be done with rightly motivated psychiatric aides and mental health professionals. The mentally ill and the psychiatrists became real people and hospitals became understandable human efforts.

Within the larger group of Mennonites a small number seemed to say, "If God has exposed *us* to this need and *we* don't do anything, how can we expect anyone else to do so?" Furthermore, nationally recognized psychiatric leaders gave reasonable confirmation that "Mennonites might have a special contribution to make."

Mennonites have had a long history as a minority. As an Anabaptist-Mennonite group that was severely persecuted and had to move from country to country as immigrants, they had a strong tendency toward isolation and strong in-group loyalties. As pacifists they felt themselves to be different from "regular Americans," a minority feeling experienced by Mennonites of all ages particularly in times of war.

Karl Menninger's analysis of the experience of the Jews as a minority in relation to psychiatry may also provide perspective for the Mennonite experience. He shows how children growing up in a religious minority experience discrimination and rejection and often have a strong desire to excel. Such experiences can give them a special sensitivity to other odd people such as the mentally ill, and provide a strong motivation to help people in need.[61] Mennonites were held back during World War II from the positive role they desired to play in relieving wartime suffering. It is understandable that they would have been looking for a special opportunity in peacetime to respond positively to the needs of society, such as mental health, even if they had to create that opportunity themselves.

Many Mennonites had experienced the values of a Mennonite Central Committee (MCC) as a wartime service agency. By 1946 there were concerns and high hopes that MCC would convert its organizational capability to serving ongoing peacetime needs. Thus the mental health cause came to the fore at an opportune time for prime consideration.

With the wartime CPS program being closed out, MCC also had experienced, young leadership ready to be tapped for this new cause. The MCC headquarters, Akron, Pennsylvania, had become a unique gathering of both young and older leadership who had learned to collaborate to bring other new ideas to fruition. Both were needed to successfully launch a new type of church institution.

Furthermore, demobilization of CPS had made available an MCC-owned farm in Maryland at a reasonable location for beginning a mental health program. In fact it was the need to dispose of it that provided the opportunity for concrete action.

Bethania, the Russian Mennonite mental hospital, was not a primary nor a dynamic factor for the post-World War II mental hospital initiative. However, it was a supporting precedent which made it easier to visualize a role for the church serving the mentally ill. This awareness was particularly evident in H. A. Fast and P. C. Hiebert, leaders who represented two of the larger groups of Russian Mennonites.

The Canadian Bethesda, a direct descendent of the Russian Bethania, played a more specific, short-term role. In effect, it served as a spiritual model as well as a pragmatic model. A visit to Bethesda by one of the Mental Health Study Committee members in 1946, along with the availability of a CPS farm in Maryland, triggered the actual beginning of Mennonite Mental Health Services in the United States.

Lessons From History

This summary of the historical context for the Mennonite mental health story has been an effort to provide some perspective to society's dealing with the mentally ill from Hippocrates to the community mental health movement, to the moral treatment approach and modern psychiatry, and to the role of the church through the centuries, particularly the World War II role of conscientious objectors.

What can be learned from this broad historical review? Several ideas stand out: 1) The continuing struggle with the stigma of mental illness must be seen in the perspective of its deeply rooted past. 2) The church cannot forget that it too can be the victim of demeaning forces of its own times. 3) The church when most true in following its Master has contributed leaders and groups who have been ahead of their times in providing better treatment of the mentally ill. 4) The conscientious objectors working in state mental hospitals during World War II made a brief but highly significant contribution (not adequately recognized in historical surveys of that era). 5) Mennonite mental health programs, the therapeutic community movement, and possibly the current recognition of values in psychiatric treatment can be seen as fresh expressions of the moral treatment approach.

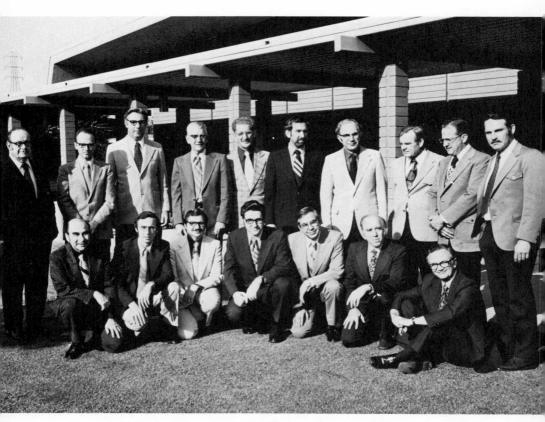

MMHS Board of Directors, 1973. **Standing** *(l.-r.), William T. Snyder, Wesley Oswald (Brook Lane Administrator), Rowland Shank, Vernon Neufeld (MMHS Director), Otto Hamm, Elvin Byler, Elmer Ediger, Arthur Jost, Norman Loux and Curtis Byer.* **Seated** *(l.-r.), Harold Z. Bomberger, Aldred Neufeldt, Larry Yoder, William Zuercher, Robert W. Hartzler, Luke Birky and Charles Neff.*

CHAPTER 2

Mennonite Mental Health Services

Vernon H. Neufeld*

As an organization, Mennonite Mental Health Services (MMHS) traces its beginning to the decision of the Mennonite Central Committee (MCC) in 1947 to begin a mental health program. To help implement the new program, MCC provided an advisory committee of seven persons "to proceed immediately with the further study of ways and means and planning" and to make appropriate recommendations to MCC. The committee, first bearing the expansive and cumbersome title of "Homes-for-Mentally-Ill Planning and Advisory Committee," was to undergo a thirty-five-year process of growth and change—from an advisory committee to a corporate body with greater responsibility under MCC, and ultimately to a collaborative network bringing MCC together with a consortium of eight mental health centers and hospitals in a new service agency.

The present chapter is a historical sketch of this evolution, following the MCC line of development, beginning with the events which led to the 1947 decision and continuing to the present time. The story is told from the perspective of MMHS, the subsidiary organization of MCC. If written from the point of view of MCC; the sponsor or parent, the narrative might well be presented in a different light, with another interpretation. Certainly the mental health institutions as well, both the five who were spawned under MCC direction and the three who joined MMHS later, would see this development with different eyes. Fortunately, each center will tell its own story later.

More than the history of an advisory committee become board, this account will deal with the overall development of the MMHS "system," which embraces the individual centers and hospitals. An

*Vernon H. Neufeld is Director of Mennonite Mental Health Services.

important part of the story is the interrelationships among the three major actors in the story — MCC, MMHS and the centers — and how these ties changed through the years, at times strong, other times nebulous or strained, yet persisting through the years to the present.

The history is presented below in four periods which represent different stages in the MMHS development and the relationships involving MCC and the mental health institutions: (1) the circumstances and events leading to the 1947 MCC decision; (2) the leading role of MCC in establishing the first three programs (1947-56); (3) the struggle for identity and greater independence by the institutions and MMHS (1957-66); and (4) the period of maturity characterized by partnership and collaboration (1967-present).

DEVELOPMENTS BEFORE 1947

Chapter 1 delineates two important historical roots to the 1947 MCC decision: the Mennonite experience in Russia and the Civilian Public Service (CPS) experience of World War II. Prompted by both influences, and his own vision and conviction, Henry A. Fast further tested the idea with the Emergency Relief Board of the General Conference of the Mennonite Church of North America, the board of which he was chairman, asking "whether the time had not come to initiate plans to establish a hospital to serve the needs of the mentally ill."[1] The board endorsed the idea and agreed this concern should be presented to MCC, which Fast did on December 28-29, 1944. The minutes record:

> Henry A. Fast spoke briefly concerning the need for a program of care for Mennonites who are mentally ill and proposed serious consideration of the desirability of establishing such a program in a central institution under the administration of the Mennonite Central Committee.

But MCC was not immediately prepared to act positively to the proposal. MCC, though temporarily saddled with the CPS program, was basically a relief agency, and not a health care or human services provider. MCC was crisis and emergency oriented, not prepared to take on more permanent, long-term tasks. MCC provided goods and services but did not establish institutions. MCC served where individual Mennonite conference groups had difficulty working alone, and institutions, such as schools and hospitals, for the most part were sponsored by individual groups. And most importantly, MCC acted only on mandate from the constituent groups, and this mandate was lacking. So MCC responded to Fast's proposal by referring this need to the several constituent groups for whatever expression they would care to make.

Apparently the only conference group to respond initially to the MCC invitation was Fast's own group and, as one might expect, at the initiative of the Emergency Relief Board. In June 1945 the General Conference Mennonite Church responded favorably to the recommendation of that board and agreed to cooperate with MCC to establish a mental institution or, if this was not possible, to establish one of their own.

Our dedication to the principle of nonresistance by itself did not inspire concern for the mentally ill. It did help to intensify our care about people and give meaning, direction and quality to the way we worked with the mentally ill.

—Henry A. Fast[2]

The Mental Health Study

With this concrete expression of interest, the MCC Executive Committee later in June appointed a Mental Hospital Study Committee "to make preliminary studies in regard to this matter." The committee, composed of P. C. Hiebert, H. S. Bender and Robert Kreider, performed a remarkably thorough job in the brief span of six months. They surveyed congregations to determine the incidence of mental illness and mental deficiency, asked ministers about the advisability of establishing a mental institution, and consulted administrators of homes for the aged and general hospitals. The committee also used the resources of the National Mental Health Foundation (NMHF) and consulted with psychiatrists and mental hospital administrators outside the constituency.

Our concern for the mentally ill was a growing, transforming experience. Working a little like leaven it appeared perhaps a little soft and non-descript in the beginning but it had life in it and slowly it began to transform our whole attitude and manner of work with the mentally ill.

—Henry A. Fast[3]

In its report to MCC in December 1945, the committee recommended that Mennonite general hospitals consider establishing psychiatric wards, that conference or regional groups consider establishing homes for the "chronically mentally ill" and the "mentally deficient," that MCC continue sponsoring voluntary service units in state mental institutions, and that Mennonite doctors and premedical students consider specializing in psychiatry. But the committee was "not convinced that the conference groups should at this time share in the establishment of a separate institution for the care of the mentally ill." The reasons were costs, difficulty of securing a convenient location, and the dearth of professional psychiatric personnel. The door, however, was left open for later action.[4]

A supplementary report of the committee on April 8, 1946, with Grant Stolzfus serving in place of Robert Kreider, offered additional recommendations: to emphasize the contribution of religious faith to mental health and encourage pastoral counseling; to encourage foster home care; to suggest that several small institutions might be sponsored; and to become involved with the national mental health movement.[5]

The Leitersburg Possibility

A new element in the developing climate of interest was introduced at the September 14, 1946, MCC Executive Committee meeting when it was suggested that the Leitersburg farm near Hagerstown, Maryland, owned by MCC and recently vacated as a CPS base, might be used for a "rest home for Mennonites needing mental care (mild cases)." MCC requested a more detailed plan, so MCC staff member Elmer Ediger presented a seven-page document to the October 19 meeting and subsequently to a special meeting of MCC on October 31. The recommendations provided detailed suggestions on how to utilize the existing facilities, the kind of patient to be served, personnel, finances, and therapy. MCC approved the recommendations in principle with the suggestion, once more, that perhaps one of the constituent groups might undertake the Leitersburg project. So far as can be determined, no group picked up the suggestion. There may not have been time.

Almost immediately the Leitersburg proposal received further scrutiny. In December MCC staff members Arthur Jost and Elmer Ediger met with Harold Barton, William Keeney and Richard Hunter of NMHF, primarily to test the proposal. Dallas Pratt, a psychiatrist on the NMHF staff, had previously provided a written response to the Leitersburg plan. This contact with NMHF was a push, to be felt more fully later, toward providing active treatment rather than merely custodial care for mental patients.

West Coast Interest

A further development occurred about the same time, when MCC received a letter on December 10 from Ben Wall in behalf of the board of the Mennonite Brethren Home for the Aged, in Reedley, California. The Pacific District Conference of the Mennonite Brethren had authorized this board to let MCC know that they were

...It's very significant how Dr. Dallas Pratt of Philadelphia, in reading through our first Leitersburg proposal, came through with a whole sheet of suggestions, not deriding what naivete there might have been there but focusing on several things, on what we ought not to do and what we should concentrate on, such as the central role of a psychiatrist in the program... Well, as I look back, that tipped the scales between the possibility of doing what a lot of other church mental hospital programs have done—fading off toward chronic care, mixing everything, mentally deficient and everybody, just having a home-type thing—and edging us toward a treatment program.

—Elmer M. Ediger[6]

ready to cooperate in the promotion of a possible home for mentally ill on the West Coast.

So the ground was laid for the significant and comprehensive action of MCC at its annual meeting on January 3, 1947. MCC agreed on a master plan to establish "three small homes for mentally ill and/or rest homes," one each in the eastern, western and midwestern parts of the United States. The offices and resources of MCC were made available for getting the programs started, CPS funds were to be used for further planning, and an advisory committee was to study ways and means, make plans, and present recommendations to MCC in implementing the program.

MCC Establishes the First "Homes" (1947-56)

With this mandate from the cooperating church groups, MCC was prepared to move ahead. And move they did, with some sense of urgency and dispatch. The experience in administering relief and service programs was put to good use and applied to the new effort. The MCC Executive Committee made most of the decisions with weightier matters referred to the larger annual or special meetings of MCC. The Akron office was well-staffed with Orie O. Miller as executive secretary and a corps of youthful administrators who had been trained by the experience of CPS. Two among them, Elmer Ediger and Arthur Jost, were to assume major roles throughout the years of the Mennonite mental health movement.

We did not start this work with an organizational chart neatly grafting another inter-Mennonite venture onto the growing MCC tree. We started with the desire to make available a service that would minister to our deeply felt needs and then set up an organization fit to carry this responsibility.

—Henry A. Fast[7]

One of the first items of business was to establish and make operative the advisory committee for the mental health program. MCC appointed Titus Books, Paul Nase, and J. Harold Sherk from the east; E. C. Bender from the Elkhart area; H. A. Fast from Kansas; and Henry R. Martens from the West Coast. These with Orie Miller made up the committee. In three weeks, on January 25, they met at the Atlantic Hotel in Chicago and elected Fast as chairman and Sherk as secretary. At this first meeting of what was to become Mennonite Mental Health Services, the committee formulated recommendations for MCC which would move the program forward on all three fronts.

The Master Plan Implemented

The eastern project, of course, had a head start because of the preliminary work done by the Akron staff the year before. MCC owned the farm, so buildings were immediately available. Before the year was over, the Leitersburg project, now named *Brook Lane Farm*, was well on its way with the farm buildings and CPS barracks being remodeled and a new hospital wing under construction. MCC had named Delvin Kirchhofer, a former overseas relief worker, as administrator and Helmut Prager as medical director, and had appointed Books and Nase of the MCC advisory committee and Walter Temple as a local advisory committee for the project. The first patients were admitted in January of 1949.

For the West Coast, the MMHS committee at their first meeting asked Fast and Martens to work with MCC staff member Elmer Ediger in launching the project. A group of constituent representatives was called together in March 1947 in Reedley. They supported the proposed West Coast home; and before midyear MCC had approved plans for a thirty-bed facility, expandable to one hundred, and a $100,000 budget to be raised in a one-year period. It had appointed Arthur Jost administrator and named a West Coast advisory committee composed of Martens, D. C. Krehbiel, and Sam Eicher. But, unlike Brook Lane, there were no buildings or land to start with, so the large amount of money to be raised in the west caused some delay before plans were realized. Construction was completed in 1950 and *Kings View Homes* was opened early the next year.

The wheels were also set in motion for the Midwest project following the first meeting of MMHS. Some thirty-eight representatives from an area ranging from Colorado to Indiana, Minnesota to Oklahoma, met in Newton, Kansas, December 6, 1947, with P. C. Hiebert and H. A. Fast in charge. It ultimately took a couple of years to move the project to completion, largely because MCC needed to devote its attention to the other two projects. MCC did appoint an advisory committee and planning continued. By midyear 1950 Newton was identified as the site, and the committee searched for a suitable spot to locate *Prairie View Hospital*, as it had been named. In 1952 plans were prepared and approved for a $200,000 forty-bed hospital, and Myron Ebersole was named the first administrator. The hospital opened its doors in March 1954.

Reasons for Success

So within a seven-year period, the 1947 master plan had been realized. One wonders what made it move so rapidly. Clearly there was a lot of momentum from earlier CPS years which pushed MCC forward. There was anticipation in some quarters for a church-sponsored program, and some excitement to get going. The studies of 1945 and 1946, the Leitersburg proposal, and the numerous visits and interviews served to spark enthusiasm and to build the necessary confidence and courage to proceed.

Thus during the war years these two generations of leadership learned to work together efficiently and with an amazing "pulling together" of rather widely divergent Mennonite groups. They had discovered ways of brainstorming, proposing, revising, decision-making and acting to get things done. The regular MCC Executive Committee meetings, spaced about a month apart, became convenient target points for a "management by results" for those days.

—Elmer M. Ediger[8]

Crucial to the success of those early years was the leadership which took charge in implementing the plan. There was a two-generation level of leadership. The established leaders during the war years like Orie Miller, H. A. Fast, and P. C. Hiebert exhibited a wisdom, organizational skill, and ability to delegate which allowed the "second line" administrators like Ediger, Jost, and Robert Kreider to stretch their capabilities, experiment, do creative planning, and make things happen. For the first four years, Ediger served under Miller as director of the mental health program, until 1951 when Delmar Stahly, at first an assistant in the office, took over.

The advisory committees which were appointed very early in the process also were vital to the success of the program. MMHS itself was clearly advisory to MCC, even after the 1952 incorporation, but this served well in the planning and decision-making process. Recommendations in effect became decisions, for rarely did MCC modify or reject them, though at times they were delayed. The advisory

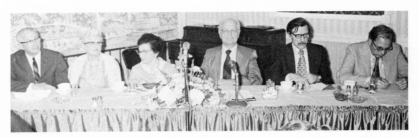

Speakers' table at the 25th Anniversary of MMHS at Brook Lane, October 1971. Delvin and Helen Kirchhofer, Mrs. and Henry A. Fast, Jacob Goering and Elmer Ediger.

committee for each hospital served to provide a local planning and recommending group in the process, and they became the nucleus of boards of directors later on.

All these persons and groups were linked together in a remarkable network as a single organism. MCC and MMHS were linked by persons like Fast and Miller, who functioned in both organizations. MMHS members also served as members on each of the three local advisory committees. And MCC mental health staff members were located at Akron and, as administrators, at each of the three programs.

The Function of MCC

During the first decade, with this network of persons and committees, MCC served exceptionally well in initiating and operating the three programs. The MCC philosophy of serving "in the name of Christ" permeated the program and strongly influenced the entire development. The emphasis was upon service, volunteerism, frugality, and witness. The leadership was strong, creative, dedicated, and resourceful. With nothing to begin with except a memory of Bethania and the difficult experience of untrained young people in state hospitals, this group of leaders managed to create mental health service programs with ever increasing credibility and respectability.

A major reason for the success of the MCC program was the sensitivity and openness to change. The leadership sought the advice of experienced and trained professionals, searched for appropriate and useful models, learned from others' success or failure, and were prepared to adapt if this seemed the best way to go.

Originally the thought was to serve Mennonites, that is, "the household of faith." The 1945 study in part was to demonstrate a need among the constituent groups in order to justify a new service program. As planning proceeded, it was evident that services were to be available to anyone, although Brook Lane at first charged a different fee for nonconstituents and Kings View attempted to "reserve" space for constituents. But this did not last and soon the facilities were open to all.

Earlier, the leaders talked vaguely about serving the mentally ill and mentally deficient. And *mentally ill* at first referred to seriously ill, hospitalized persons, such as seen by CPS men in the state hospitals. Over the first few years there was a shift in thinking from serving chronically ill, former hospital patients, in a homelike atmosphere for long periods of time, to treating acutely ill patients for a shorter time in an active treatment facility. This development in concept undoubtedly occurred as a result of the numerous contacts with psychiatrists and other professionals in the field and the influence of the first medical directors of the MCC programs like Helmut Prager of Brook Lane and Jackson Dillon of Kings View.

We started with a hospital image because care of the mentally ill at the time appeared to require hospital treatment. It is through the exploratory learning process that we discovered how to use effectively the "clinic" program.

—Henry A. Fast[9]

In a real sense this overall movement to active treatment thwarted the original idea that the three homes were to be "experimental," each a different model in providing mental health services. When Brook Lane set its direction under Prager to treat the acute mentally ill, the plan was for Kings View to serve the chronically ill and the elderly disturbed. Prairie View, located in an area with three Mennonite colleges and several Mennonite hospitals, was to focus on training and education, among other services. But both Kings View and Prairie View, like Brook Lane, also became primarily active treatment hospitals when they opened. This disturbed some in the system. As late as 1954, MMHS discussed how Kings View had diverged from the original concept, and there was concern about the needs of chronically ill patients and "our neglect of them." Fear was expressed that "we were following our psychiatrists rather than acting independently as our constituency would prefer to have us act."[10] Prairie View's advisory committee, in a report to MMHS, stressed the seriousness of needs not met, "such as the needs of the aged, the chronic and the mentally retarded cases."[11] But little was done immediately to change the situation.

A further result of the move to active treatment was the need for professional staff. The earlier vision of providing "homes for the

mentally ill and/or rest homes" suggested that these could be operated largely by untrained staff members, former CPS men, for example, with part-time psychiatric coverage. But active treatment meant
psychiatric treatment, and MCC faced the fact that no Mennonite
psychiatrists were available. Consequently, the first psychiatrists
and medical directors in each of the three facilities—Prager at Brook
Lane (1947), Dillon at Kings View (1950), and Thomas Morrow at
Prairie View (1953)—came from outside the constituency.

MCC hoped to use mostly volunteers in staffing the new programs plus a few more permanent staff members in key positions.
This worked for a while. But in addition to the need to increase
professional staff, it became more difficult to secure and hold other
staff members. And what about salaries? What should permanent
staff be paid? This became a recurring and difficult question, raised
frequently at MMHS meetings. Akron was urged to develop a more
stable remuneration policy. Stahly presented personnel policies and
a salary scale to the December 1953 meeting, but problems persisted. Brook Lane complained of a critical staff shortage and Prairie
View said low salaries were cutting them out of the local labor
market. Ultimately, the general hospital model was adopted and
competitive salaries were offered to attract competent staff.

---

*It was some time before we realized we would have to pay aides and
maintenance staff with competent skills in order to get enough to staff
the hospitals, but we had no difficulty in making that transition after
convincing the budgetary-minded MCC that these changes were necessary.*

—Delmar Stahly[12]

But the concern to keep costs down continued. MCC kept alive
the mission and service motif, and fees and budgets were increased
only reluctantly. The chairman of the Kings View board at the
October 1954 MMHS meeting expressed appreciation for the effort of
MCC "to hold down fees in spite of the pressure on the part of the
psychiatrists to increase costs." At the same meeting, E. E. Miller, on
special assignment under MCC, admonished that "we should face
more positively the matter of caring for patients who cannot pay for
services." Stahly recommended that the MCC hospitals "make provision for charity cases." This was approved by both MMHS and MCC.

As much as possible, the Akron staff carried responsibility for
informing the church constituency about the mental health program. In the early years there were expressions from the hospitals
that MCC should do more. One of the significant developments was

> *As long as I was in the framework of administration that clearly spelled out that the MCC Executive Committee had final responsibility for everything relating to the administration of the hospitals and I was responsible to the Executive Secretary of MCC, I felt I had no choice but to represent them in the administration of my work because on paper I had that responsibility. And so I did often become an irritant in all of the hospitals. This was particularly embarrassing when the hospital staff would say, "We are the church as much as you are, so how can you say you represent the church?"*
>
> *— Delmar Stahly*[13]

the decision to hold regional Mental Health Institutes for discussing and explaining Mental Health Service and the problems of mental illness and, in general, for promoting understanding of matters concerned with mental health. The first three authorized in 1949 proved so helpful and successful that a number of additional institutes were held, at least as late as 1955.

The Need for Review

After the three hospitals were established and operating, those involved realized some overall review and evaluation of the mental health program was needed. There were two primary reasons for this. One was that the original master plan of 1947 had been carried out and, in the normal manner of operating, MCC felt it was time to evaluate the program and decide what to do with it in the future.

The other was internal. The local programs were experiencing growing pains under the current arrangement with MCC, largely around the issue of local initiative and responsibility versus Akron control. The hospitals, operating with local advisory committees and local administrators on Akron's payroll, felt they carried a responsibility far greater than the authority granted them. And MCC too felt increasingly uncomfortable in being directly responsible for administering such a widely-dispersed mental health program. As the study report stated, "The program appears to be growing too large, too widely distributed, and too complex for a highly centralized pattern of administration."

At its annual meeting January 1, 2, 1954, MCC provided for "a study of general policy in regard to the administration of the mental health institutions now administered by the MCC." However, this was sidetracked for two years by a request from the North Central area constituents (Illinois, Indiana, Michigan and Ohio) for a survey and study on the feasibility of a mental health program in that area.

But early in 1956, MCC appointed a committee composed of C. N. Hostetter, Jr., chairman, Robert Kreider, secretary, H. Ernest Bennett, Reuben Short and J. B. Toews. In his instructions to the committee, Orie Miller stated the task: "The scope of the committee would be to review the original assignment of MCC in the Mental Health field, review present administrative and operating procedures, and suggest any directions that should be taken in the future." The committee completed its work that year and submitted its report and recommendations to the next annual meeting of MCC, December 27, 28, 1956. Major changes were to follow.

Struggle For Identity and Independence (1957-66)

There followed a period of struggle and pain for all three major groups — MCC, MMHS and the centers. It was not easy for MCC to release its control and transfer greater autonomy to the hospitals. A major reason for this reluctance was that MCC felt that the control of the local hospitals essentially was in the hands of the medical directors, and until Otto Klassen joined the staff of one of the hospitals, Oaklawn, in 1962, all were nonconstituent psychiatrists. This produced an ideological tension, since the founders had envisioned a Christian institution allied with and servant of the church. Psychiatry, whether Freudian, Adlerian, or whatever, was seen as more humanistic in its approach and outlook.[14] There was fear that the programs would become local clinics to serve mostly the doctors' needs and that the Christian aspect would be glossed over. It was felt that to loosen MCC ties was to loosen ties to the church.

It may have seemed that the MCC leadership resisted this change/to local responsibility/; they did from within admit that they did not want the hospitals taken from them. At the same time, I think, they would have been ready to make the change to professional help had they known how to do it. In reality, the decentralization to the local boards was essential to make this change, while the MCC administration was not farsighted enough to recognize this. Of course, the effectiveness of Elmer Ediger and Art Jost was of the essence in the actual changeover.

— Delmar Stahly[15]

Changes Made

Nevertheless, in early 1957, a number of substantial changes were made as a result of the 1956 Study Committee Report. The findings specified that MMHS should "determine the broad policies of the MCC Mental Health Services," though still in line of responsibility to MCC. The MMHS director was to become "coordinator" and serve as executive officer for MMHS. Local advisory committees were to be organized as boards of directors, with members still appointed by MCC, and be responsible for all "administrative decisions." And local administrators were to be directly responsible to local boards. MCC agreed and the recommendations were implemented.

Symbolizing the change in policy, a new MMHS board assumed responsibility in 1957. Now serving were H. Clair Amstutz, subsequently elected chairman; Robert Kreider, secretary; Otto Klassen; and Frank Peters. Norman Loux, appointed a year earlier to replace E. C. Bender, continued, as did H. A. Fast, who had served from 1947. Orie Miller retained his spot on the board as *ex officio* member and treasurer of MMHS. Leaving after ten years of service were Titus Books, Henry R. Martens and Paul Nase, as well as George Classen, who had replaced J. Harold Sherk in 1951.

At its first meeting, the new board in April 1957 moved quickly to effect the changes. Delmar Stahly, earlier director, was appointed coordinator. The board took steps to organize the local advisory committees and, going beyond the recommendations, agreed that once organized, the boards should be incorporated. Organization of the boards was complete before the end of the year and incorporation followed. Kings View, already incorporated since 1951 for state tax purposes,[16] was followed by Prairie View in 1958, and Brook Lane in 1959. The new Oaklawn Psychiatric Center was also organized in 1958.

Oaklawn had been conceived earlier when the "East Central" project was initiated during a meeting of representatives from a four-state area in Goshen, Indiana, on April 3, 1954. This led to a needs assessment by MCC in 1955 and the subsequent establishment of an advisory committee which began to develop plans for what was to become Oaklawn Psychiatric Center. The Oaklawn advisory committee was organized as a board in 1958 and MMHS accepted responsibility for the program as with the other three. Robert W. Hartzler, at first chairman of the board, became the first Oaklawn administrator in 1961; and Otto Klassen became medical director in 1962. Oaklawn received the first patients in February 11, 1963, and the facilities were dedicated in September 20, 1963.

The Degree of Autonomy

Though now incorporated individually, the four centers, with MCC and MMHS, continued to struggle on the degree of autonomy this should represent. An immediate question was, Who can serve on the local board of directors? It was obvious initially, as with the preceding advisory committees, that members should come from local MCC constituent groups. When at the July 1957 MMHS meeting the question of non-Mennonites serving on the board was raised, the consensus was that "for the present, board membership should be confined to Mennonites." But the following year Prairie View brought a specific request to MMHS for community representatives. With considerable debate, this finally was approved. The other centers in time also requested community representatives, and in 1962 the bylaws of all four programs were amended to allow for up to four members-at-large, provided that two-thirds of the board represent the constituent groups.[17] "Constituent groups" by then had been defined to include the Church of the Brethren.[18]

Another question which proved difficult to resolve was, Who shall hold title to the property? Title of property meant ownership, and who owned the hospitals, MCC (MMHS) or the local boards? The real and other property, originally held by MCC, had been turned over to MMHS following the 1952 incorporation; indeed this was the main reason for incorporation. The 1956 study clearly stated that title to all property was to remain with MMHS, and this continued to be the position of MCC as the hospitals more and more questioned the wisdom of this policy. They argued that holding title was essential to full local responsibility. A concession of sorts occurred in 1959, when non-real estate property was transferred to the local corporations, but leases were arranged for the real property, the title for which remained with MMHS. It was not until 1965 that title to all property was transferred.

Nor were we [MMHS] sure of our authority. We were the tool of the MCC Executive Committee. As C. N. Hostetter remarked, we had been given the responsibility without the requisite authority. That was why MMHS was changed to board status with more autonomy.
—H. Clair Amstutz[19]

Toward an MMHS Role

The MMHS board had its own problems. Somehow suspended between MCC and the programs, what was the task of MMHS? How could it function properly vis a vis the institutions, now becoming stronger professionally, growing in maturity and expertise, and gaining more and more independence. One obvious move was the attempt to strengthen the board itself. Of the six members appointed in 1957 (other than Orie Miller), three were physicians (two of these psychiatrists) and three were professors with Ph.D. degrees. Others appointed during this period were: Roy Just (1961), Ernest Boyer (1962), William Klassen (1962), Paul Mininger (1962), John R. Mumaw (1963), Ray Schlichting (1965), Howard Musselman

(1965) and Charles Neff (1966). It is significant that MCC appointed some of the best-trained and experienced professionals and church-men from the constituency—psychiatrists, physicians, college presidents, professors, and businessmen. The MMHS board indeed was a powerful group.

The uncertainty of role also was manifested in the position of coordinator filled by Delmar Stahly. Located at Akron, he continued tacitly to represent MCC, with that kind of line authority, though according to the reorganization he was to function under MMHS and he was to "coordinate" rather than "direct." As a layman, it was increasingly difficult for him to relate to the developing mental health centers and especially to the professional staffs. The MMHS board in 1957 even designated Amstutz as "executive officer" to make the relationship, especially to the medical directors, more compatible and acceptable, but time and distances made this an impractical arrangement. Stahly found himself occupied more and more with staff recruitment and training, and with general publicity, and less with direct contact and coordination of the programs. The fact that the institutions were paying MCC for coordination and other Akron services continued to be an irritant for them.

In spite of such growing pains, MMHS began to find a role for itself. With experience, MMHS learned better how to develop policies and coordinate the work of the four institutions and not try to manage them directly. The board worked on a number of policy questions confronting the local programs and in this way provided overall direction. How do the administrator and the medical director relate to one another and to the local board? What are the values of an open versus a closed medical staff in an inpatient service? What should be the policy on sabbatical leaves? What policies and procedures are needed for such areas as property evaluation, uniform and standard accounting practices, bookkeeping, records, depreciation, and auditing?

Much effort by MMHS went into the continuing concern, usually from MCC, about the Christian witness of the mental health programs. As the local institutions gained in competence, as non-constituent persons joined boards and staffs, the concern about church-relatedness and Christian witness did not diminish. MMHS discussed the issues at board meetings. A series of study conferences on religion and psychiatry was sponsored in various regions. Representatives attended and participated in the Academy of Religion and Mental Health. They encouraged the appointment of chaplains at each institution, and by 1965 all four had provided for chaplaincy services.

*I was responsible to Delmar Stahly almost from the beginning...
When Delmar's role was changed to coordinator, his meetings, his
visits were more of a consultative nature, obviously; when he came
down...I felt there was a big difference between working for a local
board and working for the Akron office.*

—Arthur Jost[20]

Kern View Hospital

The end of the second decade saw the fifth MCC center open its
doors to patients. Kern View Hospital, Bakersfield, California, began as a satellite program of Kings View. In 1962 MMHS agreed that
Kings View should negotiate with the Greater Bakersfield Memorial
Hospital to set up a psychiatric program on ground adjacent to and
leased from the hospital. MMHS and MCC approved the project in
1963. The Kings View board was enlarged with representatives from
the southern part of the state, and these then became the board of
directors of Kern View when it was incorporated separately in
January 1967. The first patients were admitted to the twenty-five-
bed inpatient and outpatient facility in 1966.

More Changes

In the mid-1960s MMHS undertook a series of "role" studies
which moved the centers even more toward independence and
MMHS farther from MCC. A study committee in March 1964 reported
that "the trend toward more autonomy on the part of those clinics
now sponsored by MMHS is both inevitable and wholesome. MMHS
would "engage in coordination and creative planning" and establish
"broad principles and common objectives" for the mental health
programs. MMHS rather than MCC would appoint local board members and approve the appointment of top personnel, specifically
the administrator, medical director and chaplain. The MMHS staff
position was to be changed to "director" and the office shifted from
Akron to a site near one of the programs and if possible an institution of higher learning.

The March 1964 report, recommended by MMHS, was presented to the MCC Executive Committee in April, approved and sent
on to a special meeting of MCC on May 8, where it also was approved. So MMHS was "now free to continue development of the
new structure."

But this took a bit longer. Further work on the role statement
continued through 1965 and finally was approved as a working
document. To replace Delmar Stahly, who had served fifteen years
as primary staff member, MMHS appointed William Klassen as the

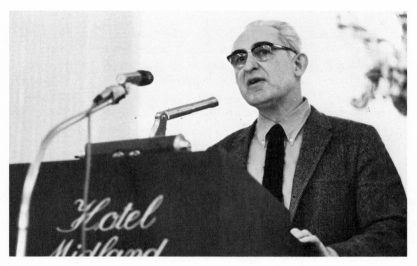

Paul W. Pruyser, Menninger Foundation, addressing the annual meeting of MCC, January 21, 1972, on the 25th anniversary of MMHS.

new director for a fifteen-month period, 1965-66. While the board searched for a replacement, Klassen continued another year on a part-time basis as he resumed his position on the faculty of Mennonite Biblical Seminary. The office shifted from Akron to Elkhart during these years. A further indication of the change was the departure of H. A. Fast and Orie Miller from the MMHS board. They had served two full decades from 1947 to 1966.

Partnership and Collaboration (1967-82)

Further attempts to clarify and implement the 1964 reorganization plan followed. A document on "The Future of MMHS", drawn up by the new director, Vernon Neufeld, was considered and revised in 1968 and 1969. It essentially recognized the quasi-independence of the member centers and noted that the strength of MMHS was derived from these programs as well as from MCC. The statement delineated the programmatic direction of MMHS toward the mental health programs and to other service areas which might be defined. The MCC Executive Committee in July 1969 supported MMHS in this clarification.

The Reorganization of MMHS

The next logical step was the reorganization of MMHS in January 1971, when MCC appointed representatives from the local programs themselves, as well as from the churches at large, to the MMHS

...The tone and content of that April [1969] meeting...had an edginess to it that I have not subsequently experienced. A variety of intangible, or at least unspoken tensions existed... It almost seemed to me as if one or two of the centre representatives were so distraught over historic linkages, that they were about ready to unilaterally take their leave of MMHS and MCC. At the same time, I was most impressed with how these tensions—spoken and unspoken—were handled. In retrospect, I wonder whether that particular meeting didn't signify the "bottoming-out" of many older and likely counter-productive agendas, and the beginnings of the rebirth of MMHS as we know it today.

—Aldred H. Neufeldt[21]

board. In MMHS, MCC and the offspring of MCC had become partners. The MCC centers or hospitals—Brook Lane, Kern View, Kings View, Oaklawn and Prairie View—were represented, as was Eden Mental Health Centre, which had joined MMHS as an affiliate in 1968. Philhaven Hospital, which had sent representatives to MMHS meetings for a number of years, joined MMHS in 1972 and was represented on the board the following year. The last to join MMHS and be represented on the board was The Penn Foundation for Mental Health, which came in at the end of 1981 after years of informal participation.

The Question of Separation

It is not surprising that during this period, the late 1960s and early 1970s, one persistent question being raised was whether MMHS and MCC had fulfilled the original mandate with reference to the mental health centers. Wasn't it time to help one or more of the centers cut the apron strings and become completely independent as a local community center? Indeed this possibility had been raised earlier in connection with the 1964 study report. MCC Executive Secretary William T. Snyder at times reminded MMHS that the long-term unwritten policy of MCC was to move into an area of need with program and personnel, and retreat at the strategic moment.

There were thoughts on separation and independence also coming from some of the centers. Arthur Jost in 1971, partly in response to Snyder's question and in view of strong community ties and the increasing practice of contracting with governmental entities, expressed an openness to the idea that Kings View might become a completely local program. Brook Lane in the early 1970s also questioned the value of maintaining ties with MMHS. In such

I think the first inkling of this [separation] from MMHS came from Bill [Snyder]. And I think I personally took a great deal of umbrage at the thought, at the idea. I remember distinctly speaking about it but it was more like a hurt child about to be kicked out of the house because I could never see how we would do it. We were getting into those contracts and immediately I could see the county appointing several board members. That's the way I saw it going and I was never really serious about it. I thought if we needed to comply and if Bill really wanted, or MCC really wanted, a pilot, I felt under certain obligations to consider it because we were at that point the farthest out on fooling around with Hill-Burton and federal monies, and county and state monies, that we should probably be the sacrificial lamb.

— Arthur Jost[22]

discussions local administrators and board members, more than MMHS board or staff, concluded that the link with the churches through MMHS and MCC was still valid and needed, and that it should continue. The alternative of becoming a local program, likely with a self-perpetuating board and subject to local "politics," was not attractive.

Canadian Ties

An added dimension to MMHS during this period came with the development of a stronger relationship to the Canadian constituency. Through MCC the churches in Canada had always been loosely tied in, but the MCC mental health program had been almost entirely a United States development. With discussions in Manitoba preceding the establishment of Eden Mennonite Mental Health Centre, MMHS became more actively involved. Orie Miller, H. A. Fast and H. Clair Amstutz visited Manitoba during the development stage, and representatives from Canada attended MMHS meetings as well. With Eden's joining MMHS in 1968, this tie was formalized and the relationship with Canada enhanced. In 1969, Aldred Neufeldt was appointed to the MMHS board as the first Canadian representative. Today there are five board members from Canada, including Eden's representative.

MMHS and Center Relationships

During the 1970s, MMHS, now the joint effort of MCC and the member centers or hospitals, searched for and experimented with ways to express the new partner relationship and fulfill its mission, with programs either center-related or aimed to meet other needs.

MMHS continued to serve the five MCC-founded centers in specific ways by appointing all board members, approving bylaw amendments and approving top staff appointments. These responsibilities came to be seen as a cooperative effort of the local board and staff with representatives of the church at certain critical points, more than as the retention of authority or veto power by MCC-MMHS. The greatest value of the legal tie was seen in the process of determining local board members, in discussing long-range implications of bylaw changes, and in the review of personnel who were to lead the local programs.

MMHS, through its director, encouraged and participated in local board retreats, orientation and training events to improve board functioning at all centers. To help with staff needs, MMHS served as a referral point for the centers. A scholarship program during the period 1968 to 1981 made grants ranging from $500 to $1000 to a total of forty-two persons. Staff members were encouraged to prepare studies and papers about aspects of their work; a total of twenty-five "Occasional Papers," a number of which were published in professional journals, were produced and distributed from 1971 to 1979.

MMHS came to be viewed as a support and counseling body for the centers, a forum where problems and issues could be shared and dealt with in a nonthreatening, fraternal way. In periods of crisis at the local level, the MMHS board and director were prepared to back up local authorities with needed changes and provide direction and guidance in planning the future. In MMHS, the administrators, particularly, found a place where they could give and receive advice and counsel on matters not dealt with in other contexts.

MMHS Outreach

Mennonite Mental Health Services as a joint effort of MCC and the centers now moved into new areas of service. As early as 1971, MMHS had expressed specific interest in working with offenders, and later with the MCC Peace Section had encouraged MCC to provide for a comprehensive, inter-Mennonite program. The eight mental health centers and Mennonite Disaster Services (MDS) cooperated in sponsoring a series of workshops during a period from 1977 to 1981, bringing together mental health and MDS workers to deal with the emotional and psychological factors of disaster work.

Another outreach program of MMHS was to work in the area of mental retardation. Earlier attempts to launch a program during the 1960s, under an MMHS advisory committee chaired by John R. Mumaw, had been tabled in 1968 and referred to MCC for disposition.

Late in 1970 MCC requested MMHS to assume the task and in April 1971 the board of MMHS acted to accept the mandate. MMHS appointed a committee to be responsible for constituency education and initiating some services. But clearly the committee was limited in what it might accomplish, so at the April 1973 meeting the MMHS board approved the recommendation of the advisory committee to appoint a full-time staff person. Jack Fransen was employed for a two-year period beginning in 1974. He was succeeded by Nancy Williams (1976-78) and Dean Bartel (1979-). The staff role was a multiple one, covering the Mennonite constituency in Canada and the United States, working with existing institutions, church conferences, congregations, MCC and schools, and helping each group in its particular responsibility for developmentally disabled persons.

Interest in a possible international program for MMHS emerged in the late 1970s. A number of circumstances contributed to this. Chester Raber, chaplain at Brook Lane, spent a sabbatical year 1967-68 in Singapore, and upon his return urged MMHS to become involved internationally. At the April 1968 MMHS meeting, Howard Musselman, board member, reminded the group of Orie Miller's long-standing concern about overseas work for MMHS. In Kansas, the newly created Paraguay-Kansas Partnership was stimulating an interest at Prairie View in that country. In April-July 1969, Julie Neufeld, a psychiatric nurse from Prairie View, spent four months in Paraguay as a consultant, primarily with the school of nursing in Asuncion. MMHS interest in Paraguay was greatly stimulated by this development.

In September 1969, the MMHS board asked its director to "investigate the possibilities, the obstacles, and the implementation of a program" in Paraguay. The feasibility of a Paraguay program was first explored stateside, which led to an investigative trip to Paraguay in March-April 1970 by Elmer Ediger, Vernon Neufeld and Augusto Esquibel, psychiatric consultant in international relationships for the National Institute of Mental Health. With these ties and contacts, various possible directions were suggested and explored during the months which followed.

Gradually two distinct service tracks emerged. One involved the Paraguay-Kansas Partnership, through which numerous staff exchanges occurred between Prairie View and a private group in Asuncion providing mental health and mental retardation services. The other was more specifically a program of MMHS and MCC, whereby various collaborative efforts were undertaken with the Mennonites in Paraguay. These efforts focused on the national

mental hospital in Asuncion and the Mennonite colonies in the
Chaco region of Paraguay.

Thus the last fifteen years have seen a marked shift in MMHS,
from a climate where some of the MCC hospitals might have become
independent, to the emergency of a new collaborative structure
which includes the contribution of both MCC and the centers as
partners in a newly defined program of service. Moreover, rather
than losing centers, MMHS gained three additional partners, Eden
Mental Health Centre, Philhaven Hospital, and Penn Foundation.
Especially during the later years, there is evidence of a renewed
interest on the part of the centers to strengthen the ties to the church
via MMHS and MCC and openly to express locally the mission of the
church. A Special Task Force on the Future of MMHS, established in
1979 and working during 1980 and 1981, clearly expressed the
desirability of this linkage with the church in years to come. MCC
continues to serve as the administrative home for MMHS, appointing
all board members, approving bylaw changes, approving the annual program and budget, and financing the major part of the
overall program.

There are three discernible periods in the unfolding Mennonite mental health story. In each there were adjustments in the
roles played by the three major groups, MCC, MMHS, and the centers, and in their relationship to one another.

During the first decade, MCC was clearly in charge. With its
organization, its staff, its leadership, and its vision and sense of
mission, MCC was in place to act responsibly in getting the programs
started. MCC carefully nurtured and guided the programs, closely
monitoring and controlling them. The programs themselves were
the mission, so their individual institutional identity and character
were emerging but not yet mature. MMHS was only advisory to MCC,
an important role though it was, but limited in expressing its own
individuality and mission.

But the offspring grew up, and during the second decade MCC
wisely loosened the strings of control, though not without fear for
the welfare of the young programs in a strange and threatening
professional world living in and associating with a "secular" community. The centers struggled for self-identity and independence,
for community involvement, for competence, at times almost in
adolescent rebellion. MCC's subsidiary, MMHS, as an intermediary
came to be a buffer and interpreter between center and MCC, center
and church, to deal with some of the questions and uncertainties
expressed by a concerned constituency.

The past decade and a half have seen further shifts. The
possibility of complete separation of the centers from MCC and

Views of the Psychiatric Hospital, Asuncion, Paraguay, where MMHS has collaborated with the hospital administration and the Paraguay Mennonites since 1972.

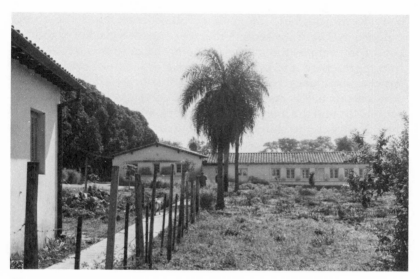

Newer women's section.

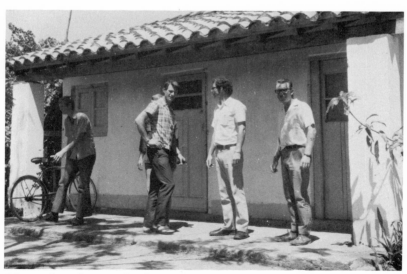

Mennonite volunteers by the unit house built by Paraguay Mennonites.

MMHS, once predicted, did not occur. The programs, like persons, became responsible individual institutions, now not anxious to sever the roots of their origin but discovering a newer relationship as partners and collaborators. Once individual identity and responsibility were achieved, the centers valued even móre the church connection, not in any sentimental sense nor as a symbol of security, but for the values, the motivation, and the purposes this relationship represented and provided. Joining in this relationship to the larger constituency were three other institutions founded under different auspices. As a collaborative service agency, joining together MCC and the mental health centers, MMHS was able to expand the ministry of the church into new areas of service. MMHS finally found its own unique mission.

How Our Centers Developed

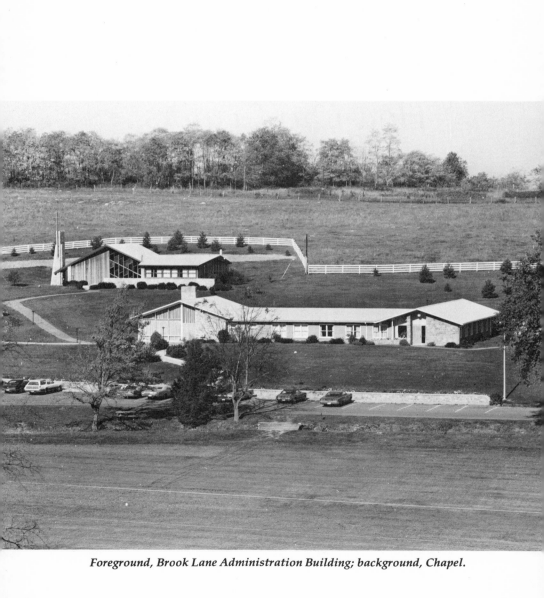

Foreground, Brook Lane Administration Building; background, Chapel.

CHAPTER 3

Brook Lane
Hagerstown, Maryland
Evangeline B. Myers*

Nestled among the rolling hills of the Blue Ridge Mountains are the attractive stone and stucco buildings which make up Brook Lane Psychiatric Center. Hidden from immediate view, the center is reached by a long lane, following the winding, tree-bordered brook from which Brook Lane received its name.

This was the first of three mental health facilities which the Mennonite and Brethren in Christ churches authorized through the Mennonite Central Committee (MCC) in January 1947. Brook Lane opened its doors to patients two years later and for more than thirty years has served the churches and the local community by helping meet the needs of emotionally troubled and mentally ill persons.

Origins (Before 1947)

Brook Lane had its beginning during the 1940s as a Soil Conservation Demonstration Farm which was operated by conscientious objectors under the Civilian Public Service (CPS) program of the Selective Service and Training Act of 1940. The farm near Leitersburg, Maryland, owned by MCC, consisted of 105 acres and was known as *CPS Camp Number 24*. The farmhouse and barn, still used in the Brook Lane program, date back to the early 1840s.

Following the war, when the CPS camps were being phased out, MCC suddenly had a farm on its hands. In the context of a growing interest among Mennonites to serve mentally ill persons, someone asked the question, Why couldn't this Leitersburg farm be used to begin a hospital program? It was in a peaceful and restful rural setting, in a Mennonite area, with a number of buildings available to be utilized. It seemed almost providential.

*Evangeline B. Myers has been on the Brook Lane staff since 1963, currently serving as a nurse. She was assisted by the editor in the preparation of this chapter.

*As a young girl of perhaps 8 or 10 years of age, I can remember coming
to Brook Lane on a Sunday afternoon with my family to visit a few of
my father's friends who were COs serving at the Farm. I can recall
seeing the many small "A" frame chicken coops or houses out on the
hill in back of the present Dining Hall. This hill is known to many as
"Chocolate Drop." Also, I can remember seeing pigs and cows in the
barn and men doing the milking by hand. The farmhouse had two
rooms with long tables and benches where the staff ate together as one
big family. The lane was a dirt road.*

— Evangeline Myers[1]

Leitersburg Proposal

So the "Leitersburg Proposal" was developed and approved
by MCC in October 1946. The seven-page document provided specific and detailed recommendations about how the program might
be implemented. The farm was to be used as a "rest home for
mentally ill, primarily for Mennonite and Brethren in Christ constituency." Both chronically and acutely mentally ill patients were to be
served, with preference given to the latter. Personnel were to include a director, registered nurse, farmer, matron, attendants, a
part-time medical doctor and psychiatrist, and a psychiatric social
worker. With the exception of the physicians, most would be on a
voluntary service basis the first year. Expenses above farm income
would be covered by contributions, families and church groups. The
anticipated cost to operate was three dollars per patient day. The
proposal named four therapies: occupational, recreational, hydro,
and electric shock. The main farmhouse was to serve as dining and
living room, offices, and two apartments. The two twenty- by forty-
eight-foot CPS barracks were to be converted to rooms for twenty
patients. The report said, "We would want to find the right combination of Christian care, home-like atmosphere, high personnel standards, reasonable financial policies, and the optimum of scientific
therapies of demonstrated value."[2]

The Leitersburg proposal received further scrutiny before January 1947. Most significant was a meeting of Arthur Jost and Elmer
Ediger with Harold Barton, William Keeney, and Richard Hunter of
the National Mental Health Foundation on December 6, 1946. The
four pages of notes recorded indicate the thorough review given the
proposal, with suggestions covering types of patients, buildings,
personnel, records, and licensing. In a written statement prepared
for this conference, Dallas Pratt, psychiatrist on the NMHF staff,
made several incisive suggestions: He warned against "mixing any
chronic deteriorated or senile patients with the more acute cases,"
and emphasized the importance of screening for admission. He

emphasized that electroshock should be given only by a psychiatrist, and must be accompanied by psychotherapy. He objected to the name "Rest Home," since activity rather than rest should be stressed for psychiatric patients. Pratt concluded:

> There is a feeling in the whole report that one can set up what is essentially a psychiatric hospital, with minor and some rather major forms of psychiatric treatment, and with patients with extremely serious forms of illness (all psychoses can be so described), yet with minimum use of the psychiatrist. No one would presume to treat the more serious diseases of tuberculosis or rheumatic fever in this way.[3]

Then followed the all-important action by MCC on January 3, 1947, a master plan to establish three mental health facilities, one each in the East, West, and Midwest. Clearly, the availability of the Leitersburg farm and the 1946 proposal to utilize it for a mental health program were vital factors in bringing MCC to the momentous decision. Indeed, the resolution stipulated "that the Leitersburg, Maryland, CPS farm project [was] to be held available for the purposes of this work in the East."[4]

Brook Lane Farm Established (1947-49)

Refining the Plan

Following the MCC decision, the Leitersburg project, named *Brook Lane Farm* later that year, moved forward rapidly. Between January 3 and 25, MCC staff members interviewed some of the most reputable professionals in the eastern part of the United States to refine the project even more. In varying combinations, Elmer Ediger, Arthur Jost, Paul Goering and Frank Wright met with H. K. Petry, superintendent of Harrisburg State Hospital (Pa.); George H. Preston, commissioner of the Maryland Division of Mental Hygiene; Robert H. Felix, Maryland Mental Hygiene Division of U.S. Public Health and later the first director of the National Institute of Mental Health; and John C. Whitehorn, head of the Department of Psychiatry and director of Phipps Clinic of Johns Hopkins University. These contacts served to confirm the direction being taken and pushed the program even more toward active treatment rather than custodial and convalescent care.

At the first meeting of the MCC mental health advisory committee, later to become Mennonite Mental Health Services (MMHS), on January 25, it was agreed, subject to MCC approval, that the Leitersburg home be approved "as an experimental project." Patients were to be of the "moderately ill type," maximum stay was to be six months, and the maximum cost $3.50 per day. The committee recommended that two of their own members from the East, Paul Nase and Titus Books, should be appointed "as advisors to the Akron

office." These recommendations were approved by MCC the following month.

Choosing a Staff

Upon the suggestion of George H. Preston, Maryland commissioner of Mental Hygiene, the planners of Brook Lane were
brought into contact with Helmut Prager, a psychiatrist in Baltimore. On April 9, 1947, Paul Goering and Elmer Ediger interviewed
Prager about the possibility of his serving in the Brook Lane program. The meeting was cordial and productive, and all agreed to
explore the possibility further.

---

*Dr. Prager gave his life story to us and then why he was interested in
working with an institution such as ours. He is a Jewish refugee from
Germany who left shortly after Hitler came into power. Although his
parents are orthodox Jews, he says that his own family has somewhat
left these traditions, although it would seem evident that Dr. Prager
was a man of high character. Dr. Preston also testified to his basic
honesty, his sincere interest in patients and that he was not the type
who particularly grabbed after money.*

—Elmer M. Ediger[5]

Later that month, Prager met with a group at Brook Lane,
which included the advisory committee members Books and Nase,
MCC representatives Ediger and Goering, Richard Hunter of NMHF,
Amos Baer representing the Hagerstown area, and others. The
group agreed on further steps for the project, most of which ultimately were adopted by MCC. Most significant was to arrange a one-
year contract with Helmut Prager for approximately two days of his
time per week. The emphasis now shifted, with Prager's influence,
from serving "moderately ill" to serving "acutely mentally ill" patients. The group agreed that the barracks and main house were to
be remodeled that summer at a cost of from $15,000 to $20,000 with
the opening of the institution scheduled for the fall of 1947.

On the heels of securing Prager as psychiatrist, MCC very early
was also able to employ a couple to serve as administrator and head
nurse respectively. Delvin Kirchhofer and Helen Moser, former MCC
relief workers in Egypt, agreed to begin serving August 1, 1947,
following their marriage. Arrangements were made for three
months of training at Chestnut Lodge in nearby Rockville, Maryland, although this was cut short by demands placed upon the
administrator to get Brook Lane ready for patients.

As plans proceeded, it became apparent that the cost of re-
modeling, now estimated at $21,000, would be too high for the

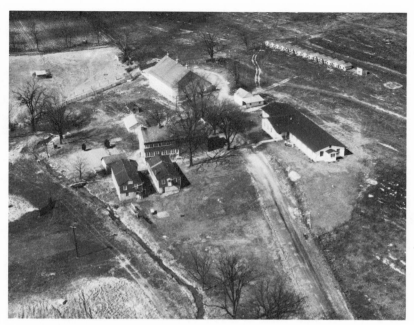

Aerial view of Brook Lane, c. 1955.

results gained. So the decision was made to construct a new twenty-three bed hospital building for patients rather than converting the barracks, but still remodel the existing buildings for other uses. The total cost reached approximately $65,000. So the opening of the facilities was delayed by nearly a year, with the dedication held in October 1948 and first patients admitted in January 1949.

Brook Lane, The Early Years (1949-57)

When the twenty-three bed hospital opened its doors in 1949, the facilities were completed, the program set, and the staff ready to go. Brook Lane was to serve acute mentally ill persons for short periods of time in an active treatment program. Though more than the $3.50 projected earlier, the charges for patients were modestly set at $5.50 per patient day; and patients from the MCC constituency were charged a discount rate of $5.00.[6] As medical director, Prager was in charge of admissions and the treatment program. The other staff members included a large contingent of volunteers in addition to salaried personnel, under the direction of the administrator, Delvin Kirchhofer. A local advisory committee of three persons, Walter Temple having joined Books and Nase late in 1947, advised Akron on developments.

The fact that Prager served part-time seemed at first not to affect the program adversely. He spent approximately two days per week at the hospital, also maintaining a private office in Baltimore and one in Hagerstown. Reports by the administrator and advisory committee consistently expressed deep appreciation for Prager's services, humanitarian spirit, cooperation, and leadership.

Inpatient Growth

Great care was exercised in admitting patients to the hospital. It was felt that mixing patients would create problems in the twenty-three-bed facility, problems for staff and patients, and ultimately lead to adverse publicity for the new hospital. Consequently, the census at first was low. But as Brook Lane became better known, referrals from within a hundred-mile radius increased. After two years, during the beginning months of 1951, the hospital was full.

Plans were made to move single staff members from one of the barracks to the newly purchased Largent house and thus provide space for eight additional patients, but this proposal was turned down by the state. So plans were initiated to build a new addition to the existing hospital. Pressure for patient space continued. In February and March 1952, for ten consecutive days, the hospital had over thirty patients (thirty-four on four of those days). Administrator Kirchhofer reported, "It was a coincidence, I am sure, that on one of those four days two nurses from Baltimore representing the State Board of Health and the State Department of Mental Hygiene came to pay us an inspection visit... They were quite annoyed at our patient census of thirty-four on a twenty-three bed licensed capacity."[7] The census was reduced and six additional licensed beds were provided temporarily by moving some offices out of the hospital and utilizing other space.

Construction on the new wing was started in 1952. It was ready for patients the beginning of 1954, bringing the total capacity to thirty-eight beds. *The Oaks*, a new kitchen and dining room building, with laundry facilities in the lower level, was completed in 1956. *The Pines*, as the administrator's home was named, was constructed the following year.

Early Staff

The staff members initially were volunteers and salaried personnel, with Helen Kirchhofer the only professionally trained full-time member. They worked long hours at many different tasks.

There were problems—one being rapid turnover of staff which put strain on more permanent members. Furthermore, volunteers and other untrained personnel were not always adequately

> *With two wash days a week and consequently heavy ironing, with the*
> *innumerable tasks in connection with cooking, baking, cleaning, and*
> *assisting with gardening, all in addition to the attendant work, the*
> *women folk are always busy. As for the men, besides the farm work*
> *already mentioned and the attendant work at the hospital, there are*
> *still so very many tasks of construction work and maintenance to be*
> *done that we never seem to accomplish all that we hope to do.*
> *— Delvin Kirchhofer*[8]

screened, so not everyone necessarily made good attendants. "We cannot afford to experiment continually on patients to see which workers are adept with mental cases," Kirchhofer complained.[9] And then there were periods, as during 1954, when there was a shortage of staff. This was partly due to substandard salary scales. In 1956 MMHS-MCC changed its policy to allow for competitive salaries.

All staff members initially lived on the grounds. Patients and staff freely intermingled. They ate their meals together, shared recreation and living room facilities, joined in religious services. This was seen as valuable to the patient to restore self-confidence. But it did create problems for staff members and their privacy. Ultimately, especially as the number of both patients and staff increased, this practice was decreased.

One continuing need, evident from the beginning, was to build bridges of understanding and support with the constituent churches and the local community. The Kirchhofers, Jacob Goering and later John Purves were particularly active in developing these relationships. The positive experiences of patients also contributed significantly.

> *The Public Relations in our community seem to have improved*
> *somewhat and a bit more interest is being shown. Part of this may be*
> *due to the fact that a relative of the Mennonite Bishop has been a*
> *patient in our hospital and fortunately improved a good deal and was*
> *discharged some time ago... One Amish bishop from western Mary-*
> *land, after visiting one of his members who is a patient at the hospital,*
> *suggested to his people from the pulpit that they help support this*
> *work; consequently, quite a few checks have been received from the*
> *members of that church.*
> *— Delvin Kirchhofer*[10]

Need for More Direction

The part-time functioning of the medical director was not without problems. Prager made heavy use of electroshock therapy, partly because of the limitation of time and partly because it was a prevailing therapeutic method. There was concern over this.[11] Jacob Goering, who joined the staff in September 1950, among other assignments, was to provide counseling and psychotherapy for patients. This was what Prager felt was needed and what he wanted. Prager himself provided psychotherapy for selected patients as he had time for this.

I recall of helping with many shock treatment patients and we gave them a section of the Barn upstairs and used cots in the Gymnasium as the recovery area. Doctors from Hagerstown usually came to Brook Lane to give the anesthesia and assist with the treatments. I recall one day a Doctor came and left the keys in the ignition turned on and the motor running and later we discovered his car was missing and so was one of our male patients. He was from out of state and gotten as far as Cumberland, Maryland, where he was apprehended by State Police and brought back to the hospital.

—Evangeline Myers[12]

The outpatient services grew, particularly after Prager closed his private office in Hagerstown at the end of 1951. As the patient

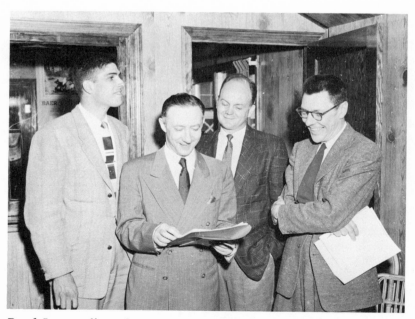

Brook Lane staff members, 1955 (l. to r.) Arthur Laemmlen, administrator; Helmut Prager, medical director; John Purves, social service director; Jacob D. Goering, psychologist.

load increased in both the inpatient and outpatient services, two additional part-time psychiatrists from Baltimore were engaged in 1953 to assist Prager, so that parts of six days each week were covered by one or another of the three psychiatrists.

But it became clear that changes were needed. It was felt that having a resident physician was a goal to be explored.[13] Prager resigned at the close of 1957, but helped bridge the gap until a full-time physician, Gilles R. Morin, came in July 1958.

More Changes

The end of 1957 brought other changes. The administrative position had undergone considerable turnover since Delvin Kirchhofer left in mid-1953 after serving almost six years. Jacob Goering filled in as interim administrator for one year, followed by Arthur Laemmlen, 1954-56, and Dennis Miller, 1956-57. D. Chauncey Kauffman began serving as administrator in October 1957.[14]

The Brook Lane advisory committee was due to be strengthened. Nase, Books, and Temple, the latter replaced by John Fretz in 1950, had served as "advisors to Akron" since 1947. Nase once complained to MMHS in his report that "the Advisory Committee feels it has made minimal contributions to Brook Lane Farm due to inexperience and distance from the hospital."[15] In 1956 a number of local members were added, so the advisory committee became more readily available. In 1957 the group was organized into a board of directors with Howard Musselman elected chairman. This board was incorporated in 1959.

The first nine years of operation, 1949-57, might well be called "the Prager years" since Prager was a major force and influence in establishing Brook Lane Farm as a respectable, recognized and successful psychiatric hospital. His concern for what was best for the patient, his sound judgment in guiding the direction of those early years, his cooperation in supporting and helping fulfill the goals of MCC, all left their mark on the institution.

Now, with greater local autonomy, with a new administrator, with a resident physician, with more professionally trained staff members, Brook Lane was to move into another era of its development.

From Hospital to Psychiatric Center

A Triad of Leadership

The transition which followed was made smoothly. A triad of leadership emerged which during the next four years served Brook Lane very well. Gilles Morin not only continued the medical program initiated by Helmut Prager, but led the hospital to greater internal strength, as will be noted later. Kauffman proved an able and experienced administrator and brought stability to the program. The most important new element in leadership came from the newly organized board of directors, with Howard Musselman as its creative and hardworking chairman. For four years these three men worked together as a team in solidifying the Brook Lane organization and program.

Morin was joined in 1958 by Roy Harnish, director of Social Work, and a second psychiatrist, John C. White. Trained in the Menninger program in Topeka, Kansas, Morin developed a team approach to patient care within the hospital:

> We have come to realize that the mentally ill patient should be approached by a variety of avenues, and that all concerned with the treatment of a mental patient should work together, each knowing what the other is doing and each one specialized in a specific facet of the total picture.[16]

Morin believed that the total milieu had an impact on the patient. The implementation of a particular philosophy of treatment "becomes the milieu within which the patients will live, interact with, and struggle against throughout his stay in the hospital." He felt the day-to-day interactions with nurses and aides had greater impact than those with the psychiatrists and social workers.[17]

Master Plan

Brook Lane's master plan, developed in 1958, projected major expansion in three areas: a new hospital wing which would increase the capacity to fifty-five beds, a new chapel building and an administration building.

Initially there was strong interest at Brook Lane to expand the hospital. With two full-time psychiatrists, the facilities were strained by full occupancy. Application was made for Hill-Burton construction funds but ultimately not accepted because of the increased cost brought by federal specifications and because of the requirement to use union labor. At one point in 1959, the board acted to double the number of beds by purchasing some existing property in the community, but this fell through.

The Brook Lane campus, however, saw other changes during this period. In 1959 a duplex staff house, known as *The Maples*, was constructed and the upper part of the barn was renovated for the occupational therapy shop and an auditorium. The projected office building, partially financed by $18,000 contributed by Hagerstown businessmen and a Ford Foundation grant of $20,000, was completed in 1960. *The Laurels*, designed as a dormitory for women staff members and volunteers, was built in 1961. And the chapel was

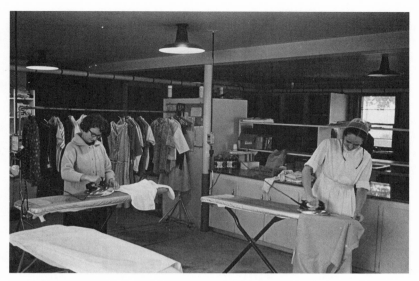

Laundry previously operated by staff and patients.

erected and dedicated in 1962, financed largely by contributions from the church constituency.

Chaplaincy Program

During this period there was a surge of interest in the religious facet of Brook Lane's program. Morin himself seemed to fit well into the efforts of Brook Lane to provide a Christian witness and ministry. He emphasized the importance of "Christian living" and the impact that staff had on patients. "I don't see this as ritualistic but more fundamental, incorporating the concept of love, understanding, tolerance and empathy. Each and every member of our organization has a very definite moral obligation in this respect," he said.[18]

One tangible indicator was the addition of Chester Raber to the staff in October 1961 as chaplain; another was the construction of the chapel in 1962. Earlier, for a three-year period from 1956 to 1959, Lamont Woelk, the pastor of the Fairfield Mennonite Church near Gettysburg, Pennsylvania, had served as part-time chaplain. But Raber, as a full-time staff member and one trained professionally in clinical pastoral care, was able to initiate an innovative program which was directed to both the internal needs in the hospital and those in the community. Musselman himself actively promoted the religious aspect of Brook Lane, even suggesting that "the Board does not look upon Brook Lane primarily as a Hospital but as the Church engaged in its daily calling to discipleship."[19]

> *This is more than adding a "preacher" to the staff to speak words of comfort to sick people. Somehow in following the Way of Christ, using the resources of mind and spirit that are given to us, we hope that we can give a more fruitful service than we have in the past. Perhaps we are naive in this but we hope that out of the MMHS hospital experiences will come a better understanding of what is involved in the mixing of psychiatry and Christian faith — a theology of healing if you will.*
> *—Howard Musselman[20]*

Change in Leadership

Late in 1961, the team of four years began to break up. John C. White suddenly became ill with cancer and died in October. Kauffman resigned effective November 1 and Lee Yoder, public relations director, was named interim administrator. Morin resigned in March 1962 and Paul Saraduke joined the staff in April as acting medical director.

This rather precipitous change in personnel had its impact upon Brook Lane. William Zuercher joined the staff as administrator in June 1962 and provided stable leadership for the next four years. But a great void existed in professional staff and leadership, particularly at the psychiatrist level. Zuercher and Musselman, reporting to MMHS in April 1963 after a year of staff shortages, sounded an exceptionally pessimistic note; both were frustrated about prospects to fill this void. Musselman referred to the "closed door" and the "blank wall" in recruiting psychiatrists.

> *Dr. Amstutz recently took issue with me when I said that MMHS finds itself in a position such as some hypothetical mission board which decides to open up a needy new field but finding itself without missionary candidates, sends out the first technically trained people it can find, whether they be Buddhists, Christians or Agnostic! I admit that the illustration is bizarre, and has dangerous overtones which I immediately repudiate, but I do maintain that its central thrust is true, namely that we are neck deep in a work for which we have not developed adequate personnel resources.*
> *—Howard Musselman[21]*

With only one psychiatrist on staff for over a year, the hospital census dropped and the plan to expand the hospital was delayed. Charles Goshen was employed as a part-time "Consulting Medical Director" in December 1962 to help plan the hospital construction and recruit a full-time medical director. However, he did not support the idea of enlarging the hospital, but rather advocated limiting the number of beds and instead planning for scattered outpatient clinics in surrounding communities.

In mid-1963 things began to fall into place. In July, David Whitcomb was engaged as medical director. Edmund Niklewski also joined as staff psychiatrist. With Saraduke remaining on staff, there now were three psychiatrists. Douglas Warner also joined the staff as clinical psychologist.

Interest in Community Services

The idea of expanding beyond the hospital into surrounding communities with clinics seemed right for the time. Almost at once invitations came from Chambersburg, Pennsylvania; Martinsburg, West Virginia; and Gettysburg, Pennsylvania. The plan to expand the hospital was abandoned. The board, which again had secured initial approval of a Hill-Burton grant, decided against the grant and agreed to limit the hospital to thirty-eight beds and rather to enlarge the administration building to accommodate the enlarged staff. The *Emma G. Musselman Clinic*, as the new wing of the administration building was named, was completed early in 1964.

The Zuercher-Whitcomb years reflected the broadening perspective which looked beyond the hospital into the community. Raber's successful efforts to relate to the clergy and churches in the community and bring them into the total mission of Brook Lane helped in this direction. Clinics were established in Frederick, though briefly for only one year, and in Chambersburg. Invitations from other communities continued to come but were turned down because of insufficient staff resources.

In his March 24-25, 1964, report to MMHS Whitcomb described this interest as the "extramural phase" of the Brook Lane program, the area where "we feel the greatest sense of excitement. This is the phase which has felt most pulled by community needs; indeed in some instances this has almost been community demand." He saw this as more than merely outpatient work provided at some distance from the hospital: here they were collaborating with other agencies with their own identity; morever, this work "promises to be much more worldly." That is, Brook Lane would now be working with "school dropouts, juvenile delinquency, vocational rehabilitation, the unwed mother, care for the aged, problems of 'hidden poverty.' "

The mood of the times was expressed by Zuercher's seven-page paper on "Community Psychiatry as Practiced at Brook Lane Farm Hospital," presented to MMHS in November 1964. In 1965 the name of the institution was changed to *Brook Lane Psychiatric Center* to better reflect the new emphasis.

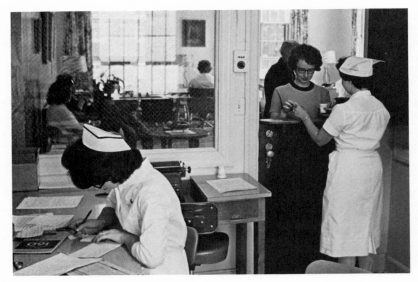

Nurses station in the early 1960s.

During 1966 another major change in the staff occurred, with Whitcomb resigning as medical director and Zuercher leaving for advanced training in hospital administration. The mood and direction was due to change once more.

Brook Lane As Hospital and CMHC (1966-80)

Difficulties with the CMHC Model

If the Zuercher-Whitcomb years moved Brook Lane on the track toward becoming a community mental health center (CMHC), the years following can be described as putting on the brakes if not sidetracking the institution from that goal. The uncertainty about Brook Lane's direction, seen in the attraction to both the hospital and CMHC models, were caused by a number of circumstances and developments.

There were problems in replacing Zuercher and Whitcomb. With the expectation that Zuercher would return after two years, the board appointed an interim administrator. Gene Schmidt, while capable, was a short-term manager with his own plans for further training after the two-year appointment. When Zuercher decided later not to return and Schmidt was not available to continue, the board asked Howard Musselman, one of its own members, to fill in as another short-term administrator, though for a three-year term. So Brook Lane obviously lacked a continuity of administration.

Edmund Niklewski replaced Whitcomb in April 1967, but he openly did not want to serve as medical director of the multi-faceted program, preferring the title *chief of staff,* after the hospital model.

The medical staff as a group at this time wanted a change in their relationship to the institution. As early as February 1966, Whitcomb himself questioned the board about the propriety of the "corporate practice of medicine" at Brook Lane, in that the psychiatrists, unlike most physicians in private practice, were working on a salaried basis. There were serious discussions in the board about the open medical staff versus the closed staff patterns, the salary basis versus fee-for-service or separate billing for services provided. The issue was brought to MMHS at a special meeting in January 1967. They advised against a fee-for-service arrangement. Nevertheless, at the urging of the medical staff, the Brook Lane board that year adopted a policy which allowed the psychiatrists to work on a private or fee-for-service basis after two years of employment. Related to this issue, several other staff members requested, and were granted, part-time employment to allow time for private practice. By mid-1967 all four psychiatrists had requested that they be allowed to practice at Brook Lane on a separate billing basis and all three psychologists and the chief social worker were employed part-time. The impact upon the institution was predictable.

This, of course, helped emphasize Brook Lane as a hospital, largely on the general hospital model, and made the effort to serve as a community mental health center more difficult. But there were other factors at work. It was noted that working with neighboring counties was becoming more difficult because "the political, social, legislative forces are working against rather than for Brook Lane Psychiatric Center." The move "toward the comprehensive community mental health center concept needs reassessment."[22] An indicator of the times was the resignation of Charles Goshen, who had joined the staff a second time as director of Community Services, when "serious concern was expressed about the validity of this work."[23] Niklewski reported to the Brook Lane board that the staff was frustrated by frequent requests to consider organized extension into the community, because "most of us are clinicians and have very little experience in the mechanics of politics and public relations."[24]

The extent of community work, however, was significant. Niklewski in his report to the board in November 1967 listed twenty-four agencies outside the hospital in which staff members were engaged one way or another. The philosophy for participation in community mental health which emerged was best expressed by Musselman at the time he was administrator: "Brook Lane does not propose to assume the total comprehensive responsibility for any of these community programs. Rather it proposes to be a contractual provider..." Brook Lane is committed to the community mental health philosophy but also "to retain its character as a private agency devoted to quality care and will limit its participation to the extent that it does not significantly dilute this objective."[25] So unlike other MCC centers, Brook Lane chose the contractor model for specified services rather than the "comprehensive" CMHC model with National Institute of Mental Health (NIMH) recognition and funding.

Growth of Services

In spite of the struggles within the staff and board over the hospital and CMHC models, Brook Lane continued to provide needed services.The staff experimented with and engaged in a variety of new programs, although some were not maintained over long periods of time. A foster home program, a work-study program, a perceptual-motor program and a halfway house are examples. The chaplaincy program, though experiencing some changes in staff and even dropped temporarily in the late 1970s, continued to provide pastoral services in the hospital and community. A psychodrama institute, a growth center, and a pastoral care institute at different times were started and administered by Brook Lane staff members. Albert Powell introduced a child-related service in 1972 and Alan Horowitz an adolescent hospital unit in 1979.

Despite all the strife that we as a staff feel, Brook Lane is still looked upon by most patients and the public to be an excellent psychiatric institution in regard to both inpatient facilities and the outpatient clinic arrangement. Apparently our internal strife is obvious only to us and is not adversely affecting patient care.

— Edmund Niklewski[26]

Church and Community Relationships

It was during this period of Brook Lane's history that questions increasingly were raised about its relationship to the constituent churches. The feeling seemed to be that Brook Lane was no longer truly representative of the church. The Mission Board of the Virginia Mennonite Conference, which since 1957 had appointed a representative to the Brook Lane board, expressed serious concern over what appeared a departure from the church. Another board member resigned late that year, partly because he questioned the church-relatedness of Brook Lane. The board responded by appointing a Special Committee on Church and Community Relations, which led to numerous efforts from 1968 to 1971 to work with the churches, by personal contacts, letters, and workshops.

As administrator, Musselman tried to increase the number of constituent members on the Brook Lane staff. He reported to the board:

> During the past two years I have made a strong effort to recruit Mennonite personnel, almost to the point of apprehension among our staff. Special efforts were directed to Mennonite physicians, social workers and nurses plus advertisement or mention in church papers for aides and service personnel. During the past two years I have not hired a single Mennonite professional with the exception of two nurses. The same situation holds for kitchen and maintenance personnel. The only significant constituent representation is among the aides and the handwriting is on the wall for these too.[27]

The Special Committee also helped the board face the question of its own composition. Paul Peachey, board member and chairman of the committee, stated that "...the ties between the conferences and the Center which the bylaws anticipate appear never to have materialized. In any case, the ties currently are rather tenuous, so tenuous, in fact, that they can hardly bear the weight of a responsible decision."[28] The board, which to this time was wholly made up of

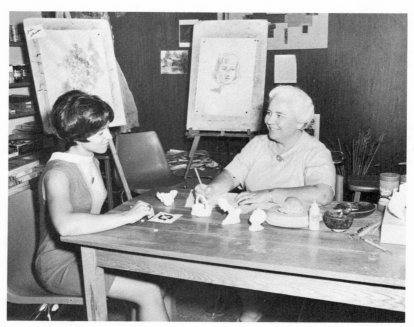

Occupational therapy.

church representatives, in 1968 agreed reluctantly to add two community representatives to the board, William Wells and John Schaf-
fer. In 1970 the bylaws were amended to allow for six community
representatives. The following year additional changes were made:
to provide for a 50-50 constituency-community ratio, to designate
church representatives "at large" rather than from specific church
conferences, to include the Church of the Brethren along with
Mennonites and the Brethren in Christ in the constituency designation, and to specify that all members should live within a seventy-
five-mile radius of the center.[29] these changes resulted in an
enlarged, stronger and more active local board of directors, and one
which did not abandon the church ties while strengthening the
community relationships.[30]

The Oswald Years

During the administration of Wesley Oswald (December 1971
to January 1980), Brook Lane for a time continued to operate under
the philosophy of a psychiatric hospital with special community
liaisons as these might be arranged individually. With the development of stronger community services by Albert Powell in the early
1970s, Brook Lane was reorganized in 1974 into two divisions, a
Hospital Division headed by Paul Saraduke and a Community
Services Division under Powell. But this did not work satisfactorily.
In his May 1976 report to the board, Oswald noted the concern of the
staff that clinical leadership in effect was spread over three
positions—the two division heads and the president of the medical
staff, the latter established when Niklewski resigned as chief of staff
in 1974. Oswald stated that there was a need "to identify more
specific clinical leadership to deal with questions of delivering of
patient care."

In early 1977 a board review of the situation indicated that the
services provided under the two divisions had not been effectively
integrated. Serious study of the situation during 1977 by outside
consultants, Ryan Advisors, Inc., and Marshall D. Fitz, M.D., led to
abolishing the two divisions. In place of the 1974 structure, the
board approved an organizational scheme with a chief executive
officer (Executive Director) supervising one director of Professional
Services for the total program, as well as a director of Administrative
Services to handle nonclinical matters. In 1978 Paul Rodenhauser
and William Baer were appointed to the new positions, with Oswald
continuing as executive director. By the end of 1979, this arrangement also came to an end when Oswald resigned, Baer's position
was eliminated, and Rodenhauser, a bit later, also resigned.

Another Change in Leadership

The year 1980 brought new and encouraging developments. David Rutherford, an experienced administrator and clinician, joined the staff as executive director in September, replacing Charles Lyon, retired business executive and former board member, who had filled in as interim executive director following Oswald's departure in January. As a churchman, Rutherford also had an interest in and concern about Brook Lane's religious dimension. So he uniquely brought together a combination of qualifications which seemed to fit the particular needs of the time.

Thoroughly backed by the board, Rutherford provided needed leadership to make Brook Lane primarily a private psychiatric hospital rather than a loosely defined community mental health center. With the help of Chaplain Clayton Moyer, who also joined the staff in 1980, the religious aspect of Brook Lane's program was openly promoted within the institution and the community. The board, under the chairmanship of Paul Horst, adopted a new mission statement clearly outlining the philosophy, purposes and goals of Brook Lane. In 1980 Brook Lane entered another period of its thirty-three-year history.

Conclusion

This is the Brook Lane story. It is the history of an institution with more than its share of trouble and pain, at times caused by all-too-frequent changes in leadership, at other times by internal conflicts or by questions over management and control. Brook Lane experienced uncertainties around a number of tormenting issues, whether to be a hospital or a community mental health center, whether to be church related or community based, whether to be private or in part publicly supported.

Though not unscathed, Brook Lane has nevertheless experienced growth and maturity, and through the years countless troubled and mentally handicapped persons have found support and help to live more useful and satisfying lives. From a small beginning on a Maryland farm, Brook Lane has become the modern mental health facility it is today, clear on its goals as a private psychiatric hospital, certain about its religious roots and purposes, respected for the quality of its services, strong in its ties to the local community, and confident about its future.

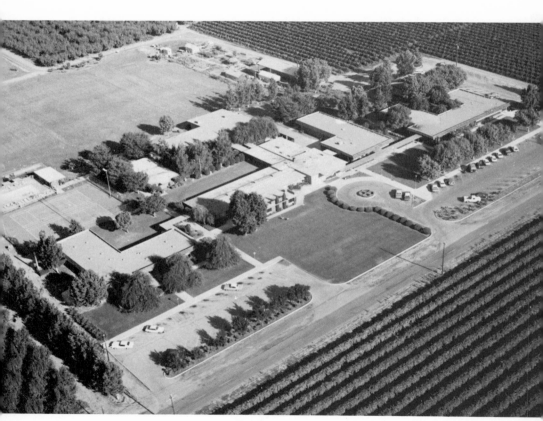

Aerial view of Kings View Hospital.

CHAPTER 4

Kings View
Reedley, California
Esther Jost*

Torrents of rain burst from dark dense clouds February 11, 1951, the dedication day of Kings View Homes, 2½ miles southwest of Reedley. The stormy weather was typical of the many difficulties of beginning a mental health facility at Reedley, California. However, just as God had helped in removing almost insurmountable barriers, the clouds disbursed and the sun broke forth in brilliant splendor, making possible the scheduled afternoon dedication services. Chairs and other equipment were soon set up in front of the building, and approximately three thousand people, including members from Mennonite churches of the Pacific area, arrived for the services. Arthur Jost, Kings View administrator, welcomed the guests; H. R. Martens, local advisory committee chairman, presented Kings View Homes; H. A. Fast, vice chairman of the Mennonite Central Committee (MCC), delivered the dedicatory address; and P. C. Hiebert, MCC chairman, offered the dedicatory prayer.[1]

The dedication services of Kings View Homes marked the formal beginning of Kings View. The original concept had been to provide separate facilities or "homes" for mentally ill persons who needed long-term or acute care, and for mentally retarded persons. Although the first building was to serve only mentally ill persons who needed long-term care, the concept had changed already before the official opening day to include people who were acutely mentally ill. The Kings View story is one of changes in concepts and patterns, with expansion in facilities and services for mental health, accompanied by issues, problems, and successes.

---

*Esther Jost is a retired public school teacher and wife of Arthur Jost, president of Kings View.

Kings View Homes

Because the Mennonite Brethren Home for the Aged in Reedley had difficulty caring for patients who were mentally ill, the need
for another facility of care was brought to the attention of the 1946
Pacific District Conference of the Mennonite Brethren. The conference was aware of a special mental hospital study committee appointed by MCC. This committee had been formed as the result of a
new concept proposed by H. A. Fast at the December 28 and 29,
1944, MCC meeting, that MCC seriously consider administering a
program for the care of Mennonites who were mentally ill (see
above, chapter 2). After the conference agreed to the need of a care
facility for mentally ill patients, Ben Wall, from the board of directors
of the Home for the Aged, wrote a letter dated December 10, 1946,
informing MCC that the conference had authorized their board to
cooperate with MCC in the promotion of a possible home for the
mentally ill on the West Coast.

The West Coast interest helped influence MCC in its decision
regarding mental health facilities. In its January 3, 1947, annual
meeting, when plans for three homes for the mentally ill were
authorized, MCC stipulated that one of the homes be located in the
western part of the United States. During this meeting, MCC appointed a Homes-for-Mentally-Ill Planning and Advisory Committee, later named *Mennonite Mental Health Services* (MMHS), to guide
the establishment and administration of the total program. To en-
sure West Coast representation, H. R. Martens, Reedley, was appointed to the committee.

West Coast Constituency Meeting

To initiate the project in the west, MCC appointed a planning
committee, composed of Martens, H. A. Fast and Elmer Ediger of
the MCC Akron office, to plan for the West Coast home.[2] They
immediately planned a Mennonite constituent meeting to be held
March 24, 1947, in Reedley. A week prior to the meeting, Ediger was
asked to come to California to confer with church leaders, explore
state official attitudes, determine counseling resources, and survey
possible locations for the West Coast facility. The constituent meeting was attended by representatives from Mennonite churches from
Reedley, Madera, Shafter, Dinuba, and Atwater, California; and
Albany, Oregon. Included in the recommendations adopted at this
meeting were: that MCC should take the initiative in establishing a
"rest home for the chronic mentally ill, mentally deficient, and such
acute mentally ill as can be given adequate treatment," and as soon
as possible, provide separate facilities to treat the acutely mentally

ill; the home should be located in California within reasonable distance of a Mennonite community; as soon as possible, MCC should appoint a full-time administrator and an advisory committee which would be responsible to the MCC executive committee.[3]

The April 19, 1947, MMHS meeting in Chicago approved the recommendations of the March 24 West Coast meeting and further recommended: "That provision be made initially for the accommodation of thirty patients, with service facilities sufficient for the eventual accommodation of 100 patients." Other recommendations included that money to the extent of $100,000 be provided within the next twelve-month period; that the staff of the West Coast home be composed of an administrator, a permanent group of well-qualified workers filling key positions, and a group of volunteer workers as attendants and helpers who would be engaged for terms of not less than one year.

A May 3, 1947, special MCC executive committee meeting approved the April 19 MMHS recommendations, and further agreed to appoint a West Coast planning and advisory committee of three members for two-year terms, to be responsible to MMHS. Fifty thousand dollars for the West Coast home were to come from the constituent groups, and finances, up to $25,000, would be provided from MCC non-peace-church CPS receivables.[4] H. R. Martens and D. C. Krehbiel, Reedley, and Sam Eicher, Albany, Oregon, were appointed to the West Coast Planning and Advisory Committee. Arthur Jost, who was serving in the mental health section, Akron, Pennsylvania, was appointed West Coast administrator.

Jost was one of approximately fifteen hundred Mennonite conscientious objectors serving in mental hospitals during World War II who sparked the beginning of the Mennonite mental health program. Serving in the Utah State Hospital at Provo, Jost was one who advocated that Mennonites should establish and maintain hospitals for the mentally ill.

While much has been done to alleviate physical suffering, very little has been done by the churches in providing care for the mentally ill... Was Christ any less interested in healing the demon possessed than he was in healing the withered hand? We have as yet made very little practical application of this single standard of Jesus' healing mission... As science makes great strides in psychiatric discoveries, now that psychiatrists realize the need for the cooperation of ministers, educators, social workers, and lay people to promote mental health both outside and inside a mental institution, there unfolds a great field of opportunity for Christian service by the churches.

—Arthur Jost [5]

West Coast Responsibility

With the appointment of the administrator and advisory committee, the focus of responsibility moved to the West Coast. Although Jost, an MCC staff member, served as administrator and attended all committee meetings, he continued to work at the Akron headquarters until January 1948, when he moved to Reedley.

On June 3, 1947, the West Coast committee met in Reedley to plan the construction of a home for the mentally ill preferably to be located in the Dinuba-Reedley area because of the heavy concentration of several groups of Mennonites, and because there was no state or private institution in this area. This meeting lacked the go-ahead spirit of the March constituency meeting, primarily because of the need to collect $50,000. Raising a definite amount of money with district conference machinery not equipped to do this posed a problem so serious that Martens, the committee chairman, reported to MCC: "It would be proper that we not go ahead at the present time."[6]

MCC continued to remain optimistic and directed that planning should proceed, though not as immediately as hoped for earlier. In October 1947, MMHS recommended the purchase of a site in the Reedley-Dinuba-Fresno area. The local advisory committee was given broader support at their November 22, 1947, meeting when Orie Miller, MCC executive secretary, P. C. Hiebert and Arthur Jost attended to help in the planning. Representatives from the West Coast constituency, who were to serve on special committees also attended. Miller reported that MCC had authorized the purchase of a site and would provide the funds, and that MCC and the West Coast committee, as a team, should raise $100,000 to $125,000. The West Coast Mennonites were to be responsible for approximately six dollars per member. Miller clarified lines of responsibility for the committees and administration: Arthur Jost represented Akron in the field, the West Coast Planning and Advisory Committee served in an advisory capacity on all matters, and the other members present acted as a liaison between MCC and representative churches in matters of raising funds and providing informational programs.

I always felt a lot of comfort in this arrangement regarding the local advisory committee, because the West Coast was very far away from MCC. On the West Coast, there was only a handful of people who had seen this vision and concept, but they were very few among the "enemy camp." I don't think I would have wanted a local board at that time. It would have been precarious, and the conviction just wasn't there; it was elsewhere, the vision.

—Arthur Jost[7]

The Plans Develop

Plans for the West Coast facility accelerated after Jost lived in Reedley and could give continuous and stable leadership to the project. MCC also had appointed him director of the West Coast MCC Relief Center, but even with the added responsibility, Jost began contacting Mennonite churches early in 1948 to raise funds and to inform the constituency regarding the mental health project.

Purchasing a building site proved difficult even though several apparently were available including one located between Reedley and Dinuba. Although money for it had been placed in escrow, the purchase needed to be canceled because people living in the area near the site had a disdain and fear for the "insane." After a fourth attempt, the committee found an acreage where the Frank Pauls family was willing to be neighbors to a mental hospital. On May 17, 1948, land located near the Kings River consisting of a forty-three acre ranch of Muscat and Thompson grapes and young plum and peach orchards was purchased for $25,000, and Jost assumed the responsibility to farm the ranch.[8]

Plans for building the West Coast facility proceeded, and a local architect produced a master plan and drawings for the initial unit. Elmer Penner from Fresno was contracted to supervise construction with the understanding that maximum use should be made of contributed labor. Martens recommended that the MCC facility be named as soon as possible to avoid the use of "insane asylum" and other undesirable terms. Since it was adjacent to the Kings River, the name *Kings View Homes* was adopted.[9] Ground breaking for the facility soon followed, with approximately one thousand people in attendance. P. C. Hiebert, MCC chairman, and Frank Tallman, Mental Health commissioner of California, gave the main addresses at the ceremony held November 20, 1949.[10]

The foundation for the 32-bed unit of Kings View Homes has been completed. Into this part of the construction have gone 500 sacks of cement. The rough plumbing had been installed prior to the pouring of the concrete floors and 28 truckloads of sand and gravel have been hauled for about ten miles by members of local Mennonite churches who donated their services. A voluntary service unit of nine men also are helping with hospital construction.

—Arthur Jost[11]

In the fall of 1950, as the building was nearing completion, construction of Kings View Homes was slowed down because of the uncertainty of adequate funds. Because of the possibility that the facility would not be completed on schedule, the West Coast committee did not want to set a dedication date. Prayer, faith, and hope continued to be positive attributes of those involved closely with Kings View, and with the hope that incoming contributions would increase during December and January, MMHS decided at its December 1 meeting to dedicate Kings View Homes on February 11, 1951.

Kings View Homes was dedicated on February 11 as planned. The afternoon services were followed by an open house, but the crowd wishing to view the modern facility for the treatment of mental illness was so large that another open house had to be scheduled for the following Sunday.[12] The exterior finish of the low-lying, flat-roofed building was rough, green-colored stucco with peach trim. The decor had been planned as part of the patient treatment and the interior was finished in bright colors on walls, ceilings, floors, and furniture, with no two adjoining rooms decorated alike. Plenty of window space admitted large amounts of sunshine to make the hospital a pleasant and attractive place for patients. Because many Mennonite women's groups had helped furnish the hospital rooms, and 30 percent of the labor for the 8,499-square-foot facility had been donated by volunteer workers, the estimated cost of $144,000 was decreased to the actual cost of $90,000.[13]

Kings View Hospital
Although the intent of Kings View Homes had been to care

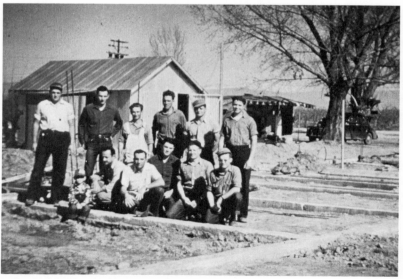

Voluntary service workers helping construct the hospital.

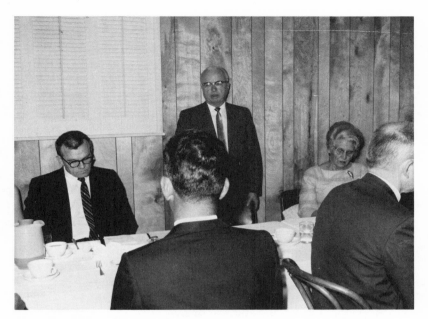

Henry R. Martens, first chairman of the Kings View board, with Arthur Jost, administrator, and Mrs. Martens.

only for long-term mentally ill persons initially, the admission policy had changed before the official opening day and four beds had been reserved for treatment of the acutely mentally ill. Since acutely mentally ill persons received treatment, Kings View Homes often was called *Kings View Hospital.* In 1960 Kings View Hospital appeared on the certificate of accreditation from the American Psychiatric Association and on the certificate of membership in the American Hospital Association, and the name *Kings View Hospital* replaced *Kings View Homes.*

The Early Years

The hospital opened with a maximum staff of twelve persons including Jackson C. Dillon, a psychiatrist from Fresno, and Ann Warkentine, a registered nurse from Canada. The salaries ranged from the psychiatrist's pay for one-half day a week service of fifty dollars, the administrator's half-time weekly salary of twenty-seven dollars, to an attendant's weekly pay of twenty-five dollars.[14] Many of the staff were voluntary service workers.

Although in its master plan MCC intended the West Coast facility to focus on long-term care, an active treatment program at Kings View Homes had not been ruled out. Immediately after dedication day, the hospital admitted patients based on medical need and also accepted its first fifteen patients regardless of church affiliation or geographical location. The remainder of the beds were allocated on the basis of specifications set by the West Coast Advisory Committee.[15]

Dillon, who had been appointed in late 1950 to provide psychiatric supervision, at first spent minimal time with the hospital since he worked full time in a Fresno clinic. As the trend toward treatment of acutely mentally ill patients accelerated, Dillon extended his time at Kings View for both inpatient and outpatient care. Under Dillon's more continuous supervision, many elderly long-term patients improved and could be discharged. Vacant beds were utilized for younger long-term patients and for the acutely mentally ill. In time Kings View Homes became an active treatment hospital.

Kings View Hospital regarded the patient to be the most important person in the program and the therapeutic atmosphere of the hospital essential to the patient's healing. Dillon reported to an early advisory committee meeting: "I believe our greatest asset at Kings View Homes is the spirit of dedication and Christian service expressed by our staff which enables us to create a therapeutic atmosphere which in turn allows our patients to reorient themselves and attack their disabling personal problems."[16]

The spiritual care ministry was part of the treatment program when Kings View Hospital opened its doors in 1951. Each day began with a short devotional period led by a staff member, and the majority of the patients participated voluntarily in the singing and at times in other parts of the service. Nursing staff read Scripture and prayed individually with patients requesting this ministry. Between nine and ten o'clock Sunday mornings, a combined class of staff and patients assembled to study the Sunday school lesson. Patients who were able to go off grounds attended worship services in nearby churches. Local ministers and religious groups presented programs at the hospital one evening biweekly.[17]

As Kings View Hospital gradually moved into an active treatment program, need for more nurses and other skilled staff increased. Many of the positions were filled by voluntary service workers. Jost reported to MMHS in May 1951, "We believe Kings View Homes could never be what it is or what it will become without our V.S. element." Yet their service, as an economic value, was minimal since the differential between V.S. salaries and salaries paid by the institutions was so small.

Needs for treating patients more effectively resulted in expansion of facilities. By November 1951 an occupational therapy building was on the drawing board. Because of the shortage of psychiatric services in the area, Kings View Hospital was granted both federal and state monies in 1957 for constructing an additional inpatient building.

Temporary Closing

Expansion was not possible immediately, however, because of intense internal problems. In a May 3, 1957, report to the Kings View advisory committee, Jost defined existing problems to be a low census, shortage of clinical and nursing staff, part-time administration since Jost had to divide his time with the regional MCC office, underdeveloped public relations, and lack in communication. Because of a low census problem, Dillon and a second psychiatrist from Fresno admitting patients informed the Kings View advisory committee in September that they no longer presumed to maintain a workable load at the hospital.

In a letter dated October 10, 1957, Jost informed Orie Miller of MCC about the conditions at the hospital. Less than a week later, on October 16, Jost received a telegram from Miller, who was in Paraguay at that time, instructing Kings View Hospital to close its doors to inpatient service. After remaining patients at Kings View Hospital had been relocated in other facilities, the doctors resigned. Proper arrangements with staff were carried out, and on October 30, Kings View Hospital terminated inpatient service though continuing to offer outpatient care.[18]

Ironically, a ground-breaking ceremony was held for a new hospital unit and a building program was in progress during part of the period Kings View Hospital was closed to inpatient services. Confidence that things would work out prevailed, and on March 17, 1958, the hospital opened its doors for both inpatient and outpatient treatment.[19] Ross Hendricks, a psychiatrist from San Francisco, was available to provide interim services to minimize the period in which the hospital was closed.

The building program, completed in 1958, increased the inpatient capacity from thirty to forty-two beds. Further expansion in 1964 brought the total number to fifty-five beds.

Charles A. Davis became full-time medical director July 3, 1958, several months after the hospital reopened. His able leadership helped develop relationships with referral sources and admissions to the hospital increased.

Davis helped to develop the "therapeutic community" concept which viewed the total hospital atmosphere as important in the care and treatment of patients. J. D. Enterline was appointed clinical director to implement the concept. Maxwell Jones of England, who

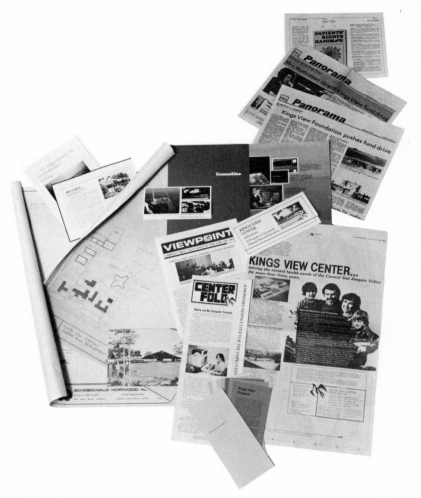

Collage of various Kings View publications.

initially developed the concept and shared it in his book, *The Thera-peutic Community*, visited Kings View Hospital in 1960 to serve as a consultant.

The importance of a therapeutic community at Kings View Hospital was underscored in the annual report of the medical direc-tor to the December 16, 1960, board of directors meeting:

> Traditional and innovative treatment modalities are supervised and implemented by a large staff of highly qualified personnel. Treatment modalities currently in use incorporate heavy emphasis on the thera-peutic community, with patients playing an important role in the treatment process... The emphasis is on extended, intensive treat-

ment while also meeting the needs for brief, crisis-oriented, psychotherapeutic intervention.

In order to promote a positive relationship between patients and hospital personnel, use of first names and direct communication of feelings if appropriate were encouraged, and both patients and staff dressed in casual clothes. Except for periods of extreme disturbance, patients were supervised in an open ward, and were encouraged to assume responsibility for their behavior.

Adolescent Program

As identifiable needs arose, Kings View Hospital was alert and ready to change in order to deal with new circumstances. Several developments during the 1970s prompted Kings View to begin a treatment program for the adolescent. More adolescents were experiencing emotional and psychological problems. At the same time, Kings View Hospital had beds available for them because adults formerly hospitalized were being treated in the outpatient program. Kings View Hospital was an ideal place to treat young people because of the hospital's location with its natural surroundings including an island nestled in the Kings River, a fully accredited high school on the grounds,[20] extensive recreational facilities, and individual psychotherapy. Soon the adolescent program, recognized for its excellence by professionals in the mental health field, had a wide referral base, and applications for admissions exceeded available beds.

Kings Valley Hospital

Although the treatment program focused on the adolescents, there was still a need for geriatric care which originally had been a strong basis for building Kings View, and Kings View Hospital again was in need of facilities. The increasing demand for adolescent treatment services at Kings View Hospital also resulted in a lowering of the mean patient age and a need to adjust services. This change, coupled with increasing need for geriatric care, resulted in the leasing of Kings Valley Hospital in Reedley, a thirty-bed nursing facility. The hospital emphasized treatment for geriatric psychiatric patients, but also admitted younger patients.

Although Kings View Hospital, secluded in the country, was beginning to be accepted by the Reedley community, several residents living near Kings Valley Hospital in Reedley complained to city hall that they did not want people with mental problems living in their neighborhood. The Reedley city council then declared Kings Valley in violation of a zoning ordinance and ordered it to operate only as a nursing home. With program goals thus thwarted, Kings Valley Hospital closed in 1970.[21]

Chaplaincy Program

Before the establishment of its hospitals, MCC envisioned spiritual ministry to the mentally ill an important part of the treatment concept. As already noted, when Kings View opened its doors in 1951, nurses and other staff carried some responsibility for a spiritual ministry. In 1953 a clinically-trained pastor joined the staff to give more direction to incorporate pastoral care services with the Kings View Hospital's treatment program.

When the program of mental health was originally begun, church leaders were sold on the fact that the spiritual aspect of this healing program would be given first place. I am sure that no one at that time really knew what this would mean in operational terms, but all were agreed that it must be so. This was to be our special genius in the area of mental health. For some time I have felt that somehow we have not been able to follow through this vision. This is not a criticism but a confession. I, too, am baffled when I face my duties as a member of MMHS. It could be that Kings View Homes is a proper place to begin. I feel that the Reedley area needs this desperately and Dr. Dillon seems open to the matter.

— Frank C. Peters[22]

In 1961, a committee of the Kings View Homes board studied the need of a chaplaincy program at the hospital. During the 1960s and early 1970s, ordained ministers in succession became part of the Kings View Hospital staff, but pastoral services were not stabilized until 1976 when Harlan E. Ratmeyer was appointed chaplain. With Ratmeyer as director of pastoral services, an accredited pastoral care program was integrated into the treatment approach to provide voluntary opportunities for worship, pastoral counseling, Bible study, and prayer for patients at Kings View Hospital. Life value classes for adolescents and adults became an ongoing part of the pastoral care program. Training in pastoral care to three or four students from either Mennonite seminaries or pastorates and other religious traditions for three-month residencies, and periodic series of half-day sessions to local pastors on pastoral counseling and ministering to the dying and the mentally ill also became available. At the 1980 November annual meeting of the National Association of Clinical Pastoral Education, Kings View Hospital was accredited to provide Advanced Clinical Pastoral Education (CPE). This accreditation made possible the training of chaplains in nine-month residencies at Kings View Hospital.

Kings View Hospital Today

Because of its high adolescent census, a need existed for a transitional treatment facility, and in 1979 the Rio Vista Transitional Facility was opened. Rio Vista, located approximately one-fourth mile from Kings View Hospital, occupies a completely remodeled building that formerly housed the Kings View Corporation Home Office. Licensed by the Community Care Division of the California Department of Social Services, Rio Vista accommodates sixteen residents, fifteen to thirty years of age, in a structured living environment that emphasizes personal experience and individual responsibility in a community setting. Rio Vista Transitional Facility and Kings View Hospital are two major treatment facilities known as *Kings View Center*.

Kings View Hospital continues to expand facilities in order to treat patients more effectively. Another ground breaking took place on August 28, 1981, for an activity therapy building. Tony Coelho, United States congressman for the Fifteenth District, was guest speaker at this occasion.

In fall of 1981, COUNSELINE, a free community service sponsored by Kings View Hospital, began operation in the Fresno-Visalia-Reedley area. COUNSELINE provides a tape library of professionally prepared recordings which can help callers better understand and cope with a variety of emotional problems. If more professional advice is desired by the person calling, the COUNSELINE operator can refer the caller to an appropriate source.

Treatment programs at Kings View Hospital are individually planned for each patient's specific needs. In a recent slide presentation, Tom Noyes, psychiatrist and current Kings View Hospital director, stated: "There are a number of things that are unique about Kings View Hospital's treatment philosophy, but I think the primary one would be in terms of the individual psychotherapy. Each patient is seen for at least one-half hour per day, and in this way, the patient does receive needed emotional support and insight psychotherapy to help him deal with his problems, not only here at the hospital but outside in his day-to-day living."[23] Kings View Hospital is licensed by the California Department of Health, accredited by the Joint Commission on Accreditation of Hospitals, and is a member of the American Hospital Association, and the National Association of Private Psychiatric Hospitals.

Kings View Community Services

In 1970, *Kings View* became the official name of the West Coast Mennonite health care services. The name represented the openness of the organization to enter various fields of health services including treatment, prevention, community education and manpower training. From the original proposal by H. A. Fast that MCC administer a program for Mennonites who were mentally ill, the concept had changed before Kings View Homes opened in 1951 to include non-Mennonites. However, almost two decades later, there were still many people who were not receiving mental health services due to a lack of both facilities and funds.

County Contracts and Community Services

In 1957, California's Short-Doyle Act made state funds available to agencies willing to provide mental health services at the community level. When leaders in adjacent Kings County hesitated to develop a program, Kings View, in 1964, took the initiative to establish a small demonstration clinic in Hanford, approximately twenty-seven miles from Kings View Hospital. Because the value of the clinic was recognized by community agencies, Kings View began a new venture into contracting for mental health services, the first between Kings County and Kings View in 1964. A one-year voluntary demonstration program in Tulare county, immediately south of Kings View Hospital, also resulted in a contract in 1964.

When the Lanterman-Petris-Short Act took effect on July 1, 1969, Kings View officials already had laid the groundwork for providing the more extensive services required by the law. The Act made it mandatory for each county with a population of 100,000 or more to provide ten mental health services: inpatient, outpatient, emergency care, partial hospitalization, precare, aftercare, diagnosis, rehabilitation, research and evaluation, and consultation, education, and information.

Since each county in the state was responsbile for providing mental health services on the local level, Kings View negotiated new contracts to provide services for Kings and Tulare counties in the 1969-70 fiscal year. Late in 1969, Merced, Mariposa and Madera counties approached Kings View about providing services, and contracts were drawn up for fiscal 1970-71. Under terms of the contracts, Kings View provided all ten of the services for Tulare and Merced counties, which had more than 100,000 people, and also for Kings and Madera counties which had populations of less than 100,000.[24] Other services provided by Kings View community mental health programs were gerontology services, pharmacy services, and substance abuse services.

Emergency services for Kings and Tulare counties gained statewide recognition. In the emergency services, radio dispatched cars were staffed by personnel on a twenty-four hour basis. They responded to law enforcement officers, jails, emergency rooms of hospitals, and private residences. Both male and female staff covered the large geographical area giving counsel or medications or both. The major goal was to prevent hospitalization. The results were impressive and many agencies visited the program to explore adaptation for their areas.

Individual contracts were designed to give each county autonomy to establish and develop its mental health program suited to the needs of the community served, with the support of Kings View financial and administrative resources. Continuity of care was reinforced by composite patient records, which followed individuals throughout the Kings View system.

Community mental health services for the counties were coordinated by a shared staff working out of the Kings View main office. By 1970, approximately 350 staff members were associated with programs of sixteen service units in five counties and in Reedley. The staff also worked with probation officers to develop alternatives to commitment to correctional institutions and with local law enforcement agencies to coordinate crisis intervention services. In addition, they lent assistance to a youth coordinating council, a committee on drug problems, a telephone service that provided drug abuse information, and conducted programs for school counselors, for indigenous workers in a health clinic sponsored by the Office of Economic Opportunity, and for county welfare department workers.

Further growth was experienced by contracting with more counties, and by 1974, the Kings View organization served nine counties, including the Sierra View program in Placer, Nevada, Sierra, and El Dorado counties. Since the 1974 peak, five counties felt capable of providing mental health services themselves and established their own local programs. Four counties, including the original Kings and Tulare, continue to rely on Kings View's expertise to provide mental health services.

The contracts with the counties and the state have been an effective means to serve many people, but postyear audit disallowances have placed undue financial liabilities on Kings View. Because of these liabilities, Kings View sponsored state legislation to make possible new contracts to prevent the liabilities. Currently Kings View is in the process of implementing new contracts, and if the venture is successful, additional geographical and population areas will be served.

Recognition for Service

In 1971 Kings View was recognized for excellence on a national level. At a special recognition service during the annual Institute on Hospital and Community Psychiatry held September 14-16 in Seattle, Washington, Kings View was presented the American Psychiatric Association's Gold Award for the nation's outstanding community mental health treatment program. Throughout its history, when planning mental health programs, Kings View has maintained its tradition of trying to reach people needing care, including poverty groups, minorities, and people in rural areas.

Kings View recognizes employees for commitment in service to others, and in 1974 adopted an annual recognition program for employees who served five years and each additional five years thereafter.

Central Valley Regional Center

In addition to its mental health programs, in 1972 Kings View was asked by the Fresno Association for the Retarded to take over its contract with the State Department of Health to operate the Central Valley Regional Center for Developmental Disabilities. (Developmental disabilities refers to handicapping conditions associated with prenatal or postnatal development prior to age eighteen, including mental retardation, epilepsy, autism, and other conditions.) The Central Valley Regional Center serves Fresno, Kings, Tulare, Madera, Mariposa and Merced counties. This part of California's regional service delivery system, in which local centers locate, assess, and arrange for the necessary services with local providers and follow developmentally disabled individuals, is the one agency through which the developmentally handicapped person can be provided all essential services.

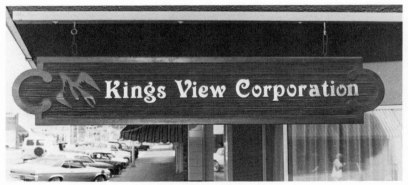

Logo with corporation sign at main offices in Reedley.

Private Programs

Kings View Work Experience Center, a privately operated program in Merced County, was started in 1975. The center provides programs of work activity, vocational development, and evaluation services to mentally and physically disabled and vocationally handicapped individuals in order to maximize physical functioning, obtain an earned income, and optimize communication skills. The center experienced considerable growth in a program expansion and physical plan design during fiscal year 1978-79, when it was relocated from the city of Merced to the Atwater Industrial Park.

Dedication of the Kings View Apartments, Incorporated, a project consisting of thirty-six independent living units built especially to serve the high-functioning developmentally disabled, was held July 12, 1981, in Atwater. The project, funded under a loan guarantee from Housing and Urban Development, is part of the federal government's national effort to develop low-cost housing for the elderly and handicapped.

Another project under Kings View Apartments, Incorporated, is a ten-bed semi-independent living facility built in Hanford in the summer of 1981 for the long-term mentally ill.

Education Program

From its beginning, Kings View has shared information and provided community education concerning mental health as well as mental illness and retardation. Over the years, media coverage with local newspapers, radio, and television has carried mental health announcements and articles submitted by Kings View staff. Seminars and workshops conducted by Kings View have been attended by members of the community as well as Kings View employees. Although several in-house communications are edited and published by individual programs, News & Views, edited by Bonnie Boldt, administrative assistant to the president, is distributed to members of the entire Kings View services.

Kings View Corporation

In addition to serving the community, Kings View strives to bring together staff, both clinical and administrative, into an effective service organization. Since it takes special organization to direct a growing and changing program like Kings View, its structural pattern has changed to meet identifiable needs and has adapted to legal and management requirements from time to time. In 1981, the name Kings View Corporation was adopted to clarify its status as an organization. All the Kings View programs are under the direction of Kings View management.

Development of the Board

At first the organization was simple. MCC in Akron, Pennsylvania, was in control. MCC had assigned Arthur Jost to the West Coast to purchase a hospital site and develop a program and appointed the West Coast advisory committee. But this simple structure was questioned shortly after Kings View opened when it was learned that under California law, the hospital could not have tax-exempt status in California unless it was incorporated in California.

Our attorney, Paul Eymann, and D. C. Krehbiel and Henry Martens, very pragmatic men on the board, said, "Well, if it takes incorporation for Kings View to get out of the tax deal, let's do it; it really shouldn't change our relationship too much with MCC." We incorporated — when Orie Miller was in South America and Bill Snyder, Orie's assistant in Akron, supported us. Not only that, the MCC chairman P. C. Hiebert, and I believe, Harold Bender signed the Reedley property over to Kings View.

Orie came back from South America and was he shocked: "We will not have this; we will not have Kings View separately incorporated." His first impulse was, "Let's unincorporate." But he didn't want us to pay property taxes either, because that was quite a big bite out of the budget. There was some discussion about amending the MCC bylaws so Kings View could be exempt from taxes, but this might have implications in other countries where MCC operated. The solution for MCC was to incorporate MMHS (1952), with bylaws copied after Kings View's since these had been prepared by Eymann to conform to California law. The Kings View property was turned over to MMHS. In the end, the Kings View corporation was not dissolved either, although it did not function as such until the 1957 reorganization.

— Arthur Jost[25]

Although Kings View was incorporated in 1952 for tax purposes, the administrator continued to report and be responsible to MCC. The advisory committee, though legally a board of directors, continued in its advisory role to MMHS until the closing of the hospital in 1957.

The hospital was closed under the old system and reopened under the new system, with a new board with full authority. The advisory committee in the end advised that we close the facility, and that was done so we wouldn't have to fire the doctors...Orie Miller and, I think, H. A. Fast and H. Clair Amstutz came down and appointed a board. Then we started operating under our own board.

— Arthur Jost[26]

After the reopening of the hospital in 1958, a Kings View board of directors was formed and the administrator became the chief executive officer responsible to that board. Members of the board were nominated by their respective church conferences, and appointed by MCC until 1966, when MMHS made board appointments. Local control of property, fiscal matters, personnel, and program greatly improved the chances of Kings View's success, and the response of the institution in a positive way was dramatic.

In 1967 Kings View, following the pattern of other Mennonite mental health programs, began to add non-Mennonite community people to the board. The number was increased gradually and, beginning in 1971, the bylaws stipulated that at least 50 percent of the members of the board must be Mennonite. In 1981, the church constituency was expanded to include the Church of the Brethren.

Managing a Large Corporation

From the outset, Kings View had a dual management model. Responsibilities for the original hospital were shared by the administrator and the medical director in their respective fields. After Kings View expanded services and began contracting health services in several counties, the dual management model continued with the executive director supervising the administrative personnel in the several units and the medical program director acting as a liaison and coordinator with the medical directors of the units. In 1974 this model was changed because the expansion into a large geographical area with clinically diverse programs required a decentralization of clinical responsibility. The administrator was given the role of corporate president and an office of the president was established which included the chief executives of the hospital, the county mental health programs and the state developmental disabilities contract program, and a home office support staff. The support staff included directors of legal services, personnel services, and finance. This model served until 1980 when the home office staff was expanded to include director of operations appointed by the president to manage the corporation. The president has the responsibility for board and government relations at all levels, planning, development, and fund raising.

Kings View Foundation

The Kings View Foundation was incorporated as a subsidiary of Kings View in 1972 for the purpose of fund development. Currently it is an autonomous corporation, whose primary mission remains the support and strengthening of Kings View Corporation, although it may support other providers of mental health and developmental disabilities services.

From a thirty-bed hospital, Kings View has grown into a corporation which currently serves a population of over one million through private and contracted county and state programs.

In keeping with Kings View's historical position that the most important person in its program is the patient, Kings View's goal is to bring to each patient a greater realization of his or her full human potential. This is best symbolized by Kings View's logo, a unified design of a dove and hands. The dove signifying the innate striving of the human mind to realize its potential and the hands the helping services provided by Kings View.

As it provides comprehensive community health services to emotionally handicapped and developmentally disabled people, Kings View maintains the premise that health services should be based upon Christian love and concern for our fellow human beings.

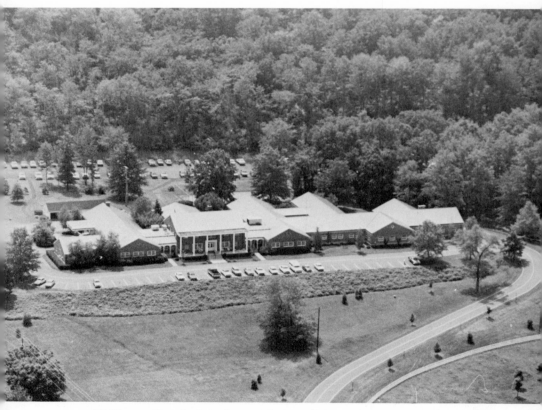

*Philhaven Hospital at the completion of the "Big Step Forward" in 1977.
Photograph taken in 1980.*

CHAPTER 5

Philhaven Hospital Lebanon, Pennsylvania
Donald M. Wert*

On Sunday, May 7, 1952, more than twelve hundred persons attended the three-hour service of dedication for Philhaven Hospital. Bishop Simon Bucher, who had served as an original member of the Hospital Study Committee eight years before, chose for his theme the verse from Psalm 127: "Except the Lord build the house, they labor in vain that build it." The solemn consecration by the bishop was reported to "ring out over the crowded, hushed hospital."[1]

> These buildings which God in His grace provided and has permitted us to build, together with all the premises and facilities known as Philhaven, we here and now, in the name of the Mennonite Church of the Lancaster Conference, do solemnly consecrate and dedicate to the glory of God for the alleviation of suffering and the distress of mankind. In the name of God the Father, the Son, and the Holy Ghost. Amen.

The dedication of Philhaven Hospital thus marked the end of eight years of careful planning and the beginning of thirty years of growth.

The Establishment of Philhaven (1944-1952)

The Concern of the Bishops

The experience of Mennonite people in Civilian Public Service (CPS) had immediate and long-range consequences for the Lancaster Conference of the Mennonite Church. Before the war ended, a new vision of the church's gifts and responsibility was growing. The published writings of Bishop J. Paul Graybill indicate that individuals within the Lancaster Conference promoted the idea of having a hospital for the mentally ill. This idea was expressed to the leaders of

---

*Donald M. Wert is director of education at Philhaven Hospital.

the church, the bishop board. Noah Risser, another bishop, was recorded as saying that members of the conference had come to him and "wondered if something couldn't be done for their mentally ill."[2] Indeed, the bishops had considered the possibility of a mental health facility prior to 1944.[3] But concrete action was first taken that year when the board of bishops established a committee to study the issue of mental health, especially the needs of members in the Lancaster Conference and "neighboring conferences." This Hospital Study Committee consisting of three bishops, Noah Risser, Simon Bucher, and J. Paul Graybill, began investigating several properties which might be developed as a mental hospital.

In 1946 the Mennonite Central Committee (MCC) offered to sell the former CPS farm near Leitersburg, Maryland, to the Lancaster Conference as a possible site, but the bishops declined to move in this direction. Also in 1946, the bishops were asked to consider the Welsh Mountain Samaritan home as another possible site for a mental hospital. The bishops deferred any decision until responses to a survey on mental health needs conducted by MCC were available. Though imprecise, this survey strongly implied the need for a mental health facility.

The study committee was not ready to recommend a specific course of action for the board of bishops. There were several reasons for this: the attention of the bishops was demanded in many areas; the subject of mental health was disquieting and strange to many; and some church members were opposed altogether to the undertaking. Nevertheless, the investigation of the study committee indicated that a ministry in the field of mental health was needed and that "such a work is worthy of our attention."[4]

I suppose I was as much afraid and unknowledgeable about the mental problem as anybody. I guess the stigma was as bad with me as anybody; but when (the Church) meant business, why, I was willing to overcome that.

—Abram Metzler[5]

In January 1948, the study committee reported that they had found at last a property that seemed suitable for a mental hospital. Although their choice was later reversed, this report precipitated a new stage in the development of a hospital. The bishop board decided to send a letter to each ordained person of the Lancaster Conference, describing the "developments to date" and inviting them to meet with the bishops on February 25 and 26 at the Hammer Creek meetinghouse. There, the bishops discussed the proposed

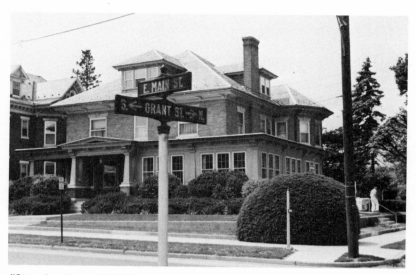

"Stepping Stone," Philhaven's halfway house in Palmyra, Pa. began accepting residents in 1972.

venture in mental health and the ministerium freely debated the proposal to found a mental hospital. The group agreed to put the matter before the conference during the upcoming spring meeting.

Conference Decides

The conference, meeting on March 18, 1948, heartily endorsed the proposal to found a mental hospital and approved the formation of a board of directors who would be responsible for such an institution. The bishops then solicited nominees and from them selected twelve men, each from a different bishop district.[6] The board of directors was elected not because of previous experience or knowledge of mental health needs, but to serve the conference. By having representatives from each bishop district, involvement of the whole conference was emphasized. The board of directors considered itself an arm of the church and responsible through the bishop board. As Melvin Kauffman remembers, "The church gave us a job to do and we...tried to do it."[7]

The board of bishops met with the board of directors for the first meeting at the Vine Street Mission (Lancaster, Pennsylvania) on April 15, 1948. The directors were introduced to one another by their respective home bishop, and charged to find a place for the church to take care of the mentally ill. They then stood together and promised to be faithful in discharging their duty. Officers of the board were elected, and in succeeding weeks a constitution and

> *This Board of Directors was unique among the institutions of the Lancaster Conference in that it was composed entirely of laymen. Although several Board members were ordained during their tenure, the Board was composed originally of men who had neither professional expertise in the mental health disciplines nor official ministry in the Church. (When the Board first assembled, not one of the men was acquainted with all of his colleagues, and several of those present had acquaintance with none of the others.) Nevertheless, the necessity of prompt action facilitated the growth of working relationships.[8]*

bylaws were written, later approved by the bishops. The board afterwards referred to themselves in their official minutes as a *Board of Trustees*, emphasizing that they held authority and responsibility in trust to the bishops and to the conference.

Three days in May 1948 were devoted to consultation and interviews. The board met with the director and other officials of the Bureau of Mental Health in the Pennsylvania Department of Welfare. Several books were recommended; all of the "most reliable and trustworthy sources of information on mental health" were tapped. Elmer Ediger of the MCC office made a presentation to the board on May 18, as did Richard Hunter of the National Mental Health Foundation in Philadelphia. Board members were encouraged by the support of state government officials and others who were working the field of mental health.[9] At this time, mental health was a new and uncharted discipline for the board. Victor Weaver recalls about their fact-finding efforts, "We went to school pretty fast."[10]

A Growing Vision

The board of trustees maintained an ambitious program of research throughout the first year of their existence. In June, the board visited Friends Hospital in Philadelphia and the Philadelphia Psychiatric Hospital. Meeting with three members of the National Mental Health Foundation, they asked questions about the kind of care to be offered, staffing patterns, and costs of hospital operation. Already, some critical issues were emerging. One was that the board was advised to consider either an acute-care facility or a residential program of care for the chronically ill; there would be many difficulties if both types of service were attempted. Furthermore, in either case, success of the hospital would depend largely upon the number and quality of staff members.

On June 24, the board consulted with the Religious Welfare Committee[11] about the decisions they were facing. From that discussion the outline of a possible program began to emerge:

1. That a program be inaugurated to benefit the acute mentally ill (those who may be restored to normal activities).
2. That community acceptance and the geographical center of the conference district be considered in choosing a location.
3. That the hospital be planned on a fifty-bed basis.
4. That, if a new building be constructed for this institution, it be located on a farm.
5. That an educational program for the membership be sponsored jointly by the bishop board and the board of trustees.
6. That steps be taken to provide for the necessary finances in relation to the former recommendations and that a location be secured as circumstances permit.

The board of trustees met twice in the month of July to develop a pamphlet to inform conference members. During the summer months, board members visited Darlington Sanitarium in West Chester, Allentown State Hospital, Harrisburg State Hospital, and later Norristown State Hospital. Several local psychiatrists and several Mennonite doctors, including Norman Loux of Souderton, were consulted. From all their visitation, the board felt they had gleaned a clearer vision of the type of institution they wished to found.

Late in 1948, the plans for a mental hospital began to take shape. The board estimated that the cost of a fifty-bed hospital would range from $250,000 to $400,000. Having considered several existing properties and explored the possibility of building, the trustees agreed that a new building was indicated. They composed the outline of a building program which they considered reasonable and effective, and presented this to the bishop board on December 15, 1948. Thus, eight months after the board of trustees was charged with finding a way to alleviate mental health needs, they returned with a well-considered plan for hospital construction.

In January 1949, the bishop board recommended that the trustees explore the "possibilities of a mental health clinic," apparently in response to the trustees' determination that an acute-care facility would best satisfy the needs of the conference. The bishops favored more careful study of the relative merits of a clinic and a hospital and of the relative need for acute and chronic care. In response, two actions were taken. First, a survey was made of each congregation in the conference to determine the number of mentally handicapped persons in homes and institutions, and to evaluate the need for a mental hospital. Secondly, the trustees visited three clinics in Philadelphia to collect data about costs, staffing patterns, and accommodations necessary to operate a clinic.

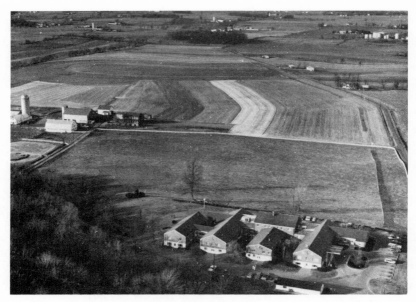

The hospital as it appeared from 1965-1977 with the farm which was donated by Graybill and Mary Landis.

By March 10, 1949, the deliberations were complete. The board of trustees reaffirmed the recommendations that they had made to the bishop board the previous June. A summary of the trustees' activities in the preceding eleven months was prepared for the bishops with copies to be distributed to each ordained member of the conference. The board was satisfied that it had "carefully and prayerfully studied the mental hospital problem." Alleviation of this problem, they concluded, would require "our best judgment and the leading of the Holy Spirit."[12]

The First Annual Report

On Thursday, April 14, 1949, several hundred Lancaster Conference church members met at Mellinger's Church to hear the first annual report of the board of directors. Members of the board discussed their experiences and the vision that they were pursuing. The afternoon and evening sessions were filled with sermons, lectures, and challenges. A physician, Merle Eshelman, assured the conference that many mental illnesses could be alleviated or cured. He urged the conference to found an acute-care facility and to undertake an ambitious work of education about mental health. Bishop Noah Risser agreed. "Begin a teaching program," he said. "We need to know that mental illness is a disease and that there is a remedy for it." Bishop Simon Bucher felt that "our first need is to educate our constituency relative to the great need" in the field of mental health. Education was, clearly, an important theme of the first annual meeting.

A second theme was introduced and developed largely by speakers who were invited from other conferences of the Mennonite church. The church's responsibility to respond to community mental health needs was considered by Elmer Ediger of MCC. Delvin Kirchhofer, administrator of Brook Lane Farm, also urged the conference to consider community needs. These brethren were among the first to suggest explicitly that the conference had a responsibility to serve the mentally ill in their communities.[13]

The themes of knowing and acting responsibly were neatly linked by Henry Bomberger in his discussion of "The Seriousness of the Mental Problem." He recognized that mental health needs were enormous and that "this great undertaking may take time"; we need to proceed in "the right direction." He envisioned "a hospital to lead patients to Jesus Christ, to give them peace and hope."[14] The evangelical nature of the church's involvement in mental health services was never before recorded so clearly.

A Site for the Hospital

Before the meeting ended, the president of the board of trustees, George Zeiset, reported to the assembly that one of the persons in attendance was moved to make a generous gift toward the foundation of a Mennonite mental hospital. Graybill Landis, member of the East Petersburg congregation, had privately informed the trustees that he would donate a farm of 166 acres to the Lancaster Conference if this would provide a suitable site for the proposed hospital. The farm, located near Mount Gretna, would be deeded "as long as grass grows and water flows."[15]

According to Brother Landis, he had purchased the farm without much deliberation, having passed the site when it was being auctioned at public sale. He and his wife stopped, learned what figures had been bid, then acquired the land by offering an additional fifty dollars. Brother Landis felt that this event, occurring shortly before the annual meeting, was divinely inspired. The Board agreed that the gift of property had been an answer to prayer.

—Monroe Garber[16]

Soon after, the board of directors visited the farm with Graybill Landis who conducted them on a tour of the property. The location was deemed eminently suitable; the board had long considered that a farm would provide the best setting for a hospital. Because the farm was rented to tenants, the board could not begin immediately to erect a building. They briefly considered the possibility of converting the farmhouse into use as a hospital building, but found that this was not feasible. Although the property was visited and surveyed on several occasions, the board did not come to a decision about the exact site of construction until the fall of 1949. At length, the decision was made to build on the hill, a site that continues to elicit much favorable comment.

Education and Fund Raising

In determining to commit the resources of the church to a program of mental health, the board realized that it must confront the stigma that was attached unreasonably to the problem of mental illness. The bishops cooperated with the board of trustees in making educational presentations to the congregations of each district. The trustees developed the themes that had dominated the first annual meeting; mental health problems were widespread, but individuals in the church and in the community could be helped through programs of therapy. While they encountered some opposition, the bishops and board members were glad to see that the church was rising to meet the challenge.

In addition to educational meetings, the bishops approved a program of fund raising. Each district designated "solicitors" who were responsible to contact every church member in their area. The trustees also served as solicitors and tackled this work with their customary zeal. Noah Kreider summarized the board's attitude, "Everyone had a will to work, and that's what it took."[17] The cost of the initial building was estimated at $180,000. The bishops considered that a contribution of seventy-five dollars for each family would be sufficient to meet the cost. A few small congregations collected the funds through an offering, but most conference members were contacted personally. By the time the new hospital building was dedicated, the building costs had been met completely.[18]

Building and Dedication

In March of 1951, almost two years after the farm was given to the conference, ground was broken for the erection of a hospital building. The original plan of the trustees to build a fifty-bed hospital was altered to construct only twenty-six of these patient rooms until the need for more beds was demonstrated. The hospital was so designed that "wings" of patient rooms could be added easily. The new building contained sufficient space for support services for fifty

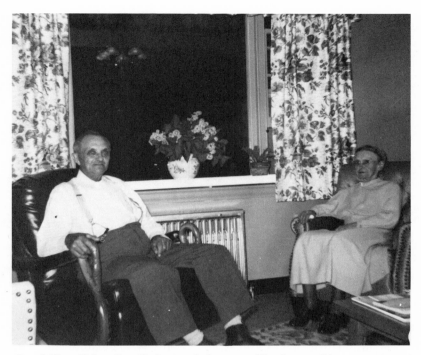

Graybill and Mary Landis during their years of "retirement" in an apartment on the campus of Philhaven.

Noah Kreider had contacted a member of his congregation who was well known to him and his family. This person, who is still a friend of the Kreiders, was "under the impression that we wouldn't be able to build a hospital and make it work." Noah explained some of the careful planning that had been done, but the doubtful friend replied, "My sister's a nurse, and she said it will never work. We (the Church) can't run a hospital." "Well," Noah Kreider said, "we're going to try." In the end, this family contributed $75 to the foundation of the hospital.[19]

---

beds and, on the second floor, staff living quarters. The trustees were agreed that the building must be well constructed and adaptable to changing uses. Abe Metzler summed up their disposition by remarking, "It is an established fact that the Mennonites must build good!"[20]

During the two years of planning, the farm had been operated for the benefit of the hospital corporation. A herd of dairy cattle was donated to the farm by members of the Lancaster Conference. Congregations, Sunday school classes, and many individuals gave a cow or the cost of half a cow. J. Clarence Garber, chairman of the trustees' farm committee, worked diligently to create a herd that would reflect favorably the support of the church. He was highly successful; the Philhaven farm still possesses a herd of superior quality. These gifts were matched in later years by numerous offerings of time and goods. For almost a decade, men and women volunteered their services in canning, clearing land, erecting fences, planting trees, and in many other work projects. There can be no doubt that members of the Lancaster Conference understood the work of the hospital as their own.

While the building was progressing, a few discouraging words were sounded by persons who lived in the vicinity of the new hospital. A letter to the editor of the newspaper in Lebanon reportedly represented the views of several residents in Mount Gretna who were alarmed by the prospect of an "Insane Asylum" in their "backyard." The letter writer wondered aloud why a small denomination like the Mennonites would require a mental hospital for the needs of its members! Fortunately, other residents of Lebanon city and county were ready to welcome the new hospital.

No one can now recall with certainty who created the name *Philhaven*, but J. Paul Graybill is most often suggested as the author.[21] The *Haven of Love* was named sometime in 1951. Elvin G. Lefever, who had agreed to serve as the hospital's first administrator, announced the name in an article he wrote for a church magazine in March of 1952. There, Lefever described the goals of Philhaven: "The best of psychiatric care . . . to be available for our patients" and "a continual atmosphere of Christian love." From the beginning, Philhaven was to be identified by a high quality of professional services offered in the context of Christian faith and charity. Lefever concluded his article by stating: "The Christian church does well to help care for the mentally sick. Our Savior, when here upon earth, took time and effort to help and heal."[22] The work of the hospital was perceived as the ministry of the church.

Now, eight years after the bishops named the original hospital study committee, Philhaven Hospital was complete and ready to receive patients.

The Development of Hospital Services (1952-82)

Early Staff Members

As indicated earlier, the trustees sought to provide good psychiatric treatment in an environment that reflected Christian faith and values. Accordingly, the board assumed that most persons providing care for patients would come from conference churches.[23] Through the first two decades of Philhaven's existence, virtually all staff members were identified with the Mennonite Church. Some persons volunteered their services to the hospital, others applied for salaried positions, and, until the early 1970s, some young men worked at the hospital as an alternative to military service. Directed by a physician and supervised by registered nurses, the staff attempted to create a therapeutic milieu.

During the first two years, the hospital experienced some "growing pains," largely because most staff members lived together on the second floor of the same hospital building where they were responsible for continuous service to the patient group. Though off duty, staff members were often called back to the unit when emergency situations arose. This occurred with discouraging frequency. Moreover, the facility was not well equipped to handle patients who were severely disturbed. Within another year, however, these problems were ameliorated by the inauguration of a building program and the recruitment of additional staff.

The board was determined to find a physician whose personal philosophy was compatible with their own, but Mennonite psychiatrists were not available. It was with great satisfaction that Philip Laucks was hired in 1952 as the first medical director. At the annual meeting in 1954, Laucks asserted that he had never worked at a place that displayed such a "Christian atmosphere" and that the work would not be possible without "the goodwill, prayer, and support of the Church." The medical director's sympathy with the aims of the board and of the conference undoubtedly contributed to the success of the hospital program.

In 1952, Dr. Philip Laucks was still subject to possible induction into the armed forces; members of the board of directors, through letters and personal visits, interceded with the selective service office on Dr. Laucks' behalf. The board sought a continuation of Dr. Laucks' draft exemption because of his indispensability to the hospital program. They were successful in their efforts during the years that Dr. Laucks was employed at Philhaven.

Expansion of Facilities

In December 1953, the board of trustees recommended to the bishop board the construction of a building to accommodate approximately twenty staff persons. In January 1954, Horace Martin, the administrator who had replaced Lefever, also presented a plan to the board for additional patient rooms. The two needs that had been identified in the first year of operation, better housing for staff and

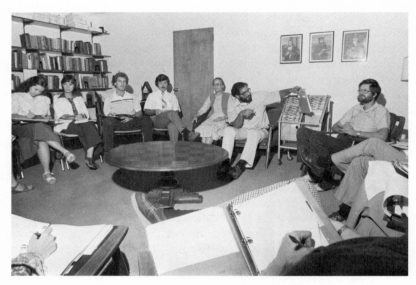

Programs of care and treatment are developed and reviewed by inter-disciplinary teams which reflect all departments of patient care.

more adequate facilities for disturbed patients, were being met simultaneously. The new annex, located at the west end of the original building, contained several security rooms and facilities for hydrotherapy. It permitted the isolation and protection of patients who were dangerously aggressive or agitated. Occupancy of the annex in mid-1954 did much to improve the safety and morale of staff members.

The next expansion of the hospital occurred seven years later when the need for office space demanded expansion and renovation of the hospital building. With the hiring of Henry Wietz as medical director in 1955 and the addition of Marjorie Morrison as a second psychiatrist in 1957, outpatient services began to grow more rapidly. By 1961, it was necessary to add a wing, containing offices, a receptionist area, and a waiting room, at the southeast corner of the hospital building. A short time later, in 1963, the board approved plans for the erection of a chapel at the east end of the hospital, which was completed in the same year. Then, in 1965, a wing was added to the west end of the building which, with the annex of 1954, provided an expanded intensive care unit (ICU). This unit was staffed independently of the original patient area which was now called the *open ward*.

For the next twelve years, Philhaven's inpatient services in the open ward and the ICU did not expand although numerous programs were developed to enrich the therapeutic milieu. Eventually, these programs began to compete for limited space. By the mid-1970s, an increased demand for ICU beds and the need for greater supportive services necessitated further building. In 1976, Philhaven launched "Big Step Forward" which included renovations in several areas of the original hospital building and construction of a new intensive care unit, creative therapy department, and gymnasium.

Therapeutic Interventions

Therapies that were available for patients in the early days of Philhaven included: psychotherapy, electroshock, insulin shock, supervision of the patients' daily activities, and reinforcement of basic living skills. The medical director was responsible for the practice of psychotherapy and for the medical modes of intervention. Otherwise, the therapeutic community at Philhaven seems to have depended upon the initiative and imagination of staff members. After 1954, hydrotherapy became available and the same year saw greater development of the occupational and recreational therapy programs. Patients were introduced to numerous arts and

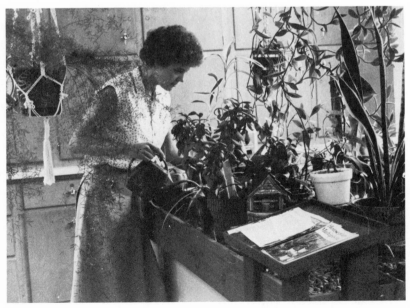

Plants and flowers are evident throughout the hospital building emphasizing the theme of growth and change.

crafts and were encouraged to participate in sports and games. Outdoor activity was enhanced by the clearing of a ball diamond in 1954. There was an emphasis upon developing hobbies or interests that could be pursued by patients after they left the hospital.

At first staff and patients shared a wide range of homemaking activities. Programs of cleaning and housekeeping, gardening and canning, were a regular part of scheduled activities for patients. Gradually housekeeping activities became distinguished as "industrial therapy," but in 1975 stricter regulations by government agencies made this too cumbersome to continue. Cooking classes, meal-planning and nutrition courses, horticultural interest groups, and patient flower and vegetable gardens succeeded the former programs.

The psychopharmacological revolution in the mid-1950s also affected treatment services at Philhaven. The staff tended to use chemotherapy as a tool to assist patients in deriving maximum benefit from the therapeutic environment, not as the primary focus of treatment. The potential benefits of the new psychotropic agents, however, were related to a gradual decrease in the frequency with which electroshock was administered. Insulin shock was discontinued entirely as a treatment.

By the decade of the 1960s a pattern can be discerned in the evolution of treatment methods. Informal activities and games became more organized into regular programs of socialization and recreation, with clearly defined therapeutic goals. Additionally, group activities, both on campus and off grounds, became increasingly diverse and specific to particular populations. Creative therapy departments had been developed in 1965 at the time that the intensive care unit was separated from the open ward. A woodshop was also established in the basement of the hospital although this was later moved to another building. These programs made possible a veritable smorgasboard of potential projects. When the creative therapy departments were enlarged and relocated in 1977, a potter's wheel and kiln were added which made possible a variety of ceramic projects. A soundproof "pounding room," complete with punching bags and other devices, was incorporated into the ICU creative therapy area.

Although the pattern was already established, the decade of the 1970s saw a rapid multiplication of the number and kinds of therapeutic activities and programs offered to inpatients. Charles Neff, who began his tenure as medical director in 1971, helped to construct a program of psychodrama. The addition of several therapists made possible the expansion of group therapy in the early 1970s. About the same time, music therapy as a professional discipline was added with the availability of a staff person in 1971. By the mid-1970s music therapy internships were being offered and a second full-time music therapist position was created in 1978. The other fine arts were not neglected and regular groups were now established in art therapy and expressive therapy. The former promoted the development of technical skills while the latter employed various media primarily as a means of self-expression. Poetry therapy was introduced in 1974. James Johnson, who joined the hospital staff in 1971 as chief of social work, offered training programs in family therapy and helped to promote more widespread use of that modality.

Among the most recent additions to Philhaven's program of treatment are self-awareness groups, life-enhancement or remotivation therapy, assertiveness training, and relaxation groups. The increasing specialization of treatment modalities has necessitated a corresponding increase in attention given to inservice education and staff development. The increasing importance of education is not limited to the staff; the great challenge of the 1980s appears in the area of patient education. During 1981, preliminary work was done in developing learning units in the areas of medication, stress, sexuality, nutrition, drug abuse, smoking, and physical exercise.

Spiritual Care

Although not identified as a particular therapy, concern for the patient's spiritual condition has distinguished the therapeutic milieu of Philhaven. From the beginning, in addition to eating and working with patients, staff members shared responsibility for leading worship services and for providing spiritual instruction and encouragement. There is no evidence that staff members ever saw mental illness as primarily a spiritual problem, but certainly they recognized that emotional disturbances might affect a person's sense of spiritual well-being, and that "spiritual health" is a component of mental health. Likewise, spiritual renewal could be an important resource to the patient in the experience of hospitalization.

Not until 1956 did the board consider hiring a hospital chaplain. He was employed not to engage in psychotherapy with patients, but to train and support the staff in their exercise of a "pastoral" ministry. This pattern has continued until the present.

Since the 1970s, the hospital staff has been recruited from a population much larger than the Lancaster Conference. Even so, a significant number of employees are Mennonites. Coordinated by the director of pastoral services, staff members continue to volunteer their assistance in preparing daily chapel meditations. Once a

week, most of the staff and patients join together for worship. This
weekly celebration often includes special musical or dramatic presentations and affirms the reality of spiritual fellowship with the
hospital. Patients have organized several Bible study groups, inspirational meetings, and song-fests that occur on a regular basis.
But, as in the past, the peculiar strength of Philhaven is the personal
Christian faith of each staff person. This faith informs and shapes
the innumerable interactions of the closely-related hospital community.

As a public service agency, Philhaven serves the needs of a
diverse and varied population. Some clients may not be familiar or
sympathetic with Philhaven's philosophical and theological presuppositions; nevertheless, the staff encourages each patient to discover the spiritual dimension of his or her personality. Philhaven
makes no attempt to disguise or minimize the importance of its
spiritual values, and believes it is vitally important that a therapist is
comfortable in dealing with every aspect of the client's experience;
the purview of therapy must include spiritual needs and aspirations. There can be no question but that Philhaven's identification as
a ministry of and within the church has fostered a tender regard for
the needs of the whole person.

Services of the Hospital

Outpatient services had been contemplated by the board of
directors even before the hospital opened in 1952. Throughout the
first two decades of the hospital's experience, outpatient services
depended upon the availability of physicians who shared this interest. Not until the 1970s, when the professional disciplines of
psychology and social services were distinguished at Philhaven,
were outpatient services to become an area of operation as great as
the inpatient function.

With Dr. Abram Hostetter's encouragement, a property in
Annville was considered for a halfway house in 1970. However,
Philhaven was unable to secure exemption to zoning ordinances
that precluded a group residence. The opposition of community
residents was a major factor in this barrier to expanded services.
Both programs, of partial hospitalization and a halfway house, were
to be realized only after Dr. Hostetter's term of service had ended,
but he was influential in their development.

Earlier efforts to develop a halfway house were renewed when
Rowland Shank was named administrator in 1971. By the end of that
year, a suitable site was identified in the town of Palmyra. The
house, a former mansion, was well constructed and could be converted into a home for eleven residents plus an apartment for house

parents. Shank and James Johnson personally introduced the halfway house idea to all of the householders in the immediate vicinity of the proposed program. In March of 1973, Stepping Stone began accepting residents into its program.

A program of partial hospitalization, initially involving day care, was implemented in 1971. This program permitted patients to engage in a full range of therapeutic activities during the daytime, then return to their homes in the community in the evening. By 1977, attention was being given to the design of a program of partial hospitalization which would function with greater independence from the inpatient activity and at a lower cost. A program for fifteen patients was licensed by the Pennslyvania Department of Public Health in 1981.

In the mid-1970s, Philhaven initiated a program of residential services for patients who could benefit from continued interaction and support in a home environment. Families within the hospital's primary service area volunteered their homes. Beginning in 1976, a director of family care worked with families and their "adopted" residents to enhance the benefits that this service provided. Within the first five years of its existence, the family care program averaged between twenty and thirty placements at all times.

The board of trustees had intended from the beginning that Philhaven should provide educational services to the constituency[24] and, by implication, to the larger community. Annual educational meetings were presented until the mid-1960s, when they began to be held jointly with the annual meeting. In 1978, the Philhaven forum committee was established with community representatives to coordinate public education efforts. The next few years brought programs for health care professionals, families; church leaders, women, parents, and single persons. Hundreds of participants visited the hospital for these forum meetings.

The long-range planning activity that began in 1980 affirmed "education and prevention" as a major function of the hospital. Thus, by 1980, five areas of service were distinguished in Philhaven's Statement of Purpose: inpatient services, outpatient services, the partial hospitalization program, residential treatment services, and education and preventive services.

Critical Issues

In the years 1969 to 1971, Philhaven struggled with issues that were critical in determining the direction and the success of future growth. After his appointment as medical director in 1969, Abram Hostetter encouraged Philhaven to build relationships with a community larger than the one with which the hospital had previously

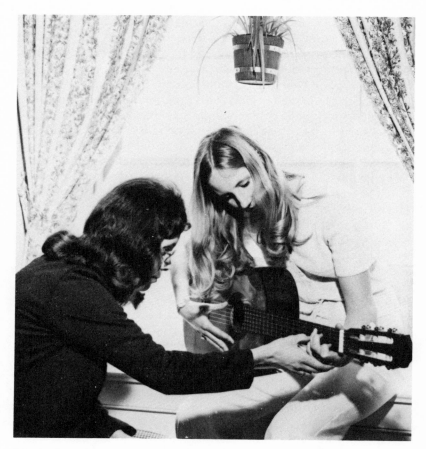

Music therapists provide individual attention to residents and leadership to many small-group activities.

related. In addition to proposing new areas of service, such as the halfway house and day-care program referred to previously, Hostetter was interested in Philhaven's potential as a community mental health center related to the local mental health/mental retardation programs.[25] Hostetter also suggested that Philhaven could widen its base of financial support by soliciting contributions from area industries. The medical director assured the board that contractual relationships or financial gifts would not compromise the hospital's independence.

These alternative patterns of development, as well as an increase in demands for service and a consequent hiring of new staff, severely tested the hospital community. Some staff were impatient for change, while others were concerned that the hospital's spiritual values were being undermined. Questions about the relation of evangelical faith to mental health work were raised as were fears that Philhaven was becoming too accommodating of secular models of mental health services. Philosophical differences easily became entangled and confused in personal conflicts. Soon, questions of authority and administrative responsibility for decision making began to interfere with the successful operation at the facility.

In an attempt to resolve some of these difficulties, the board appointed Richard Showalter as assistant administrator and personnel director in February of 1970. At the same time, the board declared its intention and desire that the hospital continually reflect "our evangelical Christian position," and approved a seven-article statement of faith. The new administrative assistant expressed his concern that greater attention was needed to develop and maintain a Christian environment in the hospital, lest the spiritual life of the institution be submerged in a mere humanitarian approach.

A month later, members of the nursing department presented a petition requesting a meeting with the board. They were uncomfortable with the policies of the personnel department as they perceived them. By February of 1971, the board needed to meet again with administrator, Horace Martin, and other staff persons to discuss personnel problems. Caleb Witmer, the board's secretary, spent many days at the hospital in consultation with any staff person who wanted to discuss Philhaven's situation. Later that spring, Martin and Showalter both offered their resignations as a step toward building a new atmosphere within the hospital. These were accepted regretfully by the board. Caleb Witmer volunteered his service as mediator and as one who might clarify the board's intention regarding the hospital. He served as acting administrator for one month. For the second time in six months, the board in May 1971 invited Rowland Shank to accept the position of administrator. After careful deliberation, he cautiously agreed to accept that offer.

The new administrator challenged the board to consider carefully what type of hospital they wanted and to persevere in moving toward that end. Shank identified three options: to close up the hospital, to allow the hospital to evolve from its original model, or to regain tight administrative control by the governing body. The board chose the latter course and began to confront more directly the questions that were being raised and to take a more active role in shaping the future of the hospital. This eventually resulted in the resignation of several persons from the staff of the hospital. The two years of intense enthusiasm and disagreement in some ways were costly to persons and to the institution, but in the end the results were positive.

By the end of 1971, Philhaven was more stabilized and again exploring new areas of mission and service. The administrator had been confirmed in his role as the board's direct representative in the hospital. Personnel policies had been clarified and strengthened. Charles Neff joined the staff as medical director. With the addition of new staff persons in many departments, Philhaven began to develop a team approach to the treatment of its clients that was truly interdisciplinary and cooperative. The long year of deliberation helped to focus the hospital's attention on what was essential to the institution. Paradoxically, the renewed emphasis upon Philhaven's "roots" actually led to increased denominational diversity among the staff, who were united more strongly in their dedication to the spiritual values of the hospital.

A Long-Range Plan

Throughout the 1960s, a committee of the board had periodically considered plans for future growth and development. As a new administrative team was developing in early 1972, the board committee was reorganized to include the hospital administrator and business manager. Even so, plans were being developed largely in response to present needs, with little attention paid to long-range development issues. Shank remembers that there was "only a vague understanding (about planning) within the Philhaven system."[26] At the completion of the Big Step Forward program in 1977, the board recognized that services were continuing to grow faster than the hospital's plan to meet them. A new emphasis upon planning began to emerge.

In the spring of 1980, Philhaven coordinated a long-range planning workshop for the Lancaster Conference Board of Brotherhood Ministries. From this experience, representatives from Philhaven were inspired to form an ad hoc planning council. Within a few months, the board approved formally the establishment of a long-range planning council for Philhaven.

The council worked slowly, deliberately, and conscientiously, devoting several hours each week to the planning process. The council recognized that its function was to initiate and supervise a

---

I believe that we ought to be alert to opportunities and deal with them. I think there's no harm in (the long-range plan) if we're satisfied to let the Lord take a hold of it anytime He wants to and tear it apart.

—Abram Metzler [27]

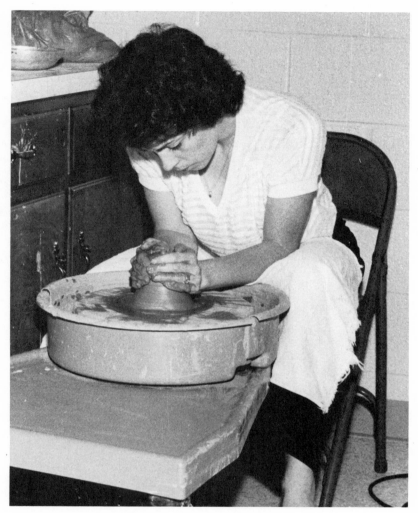

Shaping and molding with one's own hands at the potter's wheel.

long-range plan that would reflect the whole community and involve every staff member of Philhaven. A revised statement of purpose was composed with painstaking care in the summer of 1980 and presented to the board for approval in the fall. This reflected more clearly than before the hospital's involvement in a wide range of services and programs. In common with each previous statement of purpose, the new document affirmed Philhaven's commitment to professional service in a context of Christian faith and community.

By January of 1982, Philhaven was poised on the threshold of an ambitious program of construction and "retrofitting." Approaching the thirtieth anniversary of the hospital's dedication, Philhaven recognized the considerable growth it had experienced, remembered the years of struggle for identity, was grateful for the honorable tradition that it represented, and, with gratitude and hope, looked forward to greater work in years of maturity.

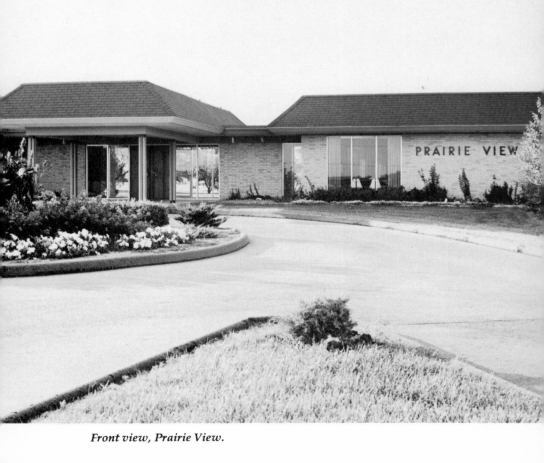

Front view, Prairie View.

CHAPTER 6

Prairie View
Newton, Kansas

Elmer M. Ediger*

Prairie View, the third of the mental health programs to be launched by the Mennonite Central Committee (MCC), opened May 14, 1954, on the outskirts of Newton, Kansas. Conceived in 1947 as a "home for mentally ill," Prairie View opened as a treatment hospital with dreams of being more comprehensive. In the years which followed, many of these dreams were realized as Prairie View evolved as a comprehensive community mental health center.

Setting the Stage (1947-1954)

Kansas offered many advantages as the MCC central area program. It had a strong concentration of Mennonites, three colleges, four church-related general hospitals, and numerous homes for the aged. A mental health interest already existed, expressed as early as 1939, which was stimulated by hundreds of young Mennonites who had worked in state hospitals during World War II and encouraged by several Kansas MCC leaders.

Central Area Hospital was the unofficial name during the first five years of planning, but *Prairie View Hospital* was the name selected in 1952. The name was modified in 1965 to "Prairie View, Inc., commonly referred to as Prairie View Mennonite Health Center."

First official name (for Prairie View) recommended to the MCC was "Central Area Hospital," but the Executive Committee meeting in Switzerland that summer fired back their response to Kansas saying, "You can be more imaginative than that!"

Names for the hospital were considered. Selection of a name was done by ballot. The names were narrowed down to the following two: Gilead Hospital 7 votes, Prairie View Hosptial 10 votes. [1]

---

*Elmer M. Ediger is Executive Director of Prairie View, Newton, Kansas.

On December 6, 1947, about forty MCC constituent representatives gathered to implement the January 1947 MCC action. This
meeting included representatives from seven states, eight different
Mennonite groups and nine general hospitals. The hospitals had
been given a special invitation to consider adding psychiatric wards,
but all shied away from this idea. Those from the homes for the aged
made pleas for the chronically ill. Others promoted prevention.
There seemed to be a call for a comprehensive program for the
central area. [2]

---

*At the Central Area constituency meeting in 1947, P. E. Shellenberg
of Tabor College emphasized, "prevention." "Why just pick up the
automobile casualties at the bottom of the mountain when you can put
up warning signs at the top and prevent the accidents?"*

A Central Area Advisory Committee representing all the Mennonite
groups was formed in 1950 and functioned until 1957 when a local
board assumed the operational responsibility.

Newton, Kansas, was a favored location, but it was not officially selected until 1950 after consideration of Hesston, Hillsboro,
and a variety of existing facilities including the Harvey and Marion
County Homes, Santa Fe Hospital at Mulvane, a large house near
Wichita, and even a state orphanage facility in Oklahoma.

The program and facility concepts crystallized through interaction of the local advisory committee and the MCC central office
staff. Insights from dozens of MCC interviews of national psychiatric leaders and the experience of the two Mennonite Mental Health
Services (MMHS) programs already begun were utilized. Planning
decisions were based on a ten-page document entitled "Envisioning
a Central Area Mental Health Service Program" prepared in 1951 by
Elmer Ediger. This included the proposal of a guidance center, a
strong emphasis on mental health education, a foster home program, and a strong case for beginning with treatment as opposed to
longer term care. The treatment view was accepted as the beginning
point of a long-range comprehensive program. [3]

Delmar Stahly of the MCC central office was the interim administrator until Myron Ebersole completed his MCC relief assignment in Jordan. Ebersole, the first administrator, arrived in Newton
just in time for the ground-breaking ceremony, October 19, 1952.

The fund raising of $200,000 was a tremendous feat for the
Mennonite constituency. Local Mennonite churches were given a
goal of six to ten dollars per member, supplied with a volunteer
speaker, and then expected to raise their own funds. Enthusiasm in

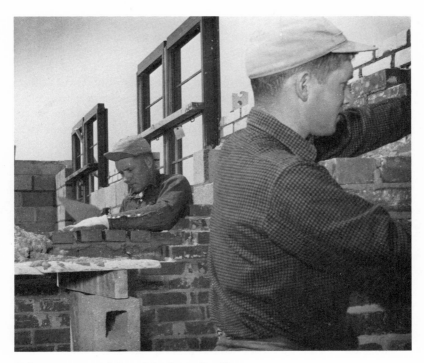

Volunteers at work in original construction.

the churches ran high and, as Prairie View painfully learned later, expectations of the new treatment program were also high. The Newton Chamber of Commerce raised $5,300 but this came only after vigorous debate as to whether the mental hospital would really be a community asset!

Formative Years As a Private Hospital (1954-1957)

The formation of Prairie View was a blend of a variety of influences which came from three groups. The advisory committee represented a cross section of the Kansas Mennonite constituency, including some strong administrative, financial, and pastoral leadership. Myron Ebersole, the local administrator, and Delmar Stahly represented the central office of MCC. A third major influence came with the assembly of the new staff.

The Doors Open

A total of about fifteen staff persons were on hand for the first patient who was admitted Monday, March 15, 1954, the day following the dedication of the new building. Besides Ebersole, early employees included Harold Vogt, psychologist, and Lucinda Martin, director of nursing. Most of the intitial hospital staff were young Mennonites recruited by the Akron office from all over North America who came for a year or two of volunteer service.

In an effort to find a competent psychiatrist who would share both the milieu therapy orientation and the dedication to church interests, Prairie View was directed to the Wichita psychiatric group of Adams, Newsom, and Morrow (AN&M). Thomas Morrow was invited to become the medical director on a part-time basis until Prairie View could find its own full-time psychiatrist.

Health leaders of the Wichita area had predicted Prairie View would be filled within a short time, but it was actually a slow process. For several months during the first three years the hospital was filled to capacity, yet the average census for the first six years was only twenty-six patients for a forty-bed capacity.

Initially Prairie View sought to serve a Mennonite constituency geographically covering roughly one-third of the United States. By 1960 this had been reduced to Kansas and parts of the surrounding states. During the first six-year period, Mennonites constituted 20 to 25 percent of the hospital admissions.

Treatment Philosophy Develops

After six months of operation Harold Vogt stated the goal of treatment as "helping the patient regain control of his emotional and mental processes as well as his behavior." This same report indicates the wide range of treatments given. Of the patients in the program at the time, five received electroconvulsive treatment, six insulin coma therapy, one subcoma insulin, and fourteen psychotherapy. [4] A year later the medical director reported a significant shift away from convulsive and insulin therapies made possible by the new "wonder drugs." There were signs of confidence and many ideas about the future.

There was also evidence of what became a growing characteristic of Prairie View—a strong belief in the validity of its own evolving treatment approach. Vogt had weekly sessions designed to place the initiative on the staff members for raising issues and clarifying responsibilities. Ebersole initiated a patient council and later an administrative council to provide opportunity for participation and responsibility. Still later an "all-staff all-patient community meeting" was established to include everyone from cooks to psychiatrists.

There were numerous innovations. By 1956 the hospital doors were unlocked, visiting restrictions were dropped, and censoring of mail and the search for sharp objects were discontinued. It was assumed that the patient always had some capacity to be responsible.

By 1958, in three important papers, staff members were able to articulate a basic philosophy to guide the hospital.[5] A common premise of these papers was that mental illness is not categorically different from normal life. "Maturity and mental health are very close to each other, if not identical."[6] Growth in maturity and in mental health comes from a combination of things that need to happen within a person—experiencing discomfort with the present, learning from past experiences, and directing one's life by specific steps of responsible action. From the "essence of helping" in the psychiatric center, the Prairie View leadership made the leap to apply these principles to other human relationships within the community.

New Programs

Among the new programs of the early years was the day hospital initiated in 1956. This program, however, did not thrive until after 1962 under the leadership of Walter Lewin and Allen Bohn.

An experimental staff-community discussion group on religion and psychiatry was started in the spring of 1956 and has continued over twenty-five years with forty to fifty persons participating in twice-a-month meetings. These groups played a significant role in developing peer relationships between community leaders and Prairie View staff.

From the beginning Ebersole and Vogt were committed to involving Prairie View with the community. The "Guidance Center" concept was kept alive through a community council study group. In 1958 psychiatric nursing concepts were marketed to the community in a nine-month "post-R.N." course. A series of conferences on aging were held in Buhler and other communities. A preprofessional program was initiated for young staff members to encourage interest in mental health professions.

Problems

Among the early problems was the salary policy. Until 1957, procurement of personnel was primarily the responsibility of the MCC headquarters. MCC as a whole was predominantly reliant upon voluntary service and "maintenance level" salaried personnel. As early as September 1954, and again two years later, Prairie View pleaded for a semicompetitive wage scale. The slowness of an MCC shift toward a competitive wage system for its hospitals became an overwhelming obstacle in hiring much needed professional staff, particularly from other than Mennonite communities.

The salary issue was intertwined with two others—the organizational relationship with the Wichita psychiatric group, and the desire for more local autonomy. In May of 1965 it was agreed that the Wichita group would assume full responsibility for procuring all professional staff. A Joint Conference Committee representing the Wichita group and Prairie View was arranged to facilitate regular discussions. For a while it looked as though this relationship might continue indefinitely. A "Prairie View Foundation" was proposed as a vehicle to unite these two groups, but the crisis years ahead eventually made the proposal irrelevant.

The discussions reflected an honest effort to look at another issue—the growing criticism from the church constituency. Initially such criticism focused on issues such as smoking by therapists during therapy, high costs, and the concern that patients should be presented "the claims of Christ" more clearly. Later the criticisms were more in regard to the slowness of the treatment program, the feeling by pastors that they were unwelcome, the assumption that professionals were being paid too much, and the concern that the hospital was run by professionals instead of the church. Many of the

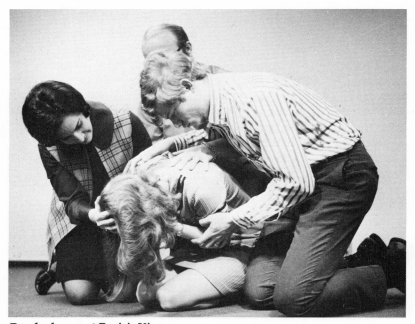

Psychodrama at Prairie View.

pastors, who initially had high hopes for Prairie View, had become seriously disillusioned.

Local autonomy was another issue. Increasingly it became clear to the leadership of Prairie View and the other MMHS hospitals that the centrally controlled administration of MCC was not suited for the operation of a local mental hospital. After a year or more of straightforward negotiations between the hospitals and MMHS, it was decided in 1957 to give local boards the basic authority needed and to allow them to become incorporated.

Late in 1957 the newly authorized Prairie View board began wrestling with the problem of high costs. Alternatives were proposed in the Joint Conference meetings. The idea of having five beds available below cost for rehabilitation of long-term patients in the community was successfully implemented. Another alternative to high costs was a "benefit association membership" that would guarantee inpatient and outpatient services on the basis of membership fees. The idea was approved but lost out in the critical years that followed. "A plan to help Prairie View pioneer" was approved and contributions were solicited from industry to make possible the "margin" required for pioneering. Though problems were accumulating, administration and board showed their continued strong belief in the Prairie View treatment approach.

In the spring of 1957 Myron Ebersole indicated his desire for a leave-of-absence for further studies. Elmer Ediger, the chairman of the board, was asked to be the administrator for an interim period of six months. Ediger accepted and later agreed to serve for an indefinite period which continues to the present.

Crisis and Redirection (1958-1962)

The low census of the hospital became a crisis in 1958. Three months in 1957 has been at near capacity of forty, but the low month in 1958 was eighteen patients. The census during these two years was like a wildly fluctuating stock market; however, by the middle of 1958 the downward trend seemed unmistakable. Fears were strong that Prairie View might have to close as Kings View, the sister program in California, had the year before.

Proposed New Direction

In mid-1958 steps were taken to trim the staff to a much lower break-even point. In addition, the staff and board asked basic questions, such as: Are we needed? and What is wrong with us? In a report to MMHS in October 1958, the administrator noted four factors contributing to the low census—too many psychiatric beds, lower stigma of psychiatric wards in general hospitals, reputation of "it takes longer," and the need for a more unique treatment role. He described the road ahead as "a painful process to educate our people to accept this 'patient-responsible-for-his-own-actions' type of treatment." At the same MMHS meeting Morrow stated that ". . . a more community-oriented program is going to be necessary. . . . This means more out-patient services, including day care, rehabilitation services, halfway houses, collaboration with social agencies, and the like. . . ."[7]

The board approved the proposed redirection of program, and a two-fold process began immediately. One was to strengthen the ties with the community and the other to consider the administrative implications of the new direction.

Contacts in the Community

The administrative leadership went to the caretakers in the community, such as the county welfare director, physicians, and ministers, to assess community needs and how Prairie View might relate to them. For approximately six months the medical director and administrator reserved a half-day a week seeking to set into motion new forms of collaboration.

The initial meetings with the Harvey County Welfare staff

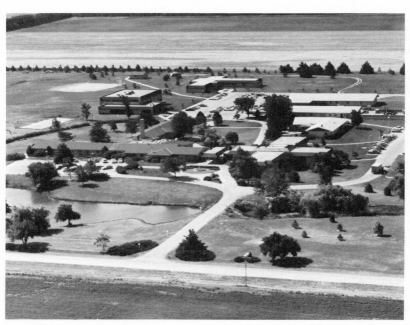

Aerial view, Prairie View.

resulted in a series of weekly consultations. Prairie View learned that "county welfare is in the real stream of community need; Prairie View has too long been sitting on the edge of town waiting for people to come."[8] The welfare department on the other hand learned to utilize professional consultation in a helpful way.

There was another round of visits to pastors in Hillsboro, Moundridge, Newton, Buhler, and other Kansas communities. Ministers said they felt "too much in the dark as to what happens in therapy." They also reported being frustrated in trying to get information from a professional staff member regarding a patient. "By implication we feel psychiatry has defined our role as non-existent," they reported. "We feel nonplused because we don't know what to do and assume psychiatry knows it all but doesn't tell us."[9] Consequently several pastoral groups with staff representation began meeting twice a month and continued for nine months.

There were immediate payoffs. By the end of 1959 the census was consistently thirty or above, the demand for outpatient services was stronger, and financial operations were above the break-even point. Prairie View had an atmosphere of renewal, despite the fact that an intense struggle was taking place behind closed doors.

Year of the Dialogue (1959)

Administrative implications of the redirection occurred in the Joint Conference Committee meeting. The committee had been enlarged to include the board executive committee members, H. J. Andres, Dan Kauffman, Ray Schlichting, and Arnold Isaac; two clinicians, Morrow and Vogt; and Ediger, the administrator. During the first months, this group struggled to define the issues. Two key issues were the "advantages and disadvantages of a full-time medical director and . . . dissatisfactions regarding finances."[10]

Considerable openness developed in the discussions. A board member noted that the current income for Adams, Newsom and Morrow (AN&M) would provide the salary for a full-time director. There were repeated discussions about Morrow becoming the medical director. Morrow sensed that something further might be wrong than his not spending full-time at Prairie View. He then asked, "What is wrong with me in the way I do things?" Board members spoke freely of having felt at times that they were being spoken to as patients in therapy instead of peers in an administrative meeting. Thereafter both Morrow and Vogt sought to deal with the board in a more direct and administrative manner.

This dialog helped the Prairie View representatives clarify their feelings about the AN&M relationship: insufficient responsibility for hospital finances by AN&M, too much feeling of "we" and "they," and too much profit going out of the operation. Board members also were able to sharpen up their sense of the contribution of the church to Prairie View.

After eight months of discussions, Morrow volunteered in a confessional spirit that he now understood the role of his Wichita group, "that decision-making rests other than here where the work is done. . . ; this makes for what you perceive as 'foreign' or 'outside.' " Shortly thereafter he indicated his long-term commitment was with his partners in Wichita, and the board accepted the finality of his decision to resign. [11]

Rebuilding the Program

As anticipated the leaving of most of the AN&M staff resulted in some pain and a greatly reduced patient load. In fact, the census at one point was down to nine patients.

By July of 1960, Prairie View had its first locally resident psychiatrist. Wilfred Gardner accepted the position of staff psychiatrist apparently in anticipation of being named medical director. When this did not happen, he resigned and Morrow again extended his time. Orlyn Zehr, social worker and former aide, was recruited as the first of the new professional team. After much searching, W. Mitchell Jones was secured as the new medical director. Later that year, Lucinda Martin returned as director of nursing; and William Wright, psychologist, was added to complete the new clinical team.

Thus Prairie View started the rebuilding venture with a new professional staff, a $13,000 deficit and some evident signs of anxiety. The year-long process of sorting out the relationship with the AN&M group had helped to bridge the separation with good feelings and built a trust that continued in the succeeding era. Mitchell Jones, who had come with good professional recommendations, was living in Newton with his family and was a member of the Baptist church. His leadership along with the rest of the newly hired professional staff gave Prairie View the feeling of "we" it had long sought.

By the end of 1962 Prairie View as a hospital seemed to be well on the way to recovery. While 1961 showed an average of 15.5 hospital patients, 1962 had 27.6, and 1963 had 32.9. The average length of stay had been cut from 100 to 50 days. The professional staff, now paid on a competitive basis, had been doubled in one year. The budget had increased by 50 percent. There was an active pursuit of Joint Commission accreditation. There was a part-time chaplain, who later became full-time. The Church of the Brethren was added as a church constituent group. The community-oriented direction was confirmed by the 1961 federal study and a new Kansas

A hospital patient from Oral Roberts University received a letter from some home friends addressed to "Prayer Review Hospital." His comment: "Prairie View was a good place to review my prayers!"

law. Prairie View even built a new activities building utilizing government surplus materials and volunteer labor. A new atmosphere of optimism and purposiveness was clearly evident.

Realizing the Community Mental Health Vision (1963-1973)

Although the hospital program continued to develop during this period, the community mental health emphasis moved to center stage. Its flowering was clearly dependent upon public funds becoming available from the counties beginning in 1963, the federal government in 1966, and the state in 1975.

Although statistics could graph the growth of this period, what cannot be charted is the change in staff who were "running scared to survive," as Mitchell Jones said, and now "having the time of their lives" creating new ways to realize their visions.

In 1961 Kansas passed a Community Mental Health Law allowing counties to set up their own clinics or to contract with an existing nonprofit agency. Between 1963 and 1967 Harvey, McPherson, and Marion counties each opted to contract with Prairie View for local mental health services. At the same time Prairie View was working with the state and federal offices to obtain a National Institute of Mental Health (NIMH) aftercare project grant providing services to state hospital patients discharged to the same three counties. This was approved for a five-year demonstration project, from 1964 to 1969. Prairie View's tri-county catchment area was official.

The concept of a private agency contracting with a unit of government to provide a public service was relatively new. The state Community Mental Health office and the regional NIMH office both gave strong encouragement for Prairie View to utilize its private base to provide public mental health services. For further input, Prairie View studies the greater Kansas City Mental Health Foundation model of contracting.

On the local level Prairie View could have contracted directly with the county in 1963, but chose instead to work with the county commissioners in creating a middleman corporation known as "Prairie View Community Mental Health Services, Incorporated." This was designed to get more citizen participation and to provide a vehicle to monitor the use of public monies in a private program. It was also hoped that it would serve to limit Prairie View's public liability. Later the middleman corporation was dissolved, Prairie View contracted directly with the county commissioners, and the citizen committees became advisory.

Becoming a "Comprehensive" Center

This movement toward a community approach, beginning as early as 1959, placed Prairie View at the cutting edge of the national community mental health movement. This leadership was recognized in 1964 when Prairie View was selected as one of eleven centers nationally to be featured in the book, *The Community Mental Health Center, An Analysis of Existing Models.*[12]

Prairie View was also in a good position in 1965 to be one of the earliest centers in the country to qualify for a federal construction grant because it had initiated a master building plan as early as 1962. However, the process of qualifying for a grant under the federal principles of community mental health was a challenge to Prairie View as a private agency. For example, the law required each mental health center to have a "catchment area" of responsibility; the principle of "accessibility" required efforts to reduce the financial, geographical, and psychological barriers; and the principle of "continuity of care" implied a public responsibility to follow the patient through various services and agencies to assure that proper treatment was received by the client. Fortunately, mental health centers were given considerable flexibility as to how to implement these principles, and over the years Prairie View was able to meet the federal expectations without unduly compromising its private stance.

The NIMH aftercare project, carried on from 1964 to 1969 as a demonstration for other communities, proved to be an excellent learning experience. Prairie View had to learn how to respond to a multitude of needs with very limited public money, which meant "achieving more with less." An emerging key concept, "the minimum effective dosage," guided Prairie View's development of clinical services. The phrase, borrowed from the medical model and Jack Wilder of New York in particular, was used to find ways of dealing with the patient's needs with the least possible professional time and cost, while still doing an effective job. Routine telephone contacts with the chronically ill patients could be utilized as a way of avoiding a relapse, and home visits could be used to deal with crises, making more costly hospitalization unnecessary. Later, when the day hospital treatment program was overcrowded, an analysis revealed that many of the patients under the "minimum effective dosage" principles could be reasonably served in a less expensive day program known as "caring places."

A decreasing reliance on state hospitals was implicit in the federal community mental health mandate, and Prairie View's history demonstrates the validity of this assumption. Studies conducted by George Dyck, the current medical director, indicate that in 1960 Prairie View had ten admissions to the State Hospital per 10,000 population. By 1972 this had been reduced to 6.7 and by 1980 to 3.6, in contrast to 6.4 for the rest of the Topeka State Hospital catchment area. The analysis above also indicated that the gains achieved by the aftercare project up to 1969 were successfully continued by the ongoing comprehensive mental health program under the successive directors—George Dyck, Orlyn Zehr, and Frances Campbell.

Making the Whole Community Therapeutic— Prevention and Growth

Prevention gradually became an integral part of the Prairie View program. In its early days, Prairie View Hospital had learned the educational value of bringing people to the hospital grounds for other than treatment purposes, with a goal of changing their attitudes toward mental illness and its treatment. This has continued throughout the history of Prairie View. In 1971, for example, there were sixty-five educational group visits involving almost a thousand people.

Mental health education became a particular challenge to Prairie View. The experience of the therapeutic community in the hospital became the model in finding an equivalent experience in the community. Prairie View applied the "laboratory training" method of the National Training Laboratory to special workshops focused on community problem solving, the improvement of marriage relationships, effective parenting, dealing with interracial conflicts, industrial issues, and other situations. The program grew, and by 1970 four to six thousand people were involved each year in a variety of "growth" or mental health education events focused largely around everyday roles in life.

Beginning in 1966, Merrill Raber devoted most of his time to community mental health education and consultation. He was followed by Wilma Toews, Glendale Norris, Jane Hershberger, and Larry Friesen. Neighborhood Family Life Advisory Committees were developed throughout the three counties to help assess needs and interests, and to help initiate educational activity in each area. In 1981 Prairie View's experience in "Developing a Mental Health

Education Program" was described in a national publication, *New Directions*.[13]

Prairie View's efforts for prevention of illness and for personal growth with tri-county organizations was designed on a "collaborative consultation" model. It focused on a series of leadership groups including the Human Service Agency Resource Council, Industrial Personnel Directors Council, Child Advocacy Committee, and meetings of student deans of colleges, church district pastors, and others.[14]

One such collaborative group, functioning in 1968 to 1974 under Merrill Raber's leadership was LINC (Leadership, Inc.). Just prior to its formation many of the Newton leaders had become discouraged by defeats of library and school bond elections and other progressive efforts to improve community life. During a period of six years, about four hundred leaders from a cross section of Harvey County participated in LINC-sponsored "Community Labs." As a result, a new climate gradually emerged in the community. A wide range of persons learned how to collaborate across their usual acquaintance circles to tackle community problems, and concrete success emerged in the form of new library and high school buildings.

With the coming of Robert Carlson as full-time chaplain in 1966, a Church and Human Relations Committee representing clergy and lay persons of various denominations was appointed, and programs were arranged to help meet both lay and pastoral needs. A wide range of services were generated to help churches in deacon training, volunteer visitation, children's work, and pastor-church relations. The Hesston Foundation has given consistent support to this program through five to ten thousand dollar grants in the past fifteen years.

...The spiritual dimension of our entire program is something that continues to be appreciated by consumers and those who represent collaborating agencies and referral sources... It is important that an agency like Prairie View not take these values for granted but seek to strengthen people in their quest for inner peace and spiritual courage.

—Robert Carlson[15]

More recently, by 1976, Prairie View's special interest in undergirding the work of churches was also expressed in procuring a second full-time chaplain to serve as a staff clergyman for the community. As a result, a community "courthouse chaplaincy" has been developed utilizing the volunteer efforts of ministers in the community. Groups providing special support to persons facing terminal illness and other crisis experiences have also been developed cooperatively with community church leaders.

In 1968 Prairie View was awarded the Gold Award by the American Psychiatric Association in recognition of its achievement in community mental health. The award was based on a combination of factors: staff had been selected carefully for professional competence; the church heritage of the center and many of its staff provided a built-in idealism; the hospital organization provided a stable base from which to launch the community program; attention was given to philosophy and goals; public funds became available; the consistent use of an outside consultant made possible some essential adjustments.

The Internal Organization Process

Although there were no major crises between 1963 and 1973, a number of disrupting situations occurred. Some staff were openly resistive to the laboratory training activity within the center. Introduction of an executive council between the top administration and the staff in 1968 was seen as a serious loss of influence by the professionals. College-age young people brought some of the campus ferment into Prairie View in the late sixties. There was a restlessness and a lack of ownership among professional staff who had been at Prairie View for five years or more. The resignation of Mitchell Jones as medical director brought new waves of insecurity.

The goal of the center at this point is to bring together the Christian vision of a caring community, the experience of mental health professionals, and the involvement of a responsible consumer community to create the dynamics needed for creative and effective delivery of a service to human needs.
— 1970 Prairie View Goals Statement

In 1967 Prairie View secured the services of an outside consultant, Vladimir Dupré, a psychologist from the National Training Laboratories. Over a period of fifteen years Dupré helped the organization look at threatening problems and to set in motion corrective steps and healing processes. Dupré came monthly at first and continues to come twice a year at present.

By 1965 Prairie View felt comfortable about its role as a community mental health center but wanted to assess how this role meshed with its total mission. Thus in May of 1965, a one-day "Workshop on Goals" was set up to face two questions: Should we have a long-range objective of turning Prairie View over to the community?, and if not, What is our vision for developing the potential of our church-psychiatry program? The board, administrative and professional staff participants came to a clear consensus of a "continued church sponsorship." They like the idealism, flexibility, and stability result-ing from church ownership. The psychiatric work could best be provided in the context of a Christian presence of faith, hope, and love.

Although the hospital continued to operate at capacity under the medical leadership of Mitchell Jones and later Vernon Yoder, the administrative energies were primarily focused on developing the community mental health potential. Both the hospital and commu-nity mental health programs had reached a point of maturity, and Prairie View seemed ready for new horizons in its development.

Accent on the Private Base (1974-1981)

During the first fifteen years, 1955 to 1970, Prairie View had a particularly strong growth rate despite a rather slow beginning. Total admissions had an annual increase of 20 percent per year. Though slower, the last ten years, 1971 to 1981, continued to have an annual increase rate of 8 percent. The increase of staff followed a similar percentage.

A variety of new efforts was introduced following 1974: a private education and consultation effort and a fund-raising office, a better management system, and renewed attention to staff selection and development. These efforts served to strengthen Prairie View's broader, private base.

Leadership

One of the keys to Prairie View's development has been its ability to accept leadership "from wherever it is" instead of follow-ing the traditional medical or other models. The top executive has deliberately been a nonmedical person who is first of all a churchman-manager. Over the years, Prairie View has been able to tap leadership with high potential and provide rewarding, creative experiences to a wide variety of persons. While there has been respect for the various disciplines, there has been an even stronger respect for persons and their potential, probably an outgrowth of the religious values and heritage of the center.

Prairie View sought to strengthen the continuity of its staff through personal growth and other benefits. As a result the current staff has five key staff members who have served twenty to twenty-five years, thirteen who have served fifteen to twenty, and thirteen,

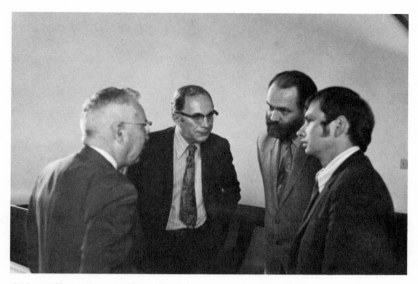

Orie Miller; Elmer Ediger, Prairie View executive director; Vernon Yoder, medical director; Larry Nikkel, administrator. Twenty-fifth anniversary commemoration of MMHS, October 1971.

ten to fifteen years. Even though some good staff persons have left Prairie View, an unusually high proportion have been retained to provide continuity and stability.

Prairie View could not have become a strong private organization without good management and business abilities. These qualities are rooted in the nature of the local board members and the expectations of the MMHS board. Since 1974, Prairie View has also evolved a clearer system of management through the assistance of a variety of consultants and training resources.

The Organization

Goal setting, including a major review of goals every five years, became an important part of the internal organizational process after the 1965 workshop experience. The 1970 process also included a major review meeting with other institutions of the church constituency. Although collaborative activities with the church institutions had increased considerably, the review revealed that the wage differential and some misgivings about psychiatry continued to be underlying obstacles in the relationship.

In a 1976 reorganization process under the leadership of Larry Nikkel, administrator, Prairie View was divided into three clearly delineated service delivery divisions and a corporate service divi-

Is Prairie View like an iceberg floating along subject largely to outside forces as to where it goes and how long it continues? Or is it more like a large ship which has difficulty in making any quick turns...but...is generally subject to change of direction and speed by humans at the controls?

—Elmer M. Ediger[16]

sion. This change made clear that the community mental health program and its dollars were a distinctive part of Prairie View, but not the whole. The Hospital Division and the Growth Associates Division were both private services to the larger geographical area, while the Community Services Division included all aspects of the contractual public service to the tri-county area.

Having experienced the value of stimulus grants from the federal government beginning in 1966, Prairie View launched its own ongoing financial development program in 1974. The purpose was to find private funds to enable a margin of financial flexibility for excellence and innovation of program. Since 1974, the development office has raised at least $100,000 a year for this purpose. In 1981 Prairie View appointed its first full-time director of development.

Emergence of Growth Associates

Established in 1971, the Growth Associates Division emphasizes personal and organizational growth for the nonpatient population. Under Merrill Raber's leadership, Growth Associates became a major part of Prairie View's private thrust covering most of Kansas and in some aspects serving nationally. Services are marketed to a variety of target groups on a full-cost basis.

The roots of Growth Associates lie in the earliest assumptions of helping to "make the whole community therapeutic." It evolved out of the tri-county consultation and education experience. The common denominator of its widely ranging activities is an emphasis on the interpersonal and emotional aspects. These are marketed, however, not as "mental health" but in the larger context of "growth" needs of individuals and organizaions.

In 1980 Growth Associates' activities included twenty-four educational events, often held on weekends, involving approximately eight hundred people in groups of ten to ninety. In other years there were as many as sixty events involving two thousand people. Subjects dealt with included Women in Management, Training and Counseling, Growth on the Job, Intensive Journal Methods, Biofeedoack, and Holistic Health.

Growth Associates provided organizational consultation in 1980 for approximately eighty organizations including five general hospitals, eleven mental health providers, nine state and federal agencies, five public schools, five colleges and universities, sixteen church organizations, and fourteen individuals. Growth Associates has also had a national role of training more than three hundred consultation and education directors of mental health centers across the country over a four-year period.

Luncheon seminars in Wichita, Hutchinson, McPherson, and Newton have become a popular medium of reaching key business and professional persons in larger numbers for a brief period of time. Likewise the Prairie View Forum, an annual series of three meetings "in search of values," has been held for the last twelve years.

After ten years the Growth Associates' total annual budget in 1981 was approximately $280,000. Although Growth Associates has made major strides toward being self-supporting, the center as a whole has provided annual subsidies to make this broader approach an ongoing part of the Prairie View mission.

Growth Associates has achieved national recognition for its program of primary prevention of mental illness and promotion of mental health. The Leadership, Inc., (LINC) program in the community was featured in the book *Primary Prevention*.[17] Growth Associates and Community Services were featured as one of six models in the recent book *Preventing Mental Illness, Efforts and Attitudes*.[18]

In the Wider Professional Community

The 1964 to 1969 NIMH aftercare project helped Prairie View assume a national demonstration role. Serving as hosts to national and foreign visitors, as many as eighty-five professional persons in 1976, provided another opportunity to share with the wider professional world. A number of professional leaders, brought together in 1979 in connection with Prairie View's twenty-fifth anniversary, called for a stronger emphasis on sharing experience through training and more collaboration with other organizations.

Training programs have gradually been on the increase but have rather consistently been secondary to the service objectives, because of financial considerations. The Clinical Pastoral Education (CPE) Program has been the most substantial training contribution of Prairie View. Beginning in 1968, this program has involved more than one hundred pastoral trainees to date. Training affiliations currently also include medical students in psychiatric clerkships, nurses, and social workers.

Prairie View staff "special leave time" has enabled an international dimension through the Kansas-Paraguay Partners program. Julie Neufeld was the first of the Prairie View staff to spend a three-month period in Paraguay in 1969. Others who have served in Paraguay are Merrill Raber, Harold Converse, George Dyck, and Elmer Ediger. As a counterpart to the above, approximately twelve mental health persons from Paraguay have spent time at Prairie View ranging from two weeks to eighteen months.

Conclusion

Some years ago Herbert Yahraes of the National Institute of Mental Health devoted a chapter to Prairie View in a publication *The Mental Health of Rural America*. He closed the chapter by quoting from a report of Elmer Ediger:

> Our program is focused on meeting human needs in the best way we can. Our staff members are selected inasmuch as possible for their skill, their character, and general sense of kinship with the church. Our language is largely that of mental health professionals and the people we serve. We are emersed in trying to use our total selves to help people. Though we do not say it often, I believe ours is a remarkably appropriate church-sponsored effort to love, to represent faith in life, in God, and to undergird virtues we believe God wants in society.[19]

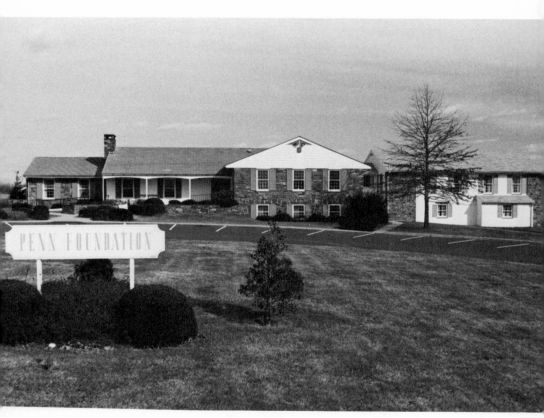

The Penn Foundation for Mental Health, Inc.

CHAPTER 7

Penn Foundation
Sellersville, Pennsylvania
Charles H. Hoeflich*

Basic Formulations

It was one of those chilly evenings which come with late winter or early spring. Four men, each solid, conservative, and in their early middle years, sat in the living room of an eighteenth- century farmhouse typical of the Upper Bucks County area of Pennsylvania. The year was 1955. The man who had suggested they meet—Dr. Michael Peters, medical chief of nearby Grand View Hospital—was not present. Each of them had been told by "Pete" to put their heads together and see what they could do about creating a psychiatric service to meet an ever-increasing need in the area his general hospital covered.

Those who sat there that evening, however, were not without something in common. Each was well known to the others, so that they could be considered friends; each had a similar religious background and commitment; each had been briefed in different ways by Dr. Peters; each had some experience or had seen the results produced by sound psychiatric treatment; and each represented a different discipline in which he had demonstrated organizational skills.

Despite the common ground, they looked at one another as they drank the coffee always present when two or more Pennsylvania Dutchmen get together and said, "Well, what are we supposed to do?" As each related what Dr. Peters said to him, a picture began to emerge, and it wasn't before the second cup was poured that the challenge of a pioneering effort was evident.

Obviously the first and most important thing was to put together a larger group. Four men used to the world of business "out there" needed the company of others with like qualifications and

*Charles H. Hoeflich is a charter member and past president of the Penn Foundation board of trustees.

145

interest and commitment. Fortunately each knew a name or two of persons who could be counted on to bring an added dimension to the possible effort and who would be equally dedicated if the project were ever to get off the ground

That was enough for one evening. Over the last of the coffee and cookies some other elements were mentioned, such as the possible availability of Dr. Norman L. Loux, a native son then serving as assistant superintendent of the prestigious Butler Hospital in Rhode Island. Also, dear to the heart of every innovator, there lurked in the background the promise of seed money to help launch a fledging community mental health clinic. Five thousand dollars — if!

From here on Providence took a hand, as has been the case to this day. Each man approached to be a possible director, providing this "mental health thing" made sense, accepted an invitation to help explore the idea. Dr. Loux appeared with a paper outlining the needs, the problems, the pioneering solutions. His truly visionary approach to the field of mental health captured the hearts and minds of all. A group of four people made it known that they had a house available for use for nearly a year in the center of Souderton, Pennsylvania.

The stimulation of Norman Loux's challenging proposal and requirements energized the expanded group, so that each of the frequent meetings which took place over the summer months saw new ideas put forth to implement the answer to the original question, What are we supposed to do now? A new query had surfaced: How fast can we move?

Basic to everything that happened was the formulation of policy:

(1) Close cooperation with the general hospital, yet corporate and physical separateness, was seen as an imperative if the facility were to be single-minded in its effort.

(2) Close communication with the medical staff, the nurses, and the administrators of the general hospital as to what the mental health group was undertaking and the meshing of its product into the needs of the practitioners.

(3) A strong public relations program informing the catchment area of the existence of the facility as a medical specialty. Basic to the program was the determination to remove any stigma which might mistakenly be in the minds of those needing help — that emotional illness was anything different from a cataract or a broken leg when it came to treatment.

(4) Definition of the service area.

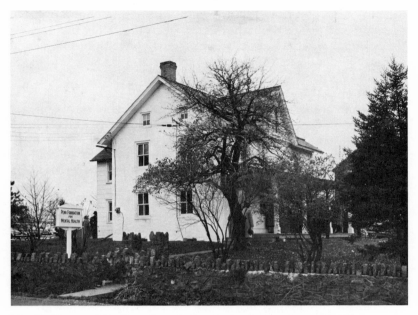

The first home of the Penn Foundation in Souderton, Pennsylvania.

(5) Criteria for qualities to be sought in board members in the future.

(6) Standards and practices to be required of professionals; i.e., they would be full-time employees and would not practice privately.

(7) Mental help in its highest and best form would be available to all regardless of ability to pay. A standard fee for service would be charged to all, but need would be met first.

(8) This would, in essence, be a mission endeavor, extending the hand of Christ and love.

A nonprofit structure was needed—but first what would be its name? Fortunately, the board included a splendid attorney who would form the corporation and steer it to its nonprofit status. But the meeting to select a name for what was, by now, everyone's favorite child was destined to go down in the books as one of the longest ever held. Apparently it was worth it all, for what was worked out that night in the proffered house in Souderton has never changed but has become favorably known in psychiatric circles both here and in other countries—*Penn Foundation for Mental Health.*

By now Dr. Loux had accepted the invitation of the group and the medical doctors to form a community mental health clinic, bringing with him from Rhode Island, Ruby Horwood, a research assistant with a wide reputation in this discipline. Horwood became the Foundation's first administrator and is now a trustee. The first formal board meeting was held on October 24, 1955.

Dedication

A more energetic or involved group of men Horwood had seldom seen. Determined to have a first-class facility, they begged and borrowed and hauled furniture and equipment. Their wives scrubbed and polished until the house, destined to serve Penn Foundation for its first breath-holding year, presented a facade it had probably not seen for a generation.

Meeting frequently during these early sensitive months to review details of operation and needs, the board of trustees soon discovered the need for more space. Various options were examined as to scope of treatment. Should an expanded facility be self-contained with the necessary rooms and equipment for overnight or extended care—or should the concept of outpatient care with the patient's family and loved ones involved continue?

Again Providence intervened. A splendid fifteen-acre tract

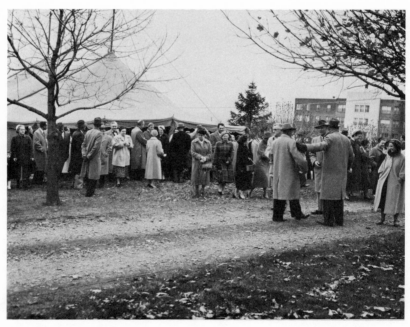

Groundbreaking ceremony at the present site of the Penn Foundation in Sellersville, Pennsylvania.

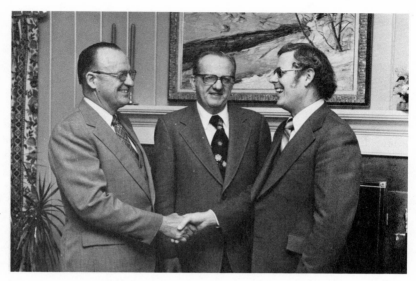

Harold M. Mininger, chairman of the board; Norman L. Loux, past medical director; Vernon H. Kratz, current medical director.

became available directly across from Grand View Hospital in Sellersville. It had a farmhouse and outbuildings which could be adapted—all that was needed was money. One of the trustees advanced the security deposit and the rest went to work soliciting.

By now the public relations program had made the name and the effort relatively well known, so that when the trustees started making their personal calls on interested people and business firms in the area, they aroused interest. If they did not, then their real enthusiasm usually produced results. At least enough money was raised to go to settlement and pay for the property—with about twelve hours to spare.

The next months were hectic. Treatment of the emotionally ill was given top priority, of course. A psychiatric social worker was added to the staff. Dr. Loux kept a full schedule, in addition to speaking to service clubs, professional groups, schools, and church groups. And always in the background encouraging everyone, were the medical doctors who comprised the original stimulus for what was taking place.

The farmhouse was renovated—more scrubbing and painting. By now an active Ladies Auxiliary had been formed which met monthly and provided many needed extra services. It was to become the nucleus of what would eventually be a highly organized and efficient operation, including volunteer work with patients, fund raising, interior decorating, catering, and a host of other activities needed to make a large organization function.

On November 11, 1956, a cold day with the sun occasionally breaking through a gray overcast, the permanent site of Penn Foundation was dedicated in a lawn tent overflowing with well-wishers and supporters. Dr. Kenneth Appel, chairman of the Department of Psychiatry, at the University of Pennsylvania Medical School, was the principal speaker. He struck just the right note of concern as he held forth the deep inner longing each person has for help as he or she passes through the turbulent emotional crises almost everyone faces at one time or another. It was a crossroads day, and the Foundation knew it was truly moving forward.

If it had been work before, it was constant effort in earnest now. An enlarged staff, plans for a new building above the farmhouse to embrace the developing techniques, fund raising by approaches to foundations and government agencies so that the needs of all would be met with first-class service, availability for round-the-clock emergency calls, new areas of counseling, and an ever-expanding case load continued to spur everyone on.

During this period especially important was the vital support of stalwarts in the mental health arena, Drs. Lauren Smith, Daniel Blain, Edward Auer, Francis Braceland, Howard Rome, Robert Felix and Kenneth Appel, to name but a few of the many prominent psychiatrists whose steady interest and ongoing advice served as foundation stones on which the sound structure was formed.

Struggle Over Federal Funding

As plans for the new building were developed, it was decided to apply for a federal grant from Hill-Burton funds to ease the burden of cost. The grant had already been approved guaranteeing one-third of the needed money, when suddenly it was discovered by the bureau administering the grant that the Foundation did not qualify because it was an entirely outpatient operation formed around a day treatment center—then a relatively new concept.

Another crossroad had been reached and another heady decision must be made. The Foundation had developed a program involving outpatient care with family, employer, and community involvement. Bulwarked by group therapy, day treatment, marital counseling, and other methods of treatment, the program was showing positive, measurable results. Should the Foundation surrender this concept and become a twenty-bed mental hospital or give up the money which was unquestionably important in the scheme of things at the time?

The answer took a special meeting and deep discussion.

Choosing a name had been child's play compared to this, for the entire future of Penn Foundation could be at stake. There was an added option—the Foundation could keep the grant if it would become an integral part of the general hospital. But its unique identity and reputation, which by now had been recognized through being the recipient of the Benjamin Rush Award, several cash awards and numerous feature articles in magazines and professional journals, would all be lost.

After an all-morning session the decision was to scrap the plans, graciously decline the government funds and start all over. The community's needs—not bureaucratic standards—must be the criteria for action.

Fortunately, the new plans were more acceptable to the staff and others involved. The ultimate cost was only 60 percent of the net estimate after Hill-Burton funds would have been applied and that included landscaping, furnishings and some emotion-warming extras.

The new building was an immediate success. The dedication was held on a day as hot as the earlier was cold. No tent was needed this time as Bishop Richard Detweiler brought a message which tied the spirit and the emotion together in a way which reflected the group's original missionary concern for people and touched the heart strings of the huge crowd which had gathered for the big step being taken.

Underlining the appropriateness of the decision to forego government funds and an inpatient hospital, a substantial grant was awarded from the Joseph R. Grundy Foundation for the purpose of establishing a pavilion of twelve beds at the Foundation's old friend, Grand View Hospital, across the road. Having long worked with their nurses and doctors as chief of psychiatry, Dr. Loux helped to establish a close working relationship between the two institutions. Therefore, such an arrangement was easily accomplished.

With this new development, as a result of a study made by the Joint Information Service of the American Psychiatric Association and the National Institute for Mental Health, a grant was awarded to the Foundation to set up a three-year "demonstration project" starting in 1967.

An early policy decision had been to confine mental health service to a catchment area of about 10½ mile radius, the thought behind the policy being that one cannot serve everywhere without the quality of treatment ultimately suffering. "If we are successful in our concept and in what we seek to do, then others will visit us and we will share with them," had been the verbalization of the reasoning. And that is exactly what happened. Mental health clinics and community leaders came from this hemisphere and from Europe to find what made this community clinic in a quasi-rural atmosphere enjoy the support of people, organizations, doctors, churches, law enforcement agencies, schools, and local governments.

The work load of handling these groups and the time necessary to share in the way the Foundation was committed to share became burdensome. The grant was to be used to relieve the burden. Ruby Horwood, who had left as administrator to return to library and research work at the Eastern Pennsylvania Psychiatric Institute in Philadelphia agreed to return on a part-time basis for the three years of the grant. During that time one of the goals of the founders was realized and a true sharing of Penn Foundation's commitment to the use of mental health as an appropriate testimony was realized.

Expansion

By 1968 more space was needed. The building dedicated by Bishop Detweiler in 1962 and which seemed vast after the Souderton house and the farmhouse, was already cramped. And there were new fields to be covered. Penn Foundation found itself needing accommodations for services to children, drug and alcohol therapy, wider occupational and recreational care, and more seminars for professionals including ministers, teachers, and law enforcement personnel, and doctors. A series of seminars for professionals, underwritten by a local drug company, and bringing a list of distinguished names in the mental health field to Sellersville, had proved popular as well as valuable.

So once more the board of trustees decided to expand. The result was a multipurpose room—the Grundy Auditorium—a wing of classrooms and offices for the ever-expanding staff, and a specially designed swimming pool donated by a dedicated constituent. The year 1969 was a busy one.

About two-thirds of the way through the decade of the '70s it became obvious that more expansion would again be required. Staff offices, meeting rooms with appropriate visual aids, and group therapy rooms were required. Plans were made, and the work undertaken. The new wing—financed through local contributions stimulated by a grant from the Pew Memorial Trust was dedicated in the fall of 1978.

During the '70s a change took place in the way mental health was handled at the county and state level. Counties dropped the system whereby they provided help to those unable to afford it through an annual grant to assist in the overhead cost. Now they took a new approach whereby the community mental health clinic

Consider...

A contribution to encourage training in mental health.

Mennonite Mental Health Scholarships help Christians train for services to the mentally ill and the developmentally disabled.

Mental illness visits persons in our acquaintance. All of us know families who have a developmentally disabled member. We want these persons to receive excellent care and service in the name of Christ.

The mental health needs in our communities and in the cities of our land call for creative forms of service and treatment.

You can enlarge the vision and ministry. Make a gift to the Fund for Mennonite Mental Health Scholarships. The interest earnings will begin working for students immediately, while the principal will remain invested to provide earnings for future students. Send your gift ($1,000; $500; $100; other amount) to Mennonite Mental Health Services, Scholarship Fund, 21 South 12th St., Akron, PA 17501.

would be compensated on a "fee-for-service" basis. Needless to say, the "fee" far from covered the cost of providing the service and a new choice faced Penn Foundation.

The Foundation believed implicitly in the philosophy of the "sound mind in the sound body" for as many people as possible in the catchment area, thereby raising the level of total happiness, health, and outlook of an entire community. So the change in government fundings presented a new challenge. The most obvious choice would be to devise two levels of service: one to be extended to those with the means to pay the bills for their treatment, the other to be extended to those on the county "fee-for-service" program but on a level below that which had brought attention for its quality to the Sellersville clinic. Another choice would be to continue the high level of quality but only serve those who could afford it. This would, of course, involve raising fees to an undesirable level since costs would continue at the same time income from the counties served would disappear.

Again there were long meetings and the purposes and goals of Penn Foundation from its start in 1955 were reviewed. But finally, the answer was clear. Commitment cannot be diluted nor can dedication disappear. Only one quality of mental health service would be offered—the best. It would be available to all persons in the catchment area who needed it regardless of their status or ability to pay. New methods of internal administration would be required,

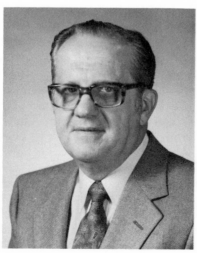

Norman L. Loux, medical director 1955-80.

productivity standards must be set, greater fund-raising efforts must be made, and new arrangements for services formerly rendered to institutions on a less than profitable basis must be undertaken. But there must be no sacrifice in the quality of service, in the expansion into new fields, or in the ready availability of the professional help Penn Foundation had to offer.

Transition in Leadership

These were lofty ideals but how, in the face of greater demand, lost income, and deep deficits could they be attained? Again faithfulness to God's direction and will carried with it solutions which were not foreseen. This time the solution came with a new administrator whose home background was from the Foudation's area, whose convictions and commitment were identical with those of the staff and board, and whose training and experience had already made their mark in the field of emotional illness. Well-located and hardly looking for a new situation, Henry D. Landes saw the challenge as well as the missionary zeal of the group with which he would work and responded enthusiastically.

Norman Loux had for several years been wanting to reduce his case load and his overall responsibility as medical director and devote his time to action in mental health areas in which he had a special interest and to which he felt called. Hardly anticipating the wider direction the Foundation would ultimately take, Vernon H. Kratz, M.D. joined the staff as a psychiatrist in 1973. A gifted man who had served in the mission field, he soon emerged as a creative leader. Indefatigable as a worker, he was the obvious successor to Dr. Loux who has been named *Senior Psychiatrist* after twenty-five years of service. Together with Henry D. Landes, the administrator, a team emerged which assures the brightness of the future for Penn Foundation for mental health.

During the year of transition significant new steps were undertaken for the purpose of increasing the impact of the Foundation. A branch facility was established in nearby Quakertown. Located about seven miles from Sellersville, it is an active community with a general hospital. Although it operated part-time at first, it was anticipated full-time service would soon be required.

Five new task forces devoting their efforts to specific areas of activity were created. Meeting regularly with professionals in each field, they provide an extension of the Foundation's work in a sensitive way which has aroused much interest throughout the total community. These task forces embrace such fields as *business and industry*, which offers workshops for area employers to instruct them in the best methods of identifying and referring troubled employees for professional help as well as being aware of the mental health needs of the executive family; *church and pastor*, with responsibility for the development of a comprehensive pastoral services program; *Continuing Care*, which has developed a community residential program for those with such needs; *Children and Youth* identifying with professionals in the child-caring field, creating and sponsoring conferences for such persons; and an *Older Adult* task force for the development of new programs in gerontology.

Coincidentally, at the time Dr. Loux assumed his new role of senior psychiatrist and Dr. Kratz became the Foundation's medical director, the board of trustees created a new effort known as the *Norman L. Loux Fund* for research and development. Funded with substantial gifts from anonymous donors, it was designed to award monies each year to an element in the mental health field which, in the opinion of an appointed jury, needed funds for further research. The initial award for 1981 went to the work for older adults — something in which Dr. Loux himself had a keen interest.

A final word regarding the board of trustees would seem in order since this chapter began with them. All members who formed the original group still serve on the board with the exception of two who have died, one who retired but continues a lively interest, and one who withdrew for personal reasons which ultimately took him out of the area. He too not only has maintained his interest but has a close contact through his son-in-law who is the administrator. Attendance at meetings usually sees a full roll call of these men and women, plus others who have joined the board through the years. The criteria for invitation to serve remains the same: commitment, dedication, and a deep conviction that a sound mental health program, properly administered, is a testimony of servanthood.

Penn Foundation: Twenty-Five Years in Retrospect
Norman L. Loux, M.D.*

When I left for my psychiatric residency in Rhode Island, there was the assumption on the part of the medical staff at Grand View Hospital that I would come back. That was not necessarily my assumption. There were a lot of other opportunities that I had that were very tempting. But Dr. Michael Peters is a leader, and he's a persistent leader, and he doesn't give up easily. Every time we would come home he would invite us to dinner and we would talk about my coming back. Frankly, he made me feel disloyal if I wouldn't have come back. I remember one time in 1954 when we came back to visit, my dad said, "I don't know what's happening. There are dozens of phone calls coming in for you." Dr. Peters had talked with others and asked them to call me and tell me they were expecting me to come back.

A New Concept

When the staff of Grand View Hospital approached me about coming back, I made it very clear to them that I didn't want to come back unless there could be an organization set up, where the organization could take the responsibility for developing a psychiatric program for the whole community, that would include case finding, that would include some preventive aspects, and that would be very much a part of the total medicine of the community.

I remember thinking very clearly that if a person with acute appendicitis came into the emergency room, there would be no question at all what would happen. That person would be admitted to the hospital. But if a person with an acute schizophrenic illness came to the emergency room, there was a much different attitude. That person would be shipped out of the community. And I couldn't

*Norman L. Loux, M.D., served as medical director of the Penn Foundation during its first twenty-five years, 1965-80. These comments were recorded on September 2, 1981, and are slightly edited, with captions added.

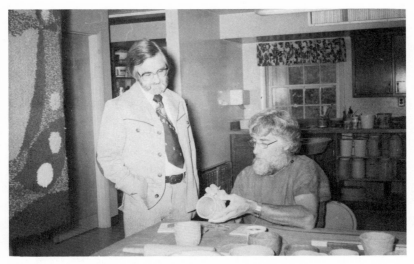

Lamont A. Woelk, Pastoral Services Director and Arthur Isaak, Recreational/Activity Therapist.

understand why that should be. I felt that here was an opportunity to bring psychiatry to the level of other branches of medicine and I felt that our community was receptive to this.

I wanted to be a part of the medical staff but I also saw that I would have to be different than the other physicians on the staff because they were in private practice exclusively. I didn't want to go into private practice because I immediately saw that that would narrow my influence because I would become only one person seeing a group of patients. There were a number of other needs I conceived as being the more important ones.

Planning a New Program

When I first came I had hoped that I would be able to spend a month or two just making some kinds of investigations, making a survey and writing a report to present to the board that was in the process of organizing at that time, which indeed I did. But at the same time that I was doing that, I was besieged with patients to be seen. I was seeing them in other physicians' offices when they weren't using their offices—surgeons, internists, family practitioners. I don't think that hurt either. And then a couple of the board members discovered that there was a house in Souderton that was going to be torn down for a parking lot, and they managed to get that for a year until we found something closer to the hospital.

The board was very troubled, I could see this. They said, "Well, Norman, what you're talking about is something that we really have never heard of before. We're thinking of a hospital that has beds, that's isolated from the community a little bit, where people can go to rest and where the community can rest from them, where they get good custodial care at the same time that they're getting treatment. Now what you're saying is that it has to be part of what goes on in a general hospital. That means that the facility would have to be close to a general hospital and there's no land available."

One of the leading surgeons in the community, Dr. Charles Wynn, said, "Well, I have an option on a farm right across the street. I hear that your board's looking for land and if they want to buy that, and if they give me a verbal agreement that they'll sell me enough that I can build a medical arts building on one part of it, why I'll release my option." That's how we got fifteen acres of prime land right across the street from the general hospital.

When we dedicated that farmhouse right across from the hospital, it was announced in the papers, but there was no great splash made. I remember we had Dr. Kenneth Appel and his wife and Dr. Lauren Smith for dinner that day. And it came to be about a half an hour before the program started. We could hardly get there, there was such a big crowd. That was a tremendous encouragement.

We were committed to having a day treatment program. And there were a lot of struggles, believe me. It's not easy to start new programs of that kind. There's an attitude that still prevails to some extent: If patients are well enough to be home at night, if they're well enough to do the things that they do in day treatment, they really don't need care. It takes constant selling.

Government Funds

There was a system whereby the Department of Mental Health of Pennsylvania would give grants-in-aid to community clinics for outpatient services. The regional director said to me, "I think you'd be eligible to get some of this money." We did then get a grant and we established quite a warm relationship with the Department of Mental Health.

I think also we have to remember that we hit a time when community mental health was popular, or the concept at least was popular. People were talking about providing services within the community and not sending people out of the community for mental health problems. And we rode the crest of that wave. Now, I have to say, and I say it as humbly as I can, that I think we were able to sustain it a bit better than some of the other centers that were federally or state supported to a greater extent, and I think that was because the people of the community had more invested in it.

One of the things I would almost have to say is that there was a kind of seduction in terms of getting government money for clinical programs. It seemed to me that we went though a period where we became a little more dependent that we should have been on government money.

Then they approached us about federal Hill-Burton funds which were used to build facilities for general hospitals. They were all bed related. But they thought that there would be a way to work this out since we were so closely connected with a general hospital. We would be eligible to get some money to help build our new building. I remember the man who was in charge of Hill-Burton funds in Harrisburg, Ira Mills, who was originally from this community and known to some of our board. It progressed very smoothly, we were promised a sum of money, and it was just a matter of working out the final details when I got a harried phone call one day from the office of mental health, saying, "My goodness, we really weren't aware of this until the federal people came, but we can't give you any money unless there are beds in your own facility."

So we respectfully declined. We felt that if our philosophy of not having beds and reduplicating facilities was correct, then it wouldn't be right to put beds in just to get that money.

Mental Retardation Challenge

One of the struggles that came along was to give more attention to the retarded program. There was a man with considerable wealth who had a retarded son, and he said, "I will give you X number of dollars as seed money to get some things started for a facility for profoundly retarded people." The board struggled with that a great deal and then decided that, while it was tempting to take that rather large sum of money, it would be much better if a separate organization were formed that could give its full attention to that need. They agreed to hold the money in escrow until what is now the Community Foundation was organized and developed. This is now a full-fledged mental retardation program which is a spin-off from us. Really, if we would have been selfish, we would have tried to do that ourselves.

Consultation and education became a real struggle. It's been a great disappointment of mine that when we went on a fee-for-service basis with the state, there was no more money to do that. You see, we had to account for our hours in terms of income. But many of us did this on our own time. I'm happy to say that we're enlarging education and consultation again.

New Frontiers

There are a lot of unplowed fields, you know.

This whole matter of the chronic care patient—we have a tremendous opportunity here because, you see, the population isn't that large that it's totally unmanageable. We have a much more supportive attitude in the community than you do in urban areas, because it's somebody's neighbor, it's somebody's brother, it's somebody's sister, it's somebody's employee.

I've been just thrilled with the way that industry has invited us to help shape their attitudes toward people with mental health problems. They're not at all unreceptive, and I'd have to say that many times industry goes farther along with concessions and helpfulness than one could reasonably expect them to do.

I think we have to pitch in and help industry. They're eager for it. We have to help the policemen, the police departments. The courts have been very sympathetic. They have just gone overboard, almost, in working with us in terms of rehabilitating people. That's a whole area that we really have not exploited the way we should.

It's also been a great inspiration to me to see how the churches have been a part of this. When there's a common goal and a common interest, it's easier to work together. It's probably easier to work with nontheologic issues than it is with theologic issues. We have never felt that the ministers have interfered, they've been helpful, they've been respectful. They've respected us and I think we've respected them. But I think we may not have given them as much feedback as we should. That's something we have to develop.

There are a lot of unplowed fields. We don't have to plow too many of them over. A lot of them haven't been plowed at all.

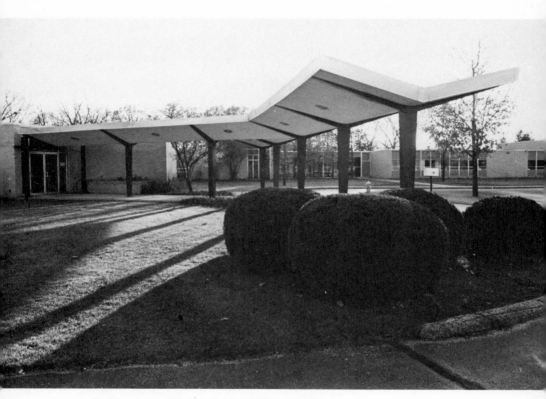

Oaklawn Psychiatric Center, Elkhart, Indiana.

CHAPTER 8

Oaklawn
Elkhart, Indiana
Terri Enns*

Tucked back among a grove of oak trees in a quiet section of
Elkhart, Indiana, is the unobtrusive main building of a church-
sponsored, community-supported mental health center designed to
meet the unique needs of the community surrounding it. Conceived
in the mid-1950's, Oaklawn Psychiatric Center, the fourth of the
institutions sponsored by the Mennonite Central Committee (MCC),
began in 1963 as a day hospital and outpatient clinic, serving the
churches and the local community. The story of the growth of the
Oaklawn Center chronicles movement from one vision to many
realities, and continues to unfold even as it is being told.

The Vision Develops (1954-63)

Early Studies and Plans

The idea for the Oaklawn Psychiatric Center, though initially
vague and undefined, was first expressed publically on April 3,
1954. On this date a group of forty-three representatives of the MCC
constituency from the four-state area of Ohio, Indiana, Illinios, and
Michigan met in Goshen, Indiana, and "generally agreed as to the
need and desirability of more Christian and professional care in the
field of mental health."[1] The meeting had been authorized and
planned by MCC as a result of the interest expressed by persons from
the Goshen-Elkhart area.[2] The representative group also agreed that
more careful study of the possibility was needed, and they asked
MCC to take the initiative, working through a study committee from
the local area.

During the next two years, MCC surveyed the constituent
churches of the area to determine what needs existed. First a study

*Terri Enns is a recent graduate of Goshen College.

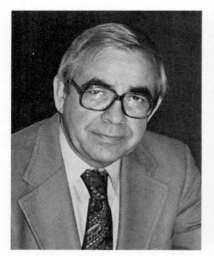
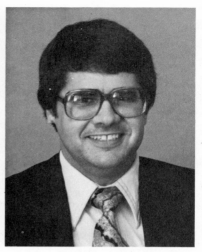

Robert W. Hartzler served as Oaklawn administrator from July 1962 to September 1978.   *Harold C. Loewen joined the Oaklawn staff in 1972, serving as administrator since 1978.*

committee, and then, after one year, an area advisory committee worked on ideas of how best to meet those needs. The East Central Area Advisory Committee, which functioned from 1956 to 1958, actively worked on questions of program and location. By the end of 1956 the committee was ready to recommend to MCC an eight-point program, which subsequently was approved early in 1957. Stated in broad terms, the program called for combining "the best of professional psychiatric service with Christian service motivation"; serving both the local community and the four-state church constituency; providing services to children, adults and the elderly; serving people indirectly through consultation services; cooperating with local medical resources; avoiding duplication of community resources; launching an educational program; and providing "complete diagnostic and treatment facilities" with an adequately trained staff in the various mental health related disciplines.[3]

Throughout most of 1957, D. Chauncey Kauffman,[4] an experienced hospital administrator, served as staff for the committee, although he functioned as an MCC staff member responsible to the Akron office of MCC. During this time Kauffman and committee members visited state officials in at least three of the four states, considered several Mennonite communities as possible locations for a mental health facility, and further refined program ideas. The eight points of the program plan were used as criteria to evaluate three of the most viable locations—Lima-Bluffton, Ohio; Fort Wayne-Leo, Indiana; and Elkhart-Goshen, Indiana. By October 1957, the committee was ready to accept the recommendation of a special site committee to explore "the medical, social welfare, and other resources of the Elkhart County area as a location for the program and facility of the East Central Area."[5]

An important reason for choosing Elkhart was its proximity to three Mennonite organizations: 1. Goshen College, with its nursing, social work, and teacher training curricula; 2. the developing Associated Mennonite Biblical Seminaries in Elkhart; and 3. the Mennonite Board of Missions and Charities, also located in Elkhart. Because of this potential of leadership and institutional relationships, and its central location, Elkhart seemed the optimal site for the fourth MCC mental health center.

The Oaklawn Board

In the reorganization of its mental health program in 1957, MCC delegated a greater responsibility to the local hospitals (see chapter 2). As part of this change in policy, MCC also appointed Oaklawn's first board of eight directors in 1958. Members were chosen from the MCC-related sponsoring churches, which included Mennonites, Amish, and Brethren in Christ. At an organizational meeting in April, this local board elected Robert W. Hartzler as chairman and E. P. Mininger as vice-chairman. These two persons were to play major roles in Oaklawn's history. The following year, Oaklawn was incorporated and the board increased to twelve members. The board was expanded again in 1961 to include a member from the Church of the Brethren after that group expressed interest in the project.

This board, "composed of Christian men determined that the Center's operation will be in line with the purposes of the church...,"[6] was concerned with how Christianity might serve the mental health field. Their goal was to benefit the churches by treating their ill, assisting ministers, exploring the relationship between psychiatry and religion, and offering services to church schools. This board planned to appoint a Mennonite administrator and a Christian staff who would implement Christian philosophies.

Mennonite Mental Health Services (MMHS), MCC's subsidiary, advisory and coordinating board, and the three other MCC-related centers also provided guidance during Oaklawn's early days. Oaklawn planned to offer care similar to the other centers, with approximately the same number of impatient beds and similar therapeutic methods. MMHS's influence connected the centers with philosophical and ideological guidance. As had the other centers, Oaklawn's board asked for financial support from the churches.

Even in choosing a name for the new center, the board followed the example of the other centers and based Oaklawn on its natural surroundings.

Church Support

Oaklawn depended on the church not only for direction and later for staff, but for solid support and money as well. A good amount of time and effort was devoted to visiting churches and informing them about the developing program.

> *Although I saw some patients, I also had to go around promoting Oaklawn. Bob [Hartzler] would say, "O.K., we're going somewhere," and we would get in the car and go give speeches. I mean we gave speeches anyplace.... When I got here he used me that way. Like he was showing off his clinician. I tell you, it's literally true, that I would get in the car and Bob would say, "I'll tell you on the way." There were times when I outlined my speech in my mind while I was being introduced. It used to drive me wild, but Bob kept observing that the best speeches were the ones I didn't prepare for.*
> —*Otto D. Klassen*[7]

Though publicity specifically emphasized that the churches would need to provide the funds to make the Oaklawn project possible, the board applied for a federal Hill-Burton grant which would supplement the church money by paying for up to one-third of construction costs. When that grant was approved, the Oaklawn board asked that one-third should come from the churches and the remainder from the community. The churches committed themselves to raising that money, especially when assured that the Hill-Burton money involved no stipulations that would limit the center in its Christian orientation. The Mennonite Church, which had three conferences in the four-state area, pledged nine dollars per member spread over the three-year construction period, and other conference sponsors promised similar amounts. The Church of the Brethren joined the sponsoring churches, although without a specific financial commitment.

Community Relations

Although initially conceived to serve primarily Mennonites, the center and its board nevertheless understood its mission to be the Elkhart community as well. The 1957 Eight-Point Program had clearly stated that the mental health facility was to serve both the four-state church constituency and the local community in which it was established. In 1959 the board requested MCC to add two non-

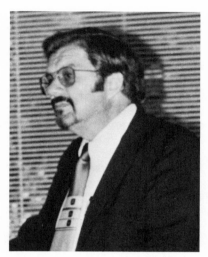

*Otto D. Klassen, was medical direc-
tor at Oaklawn until recently.*

constituent persons to the board, hopeful that they would increase
the board's sensitivity to the larger Elkhart community. This was a
strong indication of Oaklawn's increasing commitment to serve
both the church and the community. The board listened to its
community representatives for ways to relate to the Elkhart community, which had expressed receptivity to such a center. The board
gave priority to "the effort to establish, and gain acceptance of, the
place of the Oaklawn Center in the thinking of the Elkhart community."[8]

In an attempt to work with existing mental health facilities in
Elkhart, the board created an advisory committee of community
doctors and asked for approval from several key organizations in the
community. By early 1960, Hartzler reported that most community
organizations had welcomed and fully endorsed the development.
Area psychiatrists, as well as the Northern Indiana Psychiatric
Society, also endorsed the developing center. One notable exception, which was to have a major impact upon the developing program, was Elkhart General Hospital (EGH). Nevertheless, by 1962,
though there was some "uneasiness about what the Mennonites are
intending in Elkhart," Oaklawn reported to the churches that "all of
the community agencies concerned with Oaklawn are welcoming
the Oaklawn development...."[9]

Though the medical staff of EGH had endorsed the Oaklawn
project, the administration and some of the board members seemed

to have reservations. This stemmed from the fact the EGH had a ten-bed psychiatric ward which operated at less than 50 percent capacity, so obviously the prospect of a new mental health facility with beds appeared not only competitive but unnecessary as well.[10]

We agreed not to have beds because the hospital was protective. They wanted to be the hospital agency in the community.... Hospitals need to protect their turf. They were interested in that because they already had a psychiatric ward.

—Otto D. Klassen[11]

It fitted in well with the day hospital idea and freed us of the necessity to have 24-hour round-the-clock program. We shut down at 5 o'clock at night and didn't open up until morning. The poor guys over at the hospital had to be having nurses, cooks and janitors around there night and day, seven days a week. Boy, it certainly was fantastic. It was fortunate that it developed that way for Oaklawn.

—Robert W. Hartzler[12]

Oaklawn's application for a Hill-Burton grant was approved at the state level in December 1959, but on condition that the Oaklawn and EGH boards would agree "on the nature of the development to take place at Elkhart." Negotiations continued, with considerable help from the professional advisory group, and late in 1960 there was a breakthrough, with the EGH board pledging full support for the Oaklawn program, even offering land adjacent to the hospital for constructing the facility. In 1961 Oaklawn joined EGH in a joint fund-raising effort in the community, with a goal of one and a half million dollars of which Oaklawn was to receive $250,000 or one-sixth of all contributions.

The Oaklawn board had already purchased land, so the EGH offer was not considered seriously. Yet, the choice of Oaklawn's location was another indication of its commitment to serving the community as well as the church. Unlike the other MCC mental health centers, Oaklawn was located in the city, near the people it was to help. The site committee, early in 1958, first had expressed preference for a location ouside the city limits, in an attractive natural setting with substantial acreage, yet accessible to EGH and agreeable to Hill-Burton officials. But later that same year the board purchased a sixteen-acre plot at the edge of Elkhart within the city limits. The higher expense of a sewer hookup in a more rural area influenced the site selection, but it also reflected the board's desire for the center to relate closely with the community. Community approval of this desired closeness came early, in the zoning board's unanimous recommendation that Oaklawn be allowed to locate in the residential area it had chosen.

A Changing Concept

The early planning for the mental health center proceeded on the asumption that it would be modeled after the traditional hospital concept, based on inpatient services. In 1958 the board engaged Wiley and Miller of Elkhart as architects, and planning continued. Miller and the board chairman, Hartzler, visited Prairie View and the Menninger Clinic in Kansas for ideas, and the Beatty Memorial hospital superintendent, as experienced builder of mental hopsitals, served as consultant and advisor. Initial plans included thirty beds at Oaklawn, based on the Mennonite population in the area.

But the encounter with EGH changed that. By 1961 the architects revised building plans to emphasize day treatment and outpatients rather than inpatients. It was no longer assumed that Oaklawn would be the typical mental health center with beds. Bed space for those patients who required hospitalization would be at EGH. Thus the controversy over inpatient plans and the resulting relationship with EGH actually strengthened Oaklawn's community involvement.

There were offices that were originally designed by a consultant to the building program as showers. The object was to bring people in who were dirty and ill kept and shower them off. That was a state hospital attitude. I objected to that and they changed the plans and instead put in play rooms for children and offices for family treatment. This was before 1962 when family treatment was hardly known at all.

— Otto D. Klassen[13]

Though prompted by the EGH discussions, the idea of a mental health program without beds was not entirely new to the Oaklawn board. The Eight-Point Program itself did not expressly call for beds. The MMHS board, in discussing this projected program in 1958, considered "the question of whether an outpatient and day-care program can be undertaken without an inpatient program."[14] But following the EGH episode, the no-beds concept received closer scrutiny and its most articulate expression came from the Oaklawn team of leaders which emerged in 1961 and 1962. Hartzler had been named administrator in 1961, with Mininger taking over as chairman of the board, and they were joined by Otto D. Klassen as medical director in July 1962.

Klassen and Hartzler visited several day hospitals in the east to investigate that treatment method as an option for Oaklawn. A few innovative mental health centers were initiating programs that created supervised environments during the day yet allowed pa-

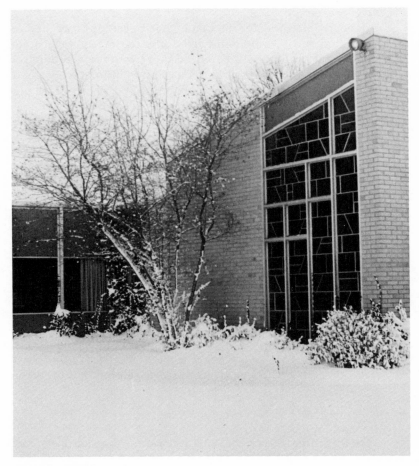

Chapel at Oaklawn Center.

tients to return to their homes at night. The Oaklawn leadership accepted the idea that the traditional rural institution created isolation not necessarily conducive to mental health, and that it was beneficial in many cases for people to remain involved with their families, churches, and jobs even as they received treatment.

The Building Completed

Plans for the building were completed and bids opened in September 1961, with costs for the facility pegged at $725,000. Ground breaking was held in November with completion scheduled for early 1963. The first outpatient came to the center on February 11, 1963, although Klassen had seen patients in a temporary office almost from the moment he had arrived in July 1962. The new building was designed to reflect the dual commitment to church and community. The architects created a building that looks more like an educational facility than the traditional mental institution. No fence surrounds the building, making it inviting and accessible. Inside, hallways are open, and glass gives a spacious feeling and allows the surrounding oak trees to be visible. The centrally located chapel reminds one of the center's commitment to the church; the courtyard's statue of the Good Samaritan, of the interdependence of all people, both helping and helped.

With the formal dedication of Oaklawn Psychiatric Center on September 20, 1963, the vision, first perceived nine years earlier, became a reality.

The Many Realities (1963-1981)

Once the center's doors opened, its programs and philosophies developed rapidly. Initially there was a two-pronged program—outpatient services and day treatment—but this was soon deployed to a multi-faceted ministry.

Outpatients and Day Patients

The outpatients came, first to the temporary office on West Franklin Street and then to the center at the corner of Hively and Oakland. Even though the number of therapists increased to eight by September 1963, the outpatient service was "literally swamped." Waiting lists developed soon after the first outpatient came, and those lists plagued the center until 1967 when streamlined operations eliminated them. Adjusted admission procedures allowed for walk-in and emergency cases also. Outpatient treatment aimed to lessen the trauma of the "removal from...community, family living and the normal routines of daily life."[15] Because outpatients can remain in their usual environments, this method became Oaklawn's preferred treatment.

It seemed to us that we had a really nice building and a nice place. People were astonished. Psychiatrists were even astonished at how nice a place it was and they predicted it would be torn down fast by the patients. Rather, the patients responded in a different way. They felt respected, well treated and returned that kind of treatment.
—Otto D. Klassen[16]

The first day patient arrived on February 21, 1963, and was cared for in an activities wing so new it was not yet fully equipped.

The day program was slower in developing than the outpatient service, although after one year the day hospital had reached its capacity to provide services with the current staff. Day treatment was based on "milieu therapy," which aims at creating a supportive, interdependent environment with a strong emphasis on group relationships. Patients give much input, and a healthy relationship between staff and patients results. Patients spend time at Oaklawn during the weekdays and return home each night and on weekends.

Two Other Programs for Patients

Implicit to the day treatment program were two other programs which helped augment services to patients. Elkhart General Hospital, from the beginning, provided twenty-four-hour hospitalization for those requiring this form of intensive care, although the number never was large. Some of those hospitalized spent part of their time in the activities program of the Oaklawn day hospital.

The other service was the community home program, which "grew out of the necessity to conceive a way of serving the outlying church constituency even though we had abandoned beds."[17] One of Oaklawn's most unique aspects, the community home program, places day treatment patients into private homes in the Elkhart community. Area ministers usually recommend these host families, after which the family goes through orientation. Candidates for the community home program are patients who live too far to return home at night or those whose home situations are not beneficial to treatment. In 1963 the program had fifteen to twenty homes, usually Christian families who chose to host people out of a commitment to serving others. Originally, rural Mennonites comprised most of the families that accepted patients, but Oaklawn now uses a variety of homes. Participating families have found the experience beneficial for themselves as well as for the patients.

Community Organizations

Several community organizations which proved to be strong support groups for Oaklawn developed early in the history of the center. The Oaklawn Auxiliary increased church and community participation in the working of the center. In hopes of improved public relations and increased numbers of volunteers, plans originally called for two separate auxiliaries. The unnecessary division between church women and community women was dropped and a single group developed. The first group, composed only of church women, first met in 1965 and a core of about twenty dedicated women set up five committees, with hopes of eventually retaining a membership of around two hundred. By 1970 the unified auxiliary

numbered sixty-two, with an active schedule of programs, conferences, and workshops. High attendance still characterizes these
events, and a continually growing mailing list indicates the increased visibility of the center through the activities of the auxiliary.

Another community group is the Oaklawn Foundation. This
nonprofit organization was incorporated in 1965 to boost Oaklawn's
programs and financial situations. It was also a legal entity capable
of owning property and borrowing money. The Oaklawn Foundation created a patient-assistance fund for those who could not afford
Oaklawn's fees, and played an important role in the development of
Lexington House, a halfway house program. Both the foundation,
which is mostly made up of community leaders, and the auxiliary
function as links between the center and the people it serves.

Helping Church and Community

Consultation and education programs emerged early as part of
Oaklawn's concern for preventing mental illness as well as helping
people after problems develop. In 1963 efforts initially were directed
primarily to the churches in the area. A number of staff members,
especially the administrator, Robert Hartzler, maintained a steady
stream of visits to the churches.

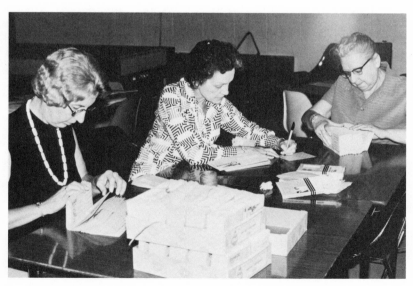

*Approximately 85 volunteers comprise the Oaklawn Auxiliary, an active
organization which assists staff in both clinical and administrative capacities.*

Staff members also arranged their schedule to allow time to counsel pastors, because troubled people often approach ministers before seeking other professional counseling. Workshops for ministers offered intensive courses in effective communication, intervention, and counseling. Monthly consultation with groups of ministers, beginning in 1967, expanded pastoral services. The usefulness of a clinical training program for pastors became evident, but Oaklawn postponed development of that program until 1969 when they hired their first chaplain.

The Elkhart county schools, as well as several Mennonite colleges, also supplemented their counseling services through the center's consultation program. Every two weeks, beginning in 1965, a staff person spent a day at Bluffton College (Ohio); similarly, Elkhart public and parochial schools have received consultation since 1966. Oaklawn has provided consultation for the schools and their guidance personnel, the county welfare department, courts, police department, and area nursing homes. The Elkhart community has benefited from this far-reaching service that reflects Oaklawn's concern for the quality of mental health care in the area.

Chaplaincy Program

The issue over a chaplaincy program shows Oaklawn's changing views of itself and its relationship with the church. Following the examples of the other MCC centers, Oaklawn intended to provide chaplaincy services and therefore included a chapel and a chaplain's office in the building. However, the board postponed hiring a chaplain in order to think about how a chaplain would fit into the overall organization of the center. "It would be unthinkable to present to the ill a man neither a real minister nor a real therapist,"[18] and a person filling both requirements was difficult to find. Additionally, the center considered itself representative of the church even without a chaplain since the center's motivation originated in the church, and the staff itself was Christian. In lieu of the final decision, in 1962 the board appointed administrator Robert Hartzler, who was a minister, as interim chaplain.

A period of discussions of the various options for the chaplaincy followed that temporary appointment. In 1963 the board formed a committee designed to explore the issue. The directors felt it important that a chaplain expand the relationship with ministers and the churches, for there continued to be a need for their input. Oaklawn's emphasis on retaining patients' normal relations as much as possible meant that patients also should be encouraged to relate with the pastors of the churches they regularly attended.

The board of directors finally tabled the issue in 1966 to allow

Well, I once went to the Beachy Amish Church east of Goshen, and they asked me to give a talk. I can't remember what I talked about, but the men were on one side and the women on the other side. The deacons were up front and I was up there with them and they had a service and sang songs. Then the chief deacon asked me to close the meeting. You don't say "no" there, so I thought, "How do you close a meeting here?" So I got up and said something and it didn't work. The Bishop got up and said to sing another song. Then he looked at me again and I said I would do it again. So I said, "As the hart panteth after the eagle that rises out of the waterfall." I was plugged in, I was desperate now. Three times I tried to close the meeting, no time did it work. Finally, he closed the meeting.

—Otto D. Klassen

With a prayer....he just wanted you to lead in prayer.

—Robert W. Hartzler

Well, I said something sort of prayer-like. I thought I did. But at any rate, by that time I was so nervous and anxious that I don't remember to this day how I got it closed. I was so nervous that I couldn't see how he did it, so I still don't know how to close a meeting.

—Otto D. Klassen[19]

even more time for study. This meant postponing the clinical training program for seminary students and pastors for various reasons including the fact that the staff already claimed four trained clergymen plus two persons with theological training. Also, the churches and therapists desired a direct relationship with one another without an intermediary. This forced the staff to maintain a large degree of responsibility to the churches. Instead of a specialized person exclusively responsible for the religious part of patients' lives each of the staff was concerned with the whole patient. Additionally, the added cost of a chaplain's salary was thought to detract from Oaklawn's desire and ability to treat the poor.

In responding to the churches' continued requests for a clinical training program, which required a chaplain, Oaklawn reconsidered the chaplaincy issue. In 1969, as a first step toward implementing that program, Oaklawn hired Chester Raber as its first chaplain-therapist. Raber, who had served in a similar position at Brook Lane from 1961 to 1969, fit Oaklawn's requirements that their chaplain be both a therapist and a person with religious training. Recently acquired county monies assisted poorer patients so the cost of hiring another staff person did not so directly affect those the center hoped to serve.

Then Chet Raber was bugging us to get a professional chaplain and he did that for quite a long time. He really wanted to work here, I believe, and we resisted. I was part of the resistance. You can't believe how many ministers we had on our clinical staff. There really were a lot of them. They were the heart of the staff. I feel I represented a kind of resistance to that idea....I thought that the staff ought to be fully ready to take up issues like that with their clients. But in time we were persuaded and Chet joined the staff. He developed the chaplaincy and then the chaplaincy training.

—Otto. D. Klassen[20]

Community Mental Health Programs

Concern for reaching maximum numbers of community people led to the creation of several satellite operations. Beginning in LaGrange and Steuban counties in Indiana, Oaklawn set up outpatient clinics in 1965. Noble and DeKalb counties followed when they received public funds to allow service in those counties on an ability-to-pay basis. The state Department of Mental Health gradually ended that funding in 1968, which led to the independence of the Northeastern Center, which included the four counties. It became a seperate institution in 1978.

In 1968 Oaklawn began offering services to Elkhart County residents on a sliding fee scale because the county granted Oaklawn public funds to subsidize needy patients. Even though three other MMHS centers—Prairie View, Kings View and Kern View—had received federal funds through the Community Mental Health Centers Act of 1962, Oaklawn had decided not to seek these funds. Initially Oaklawn hesitated to apply because their facilities were not yet fully utilized and such a designation would require some expansion, and because Oaklawn, then private, feared that relations required with public agencies might be difficult. Elkhart County initiated an application process for those federal funds in 1966. But, since Oaklawn already provided so many of the services required for such a designation, in 1968 the center decided to proceed with an application itself but with the support of Elkhart County. County representatives and Oaklawn worked together during the application process.

The separately incorporated Oaklawn Community Mental Health Center (OCMHC) resulted. Since 1973, OCMHC has provided mental health care for Elkhart County residents on an ability-to-pay basis. OCMHC rents space and contracts for staff from the now wholly private Oaklawn Psychiatric Center (OPC). Initially OCMHC

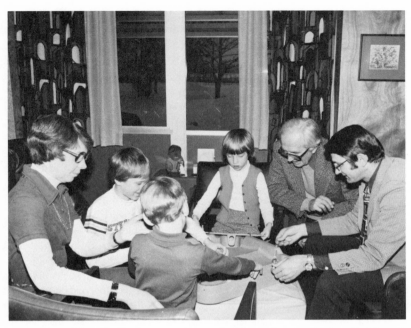

A simulated family therapy session at Oaklawn Center depicts Oaklawn's philosophy that families benefit from working together to resolve difficulties and build relationships.

used sixty-five percent of the staff's time and the center's space, but increased demands changed the ratio so that now nearly ninety percent of the time and space goes to OCMHC and ten percent to OPC. The OCMHC board is made up of those members of the OPC board who live in Elkhart County, making communication and organization as smooth as possible between the two governing bodies.

Staff and program changes resulted from Oaklawn's new role. Now required to serve all of the Elkhart County residents needing their services, Oaklawn opened offices in Goshen, Middlebury, and Nappanee. Oaklawn agreed to provide aftercare for the state-run Beatty Memorial Hospital's patients from Elkhart County, and in 1975 the center added nineteen staff members in order to accommodate the greater number of people passing through its doors. OPC now serves only out-of-county patients, and has kept OCMHC as a subsidiary organization in order to "help protect our total operation from unwarranted encroachment by public bodies...."[21]

Increasing Services

There were a number of other new programs which Oaklawn operated in more recent years. A children's day treatment program, known as the *Tree House,* opened in 1972, the result of six years of planning. In order to devote energy to this program, Otto Klassen resigned as medical director, though he later resumed that directorate. Designed to work with groups of eight elementary school children at a time, the program sought to return the children to their regular school environment as quickly as possible. Though successful, the Tree House program ended in 1978 when pressure from the state placed responsibility for the education of disturbed children on the public schools.

After a long period of planning and several aborted attempts, in 1972 Oaklawn purchased a former YWCA building for its transitional housing program. Named *Lexington House,* this downtown building contains clinical offices, a public cafeteria, the sheltered living program, and the adolescent day treatment program.

Oaklawn's increased awareness of substance addictions led to further expansion of the center's services. Initially confused about how to relate to alcoholism because it was difficult to treat and not often a Mennonite problem, Oaklawn in 1973 began to develop an alcoholism treatment program.

In our early days people used to come down from the Department of Mental Health and ask us how many alcoholics we were admitting, and our statistics were really low. They said we must be missing them. I remember people saying that. I think we tended to say we didn't know why, but they weren't coming to us. They were right and we were wrong. We were missing them like everywhere else. General hospitals in this country diagnosed one half of one percent of their cases as due to alcoholism. The proportion was vastly higher, and everybody was missing them. Hiring Jim Reiff was the beginning of the education of us all with regard to the disease. So that has been dramatic. It's not wholly a resolved issue, but there is no going back to missing diagnoses anymore. Once you start doing that you can't go back to the old days when all you saw were the psychiatric problems and not the alcoholism.

—Otto D. Klassen[22]

Now, eight years later, in addition to an addictions day treatment program, Oaklawn plans to be involved in a continuum of services for alcoholics. Administrator, Harold C. Loewen, who succeeded Robert Hartzler in 1978, stresses alcoholism treatment and education as one of the frontiers of the 1980s.

Increasingly sensitive to the unique needs of minority groups, the center's staff began focusing on interests of both blacks and the aged. Joann Bethea and others were instrumental in developing several highly successful programs aimed at the black community. Oaklawn also provided impetus behind the development of the Elkhart County Council on Aging, and since then outreach efforts and consultation with nursing homes have improved connections with the elderly of Elkhart County.

The most recent new program is aimed at chronically mentally disabled persons. Growing out of the Lexington transitional housing project, the "apartment project" was approved in 1981 by the Oaklawn board. With a loan guarantee from the federal Housing and Urban Development Department, Oaklawn constructed an eleven-unit apartment complex, located on grounds next to the center, to provide supervised living accommodations for the mentally disabled.

Maintaining the Church-Community Balance

The history of Oaklawn reveals the continuing concern and determination of the board and staff to serve both the Elkhart community and the constituent church groups, and to avoid any conflict with either in the process of serving both.

Fees

When it came to charges for services rendered, Oaklawn took care to consider the sponsoring churches when it raised its fees. To maintain understanding between the churches and the center, groups of ministers were invited to hear about fees and reasons for changing them. In order to accommodate more patients from the church who might have trouble paying for treatment, beginning in 1969 Oaklawn took Mennonite and Brethren patients on a sliding fee scale, making up the differences from church contributions. This increased the center's accessibility to the churches. For the local community, as has already been noted, Oaklawn provided services on an ability-to-pay basis for county residents, first from county funds provided and then as Oaklawn Community Mental Health Center.

Staffing

The church constituency has played a major role in Oaklawn's staffing process. The staff all came from the sponsoring churches when the center first opened, thus promoting a cohesiveness between philosophy and programs. However, a dearth of mental health professionals among the sponsoring church members led the center to hire additional staff on the basis of wider Christian commitment as well as professional qualifications. Until 1968 Oaklawn carefully screened potential staff persons through slow and deliberate negotiations, giving a unity among those connected with the center. An increase in patients after 1968, due to a substantial increase in Oaklawn's receipt of public money, encouraged a major staff increase. Since then staff has been hired for professional excellence, though still compatible with Oaklawn's philosophy, and the balance has shifted from a heavy predominance of staff from the sponsoring churches to a more widely representative group.

Board of Directors

The history of the board of directors is one of increased community participation. In the early years MCC appointed board members and the first board in 1958 were all from constituent groups. The next year, when the board was enlarged, two community at-large members were added. In 1962 the bylaws of all four MCC centers were amended to allow for four community representatives, provided that two-thirds of the board represented the church constituent groups. In 1969, after MMHS was delegated responsibility for appointing board members by MCC (1965), the bylaws were amended once more to require 60 percent of the board to be from the sponsoring churches, with the other 40 percent to be appointed by MMHS from the community. The board also was enlarged at that time to allow for more community representatives. There was talk of expanding the list of sponsoring churches to include Catholic and Methodist churches, since many patients came from those churches, but that has not taken place. In 1973 Oaklawn and MMHS agreed to remove any mention of constituent church membership as a prerequisite for board membership. At present, the only requirement is MMHS approval, although in actual practice a 50-50 balance between constituent and community representatives has been maintained.

Publicity

Publicity from Oaklawn has tried to cut to a minimum the public's occasional misunderstandings of the center's connections with the church. After being described negatively as sectarian[23] during negotiations with Elkhart General Hospital, Oaklawn has emphasized its place as a community agency. Only one of Oaklawn's regular publications, the *Newsletter*, has been specifically aimed for the churches. The rest of Oaklawn's publicity methods de-emphasize ties with the church. One unfortunate misunderstanding, during which Elkhart citizens petitioned against the center because of Oaklawn's religious connections, drew this understandable response from Oaklawn:

> "The Mennonite church was largely responsible for creating this facility." From a limited point of view this may be an accurate statement. It is grossly misleading, however, in that it fails to recognize the enormous involvement of the Elkhart County community in its creation and its almost total present control of it. . . . The Mennonite contribution has been significant but perhaps no more significant than the county's.[24]

Oaklawn recognized the Elkhart community's vast contributions and preferred to "polish their image of professional competence"[25] rather than emphasize their church connections.

Most publicity about Oaklawn, however, has been very positive, indicating its acceptance by both the community and the sponsoring churches. In 1963 an area church publication described the center as a "history-making cause" that the community should be honored to support.[26] The *Goshen News* lauded the center's willingness to be flexible in order to best meet the area's needs.[27] In 1964 a United States Department of Health, Education, and Welfare pamphlet cited Oaklawn as one of the first examples of the new community mental health center concept.[28] Its cover shows a sketch of Oaklawn's main entrance, and the pamphlet praises Oaklawn for its community involvement. The *Elkhart Truth* gave extensive coverage of Oaklawn's events, and published positive editorials in support of Oaklawn during some periods of conflict with factions of the community.[29] Nationally known mental health leaders also praised Oaklawn, saying that they were bowled over by Oaklawn's excellent programs.[30]

Professional Standards

The bringing together of church and community is also seen in another area. Oaklawn has been committed to high professional standards and attributes that commitment in part to the center's Christian roots. Former administrator Robert Hartzler viewed psychiatry as the "best tool available" to help with some major human problems, and mental health centers are "truly in behalf of that human dignity which the church seeks to enhance."[31] A pamphlet from Oaklawn emphasizes that

> The unique sense of values arising from this [church] sponsorship make imperative the development of the best possible program. The highest standards of personal as well as professional dedication are expected of its staff.[32]

*Did we down-play the churches? I think we "up-played" all the
churches, myself. Community homes contributed in major ways. I
think that's playing up churches in an important way. Our community homes were always solidly from the churches.... The churches
were our source of what we think of as excellent staff. The development of the Community Mental Health Center, with the laws and
public policies that constrain such a place, necessarily make a kind of
down-playing of religious ties. Yet in this community all of the staff
are hired by the Oaklawn Psychiatric Center, which has a church-
appointed board, so that in another way, for a mental health center,
that's playing up the church. I think that we have by no means lost
sight of the strength of the churches...; that has always been important to us.*

—Otto D. Klassen[33]

A "close-knit relationship... along with a sense of mission in
doing 'our thing'" motivated the staff to accept salaries lower than at
public institutions until 1969, but as that intimacy was "replaced by
an organizational reality which... is sounder,"[34] Oaklawn adjusted
salaries and personnel policies to more closely match comparable
professional institutions. Thus, as Hartzler wrote, "in the mental
health business, to be professionally excellent is at least as 'Christian' as words without deed."[35] This emphasis on professional excellence won respect for Oaklawn throughout the county, state, and
nation.

*The short range future is very clear in that there is a plateauing and
probably a decrease in public funding for mental health purposes.
Thus the wisdom of our having begun and having a 10-year experience as a private center, and of not relinquishing our private corporation in order to become a community mental health center, I think
comes to light now. I think we will have to resort to reviving our
private survival skills. That certainly seems true for the short term.
We don't fear that.... You work toward excellence.... The only way you
are going to get clients is that you provide an excellent service, and
that's what you work toward. And you don't have the luxury of
escaping from that marketplace requirement...; and I think that is
good for us.*

—Otto D. Klassen[36]

"From one vision to many realities." This is the story of
Oaklawn. While playing a vital role in the Elkhart and wider community, the center continues to explore new ways to serve. From its
inception as a small church institution through its development into

a far-reaching and still expanding center, Oaklawn has kept the needs of the people it seeks to help in the forefront of its philosophy. This remains its goal.

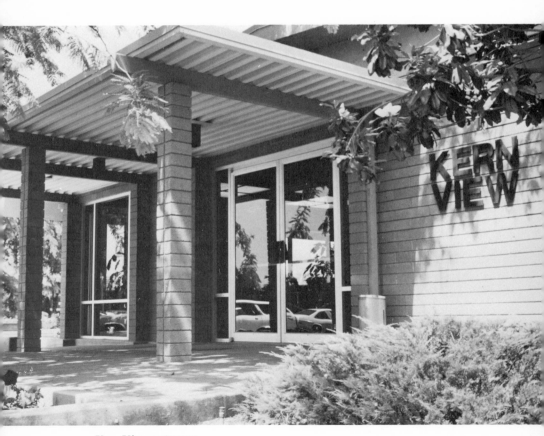

Kern View entrance.

Kern View
Bakersfield, California
Larry R. Yoder*

Kern View Community Mental Health Center and Hospital, the fifth and youngest center sponsored by the Mennonite Central Committee (MCC) and Mennonite Mental Health Services (MMHS), was opened in 1966 through the joint efforts of Kings View, MMHS, and Greater Bakersfield Memorial Hospital. Its attractive facilities are located next to Memorial Hospital in the heart of Greater Bakersfield, California, a community of approximately 200,000.

Early Negotiations and Planning
(November 1961-July 1966)

Local Explorations and Discussions
In late 1961 exploration to develop a mental health service in Kern County was begun between Arthur Jost, adminisrator of Kings View Homes, Reedley, California, and the administrator of Greater Bakersfield Memorial Hospital. Several circumstances prompted this exploration. First, Memorial Hospital had decided not to build a psychiatric ward as part of the general hospital setting. Secondly, Kings View did not want to expand its own facilities beyond fifty beds, and over the years had received a number of referrals from the Bakersfield community. Thirdly, there was an interested Mennonite constituency, though small, in the Kern County area.[1]

Memorial Hospital expressed a willingness to work with Kings View in establishing a psychiatric service and strongly encouraged Kings View to apply for federal Hill-Burton funds to assist in financing the construction of a hospital. Memorial Hospital was not willing to mortgage its facilities or to conduct a solicitation drive on

---

*Larry R. Yoder was administrator of Kern View from April 1969 to July 1982. He was assisted in preparing this chapter by Patrick C. Barker, Kern View clinical director.

It was at a casual meeting between the administrator of Memorial Hospital and the administrator of Kings View Hospital that the need and possible building of a hospital on memorial property was first discussed, and Arthur Jost was immediately enthused about it. I was not at the time because we had enough problems at Kings View. But I had an open mind on it so there followed a number of meetings between Arthur Jost, Ralph Smith, Chairman of the Memorial Hospital board, and myself. We explored the possibilities thoroughly from all angles.

—John C. Penner [2]

behalf of the Kings View project, but it was willing to develop a long-term lease for land on which to build the new facility.[3]

While legal relationships between Kings View and Memorial Hospital were easily defined, professional relationships and questions related to the scope of the program became much more difficult issues to resolve. The psychiatrists in private practice in Bakersfield favored the project, but, as an MMHS delegation reported later, they stated clearly the following expectations: "(1) an open staff, where all psychiatrists can treat their own patients in the facility; (2) that there be no outpatient department—this would appear to them to be competitive to private practice; and (3) a salaried medical director appointed by the Kern View Board, to be responsible for developing milieu as well as directly treat the patients from a distance, or direct such treatment as the local psychiatrists wished."[4]

Support for the proposed Kings View facility was also obtained from the Mennonite churches in Kern County, who expressed their concern that the staff be clearly Christian service-minded so that the witness of the center would not be clouded. Although they expressed a willingness to be identified as sponsors of the project, they also indicated early in the discussions that the local churches should not be asked to contribute capital funds.[5]

Even though the Kings View board of directors preferred to own the property on which the hospital was to be built, they could not identify a better solution than to enter into the proposed lease agreement with Memorial Hospital, which would provide land for a very nominal cost. Moreover, such a lease would fulfill the requirements of potential funding sources—Hill-Burton and the state of California, which required an applicant be associated with a general hospital.

As I was the only representative from Kern County on the Kings View board, Mennonite Mental Health Services would not be interested to build unless their representative would support the project. After many meetings by only us three it was first presented to the Kings View board and then to Mennonite Mental Health Services. Yes, much work, travel and persuasion have gone into making Kern View Hospital a reality.

—John C. Penner [6]

MMHS *and* MCC *Involvement*

Since MMHS was ultimately responsible for approving the development of the proposed Kings View project, its board was apprised of the various issues and concerns of the local psychiatrists and church groups.[7] Several MMHS-MCC delegations visited the Bakersfield community to evaluate the proposed project. The last visit was prompted by the Bakersfield Medical Society's opposition to an outpatient clinic, the limited authority of the medical director as defined by the local psychiatrists, and the proposed relationship between the project and the psychiatrists practicing in the Bakersfield community.[8] Specifically, MMHS directors felt that they should approve a project only when there was appropriate freedom and flexibility, and that "insofar as possible, all MMHS facilities should be free to develop programs that integrate our historic religious convictions regarding the nature of man and his needs and our professional convictions regarding the need for experimentation in the field of mental health."[9] MMHS raised questions regarding the degree to which this project might be forced into a mold that would deny it the latitude and the degree of independence considered essential.

In a report dated April 24, 1963, Ernest Boyer, a member of the MMHS board delegation, stated that the concerns of MMHS and reasons for further negotiations were set forth clearly in a meeting with representatives of the Bakersfield Medical Society, and that everyone on both sides of the table recognized that the proposed Kern View Hospital would be legally independent and have full authority to develop its programs. It was agreed that the program would not ignore the expectations of the local professionals, but neither would it be answerable to the local medical society, but to the Kings View board of directors and ultimately to MMHS.

Finally, outpatient services were seen as a justifiable, if not mandatory, part of a good psychiatric program.

While the local professionals still urged caution, they seemed to understand and support MMHS convictions that freedom and flexibility were essential. Boyer felt that the physicians present accepted the position of MMHS as responsible and one that they could support. His report concluded:

> While the Bakersfield community might not be ideal, I cannot honestly say that the professional attitude there is repressive or one in which community needs are ignored. In my judgment it would be unfair for the Board of Directors of MMHS to push this "freedom flexibility" issue further. We have established our position and the medical staff has responded in good faith. They have probably gone as far as we can expect them to go at this time. While some restrictions will be encountered, yet I do not believe such restrictions would be any more severe than those we would meet in a similar project elsewhere.[10]

On May 4, 1963, MCC unanimously approved the recommendation of the MMHS officers that Kings View Homes be granted approval to establish Kern View Hospital in Bakersfield. The officers of MMHS understood Boyer's report to mean that responsible leaders of the Bakersfield medical community had assured MMHS of their readiness to guarantee "the flexibility and freedom" necessary to operate the Kern View Hospital program in the spirit of MMHS'

Early Saturday morning [May 4, 1963] Dr. Amstutz arrived. At the MCC meeting, it was decided that the brethren Amstutz, Fast, Miller, Stahly and I should discuss our Kern View Hospital project in the light of Dr. Boyer's statement and at one o'clock Dr. Amstutz should present a recommendation to MCC for approval.

We met in our room and spent the entire morning for our discussion. I sensed a spirit of brotherly love and understanding. The result was that Dr. Fast was assigned the task to write up the recommendation. . . . Meeting at one o'clock MCC discussed the recommendation for about an hour and fifteen minutes after which it was approved unanimously. I thanked the brethren and then I had to hurry to the Santa Fe depot to catch my train.

—John C. Penner [11]

---

traditional commitment and to develop services felt to be consistent with good professional practice and apparent community needs.[12]

Early Administration

From its inception, all planning and coordination for the Kern View project was the responsibility of the Kings View board of directors and its administration. Arthur Jost, administrator, was relieved of some day-to-day responsibilities at Kings View to spend time on the project. In addition, the Kings View board established a Kern County Coordinating Committee in December 1963 to represent the local community and to assume more local and direct responsibility for the Kern Veiw project.[13] It was not until March 1965, when Henry Hooge was employed as administrative assistant, that Jost received some local staff assistance. Hooge later was appointed Kern View's first administrator.

Funding and Construction

After having received approval from MCC in early 1963, the Kings View board signed a ninety-nine year lease with Greater Bakersfield Memorial Hospital for four acres of land for a nominal annual fee.[14] Shortly thereafter Kings View was successful in obtaining a Hill-Burton grant and, as a result, the state of California matched the grant for the construction of the original Kern View facility. One-third of the facility remained to be financed through a long-term bank loan. In addition, by 1966 approximately $51,000 had been raised from the Bakersfield business community for the project.

One of my most rewarding experiences was working with Arthur Jost in contacting businesses in the community to raise funds. We needed financial help for landscaping, the pre-opening, and operating costs not covered by government grants and bank loans. I was struck with the interest, support, and encouragement of the business community—especially since the project was sponsored by the Mennonite Church. It was particularly rewarding to see over 380 persons representing a cross secion of the Bakersfield community attending a special fundraising event on September 10, 1964. The support the community gave Kern View in its early years has remained. Kern View continues to enjoy good support from the community at-large.
—Henry F. Brandt[15]

Once the Hill-Burton grant was approved, immediate attention was focused on planning the facilities. Kern View was envisioned ultimately as a fifty-bed facility of which the capacity for twenty-five beds would be built initially. The dining room, kitchen facilities, related offices, and recreation areas, however, would be built to sufficient size to accommodate the fifty patients. Since Hill-Burton funds were related to the construction of hospital facilities, the original building was designed primarily for inpatient programs. Ground breaking took place on January 17, 1965, and on July 19, 1966, the Kern View Hospital facilities were completed.

Initiating Services (July 1966–June 1969)

Designed as a hospital, Kern View admitted its first inpatients shortly after its completion on July 25, 1966. Phillip Leo Kelly, Kern View's first medical director, nursing and other staff members were on hand. But almost immediately a new concept of service was thrust upon Kern View.

NIMH Staffing Grant

As the board of directors of Kings View considered the cost of operating the new Kern View facility in Bakersfield, the National Institute of Mental Health (NIMH) staffing grant funds, which had just become available through federal legislation, became very appealing. On March 26, 1966, the Kings View board endorsed applying for such a grant and designated Arthur Jost as project director for Kern View. By submitting this application, the Kings View board was committing Kern View to become a community mental health center. Kings View was successful in obtaining the NIMH grant which became available to Kern View September 1, 1966, approximately six weeks after the first patient was admitted.

Just as the design of the original facility was influenced by the requirements of Hill-Burton funding for inpatient services, so also was program development to be governed by this NIMH grant. In fact, receiving the NIMH grant required that Kern View develop a much broader program immediately than originally had been envisioned. Kern View was committed to provide five basic services: inpatient, day treatment, outpatient, emergency services, and consultation/education. Thus, by the time of Kern View's dedication on October 16, 1966, the original facility, designed primarily for inpatients, was already inadequate to meet the space requirements for the full program of a community mental health center as defined by NIMH.

Problems Resulting from the NIMH Grant

An immediate reaction came from the medical community. It is important to note that Kings View and Kern View had received some of the first NIMH staffing grants in the state of California. Since federal community mental health legislation was so new, there were very few precedents to which the local medical community could turn to understand the implementation of the community mental health center concept. Thus, the establishment of an outpatient department as required by NIMH presented an initial and major public relations hurdle that had to be crossed. In spite of the earlier discussions, the medical community of Bakersfield could not accept this development favorably. The outpatient department was immediately seen as a government subsidized program in competition with the private practice of psychiatry, and an atmosphere of suspicion and stress prevailed.

Another problem was presented by the need to implement the five services almost immediately. Unless funds were used to achieve the required commitments of the grant, opportunity for financial assistance in program development would be lost. Consequently, there was mounting pressure to have the five basic services of the community mental health center in place and operating. But staff was limited. The growing demand for inpatient services consumed the entire time of the one employed psychiatrist, Phillip Leo Kelly. It was not until July 1967, when the second psychiatrist and additional staff were employed, that adequate attention could begin to be given to the development of the other four services. Even then, the initiation of services suffered significant growing pains.

For example, the outpatient department was first designed to be staffed with employed psychiatrists, psychologists, and social workers. However, by late 1967 the psychiatric staff had negotiated a special contract which allowed them to be in private practice and pay Kern View for office space and reception and bookkeeping services. This contract reduced the time available to serve Kern View and defined this service as consultation to the mental health center. In essence, the psychiatrists, who began as full-time employees of the center, were permitted to develop their private pratices and designate these as the outpatient department of Kern View. The result of this arrangement was that Kern View had only part-time physicians who nevertheless were employed in leadership roles.

At the same time, Kern View administration was faced with the fact that the NIMH staffing grant was considered "seed money," funds available under the grant would decrease annually. So it was imperative for Kern View to try to develop local contracts with Kern County to reduce the financial burden of providing the five basic services in the face of a decreasing federal grant. This process was difficult and slow, and it was not until late 1968 that the Kern County Board of Supervisors was willing to develop a small contract for day treatment services. By then a separate day treatment facility had been established in a leased building away from the original hospital facilities.

Along with its strong influence on program development, the NIMH grant also tied Kern View to a geographical area called the *West Kern Catchment Area*—primarily the western part of Kern County with the eastern border running through the heart of Bakersfield. Only Kern View, as an NIMH-designated center, was required to pay attention to this catchment area concept, not the county or the state.

This not only complicated Kern View's operation, since the community to be served and the catchment area were not the same, but Kern View's decisions were sometimes misunderstood by various segments of the community.

Concurrently, the initial attempts to establish services for children and adolescents, as well as a consultation and education service, encountered roadblocks. There was either resistance from existing community services (e.g. the twenty-year-old Henrietta Weill Child Guidance Clinic) or misunderstandings of Kern View's intentions. The approaches by Kern View were frequently misinterpreted and signs of distrust began to appear on the part of the professional community, the Child Guidance Clinic, the County of Kern, and other community agencies. It seemed to many in the local community that Kern View was attempting to take over the mental health services of Kern County.

A Separate Kern View Board

By March 1967 Kern View Hospital was incorporated as a separate entity and the Kern County Coordinating Committee of Kings View, along with all Kings View board members who lived in southern California, became the first Kern View board of directors.[16] Initially all board members were members of the Mennonite constituency. Henry F. Brandt was elected as the first chairman and served a full nine years in that capacity.

As the NIMH staffing grant requirements continued to dictate policy and program development, there was also less time for building relationships with the local Mennonite churches. In fact, the churches' involvement soon became that of primarily providing directors for the Kern View board. Since the local churches made no financial commitment to the center, the initial identificaion with Kern View soon waned.

Approximately 2½ years after the opening of Kern View, in late 1968, the board of directors began voicing considerable concern regarding program development, the conflict of interest of employed psychiatrists, a lack of local identity with the West Kern Catchment Area, and increased tensions among employed personnel. The team approach was not working. Physicians appeared to be using the facility as a stepping-stone to promote their own private practices. In addition, the administrative structure of having a project director in Reedley and an administrator in Bakersfield seemed unworkable; so the two positions were combined and a full-time director was recruited.

Six months after the board began voicing its concerns, NIMH made a site visit and reported to the board its own disappointment

> *It is doubtful that three part-time psychiatrists who devote a substan-*
> *tial part of their time to private practice can be as effecive as two or*
> *perhaps even one full-time psychiatrist. Conflict of interest questions*
> *are apt to arise where Centers employment and private practice are so*
> *closely related. It would seem that the Clinical Director's position in a*
> *newly developing Center involves so much basic groundwork and*
> *program development that full-time assignment is imperative.*
> *— NIMH Site Visit Report*[17]

in the lack of program development. The five basic services were available to some degree, but, they commented, it was difficult to distinguish between Kern View's outpatient service and the psychiatrists' private practices. As a result of these comments, the Kern View executive committee requested a review of the contractual relationships with the psychiatrists and clinical leadership issues. NIMH consultants encouraged Kern View to have one or two full-time employed medical staff rather than three or four part-time staff in private practice on the premises.[18]

Serving the Community

Although tensions had developed with various segments of the community, primarily in administrative and professional realms, a dedicated staff continued to develop the services of a community mental health center. By April 1969, 916 patients had received treatment. Kern View had established a reputation for good treatment in a very pleasant setting, which provided a significant contrast with the services provided at the psychiatric ward of the local county hospital. Overall, Kern View began having an influence on the way psychiatric clients were treated in Kern County, and the general community continued to be supportive of Kern View.

Period of Growth (June 1969-November 1979)

Operational objectives continued to be strongly influenced by MMHS and the funding bodies of the National Institute of Mental Health and the California State Department of Mental Health. The California Mental Health Act of July 1969 also influenced Kern View's development. The availability of federal and state funds continued to be a mixed blessing. Kern View was able to expand its services much more rapidly than would have been possible without these funds, but in the process Kern View also became a quasi-public agency which affected attitudes among staff members and the public. In addition, it was frequently difficult to meet all of the

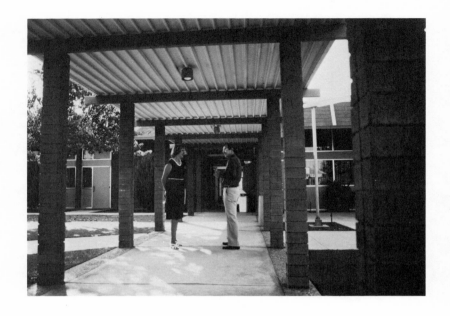

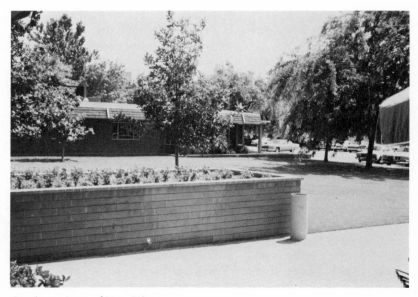

Outdoor views of Kern View.

> *The relationship with the news media in Bakersfield was excellent. The Bakersfield daily paper printed all the articles on the development of Kern View verbatim as they were presented and many trips were made to the city desk. At the point where Kern View Hospital was opened, the administrator asked for a series of editorials leading up to that opening. Again the editor invited Kern View to write editorials and they were used as presented. Radio and television stations were visited frequently and prime time was given to Kern View staff and community personnel on several occasions for forums and discussions. Frequent television shows were aired where Kern View officials appeared live. The entire news media relationships during the development period were satisfactory and conducive to a spirit of wide acceptance in the community.*
>
> *—Arthur Jost[19]*

expectations of the different funding, regulatory, and sponsoring bodies. Nevertheless, the decade of 1969-79 was one of significant growth.

A New Administrator and an Expanded Board

In April 1969, Larry R. Yoder assumed the administrator's role at Kern View, taking a leave of absence from his position at the Oaklawn Center in Elkhart, Indiana, initially for one year. He later resigned the Oaklawn position to remain as administrator for thirteen years. Later in 1969 the board of directors was enlarged to fourteen members to allow for a one-third representation from the community-at-large. Most members still represented the church constituency, which for the first time included representatives of the Church of the Brethren. With this enlargement of the board, a number of members became involved who had little knowledge of Kern View's history. Both the new board members as well as the new administrator were trying to grasp the issues which seemed to be troubling Kern View. The administrator developed a historical perspective for the board in early 1970 in which he concluded that "Kern View seems a place where the best intentions have gone awry and the services for which it had been established have not developed or matured."[20]

In March 1970 the board of directors adopted a resolution to clarify its position and to address past misunderstandings with the medical community. It clearly defined Kern View's commitment to develop a full-service community mental health center, providing the five basic services, as supported both by NIMH and MMHS philosophy. This resolution reiterated that local psychiatrists and other physicians might have admitting privileges provided they agreed with the treatment philosophy of Kern View and were willing to coordinate patient care as defined by the center's policy and developed by the Kern View medical director.

Another important action taken by the enlarged board of directors was not to allow private practice on the Kern View premises. As a result, the psychiatrists moved their practices to private offices in the community. Kern View negotiated limited psychiatric consulting contracts primarily for program consultation. Consequently, Kern View was without any resident physician on the premises for a full nine months until Sigmund A. Kosewick, a psychiatrist, joined the staff full-time in April 1970 as medical director.

Medical Staff Problems

Kern View's professional organizational model at that time followed an acute general hospital model with an open medical staff. This meant that physicians who formerly had a contractual or employment relationship with the center, though relieved of administrative duties as an employee, could still remain on Kern View's active medical staff with admitting privileges and policy setting roles. This organizational design created a situation in which community physicians who were members of an active medical staff, unhappy with the board of directors' policies and decisions, together with physicians previously employed by the center whose contracts had not been renewed, were now in a position to take action on professional policy matters outside of Kern View's administrative structure. The seriousness of this problem quickly became evident when Kosewick's application for active medical staff status as medical director of Kern View was not approved by Kern View's medical staff. In fact, Kosewick was appointed to the medical staff only after the board of directors took action to override the medical staff's recommendation.

Questions related to the medical staff's scope of responsibility continued to be a source of constant debate. In fact, the members of the medical staff could not agree among themselves regarding the extent of their involvement. Over this ten-year period of time (1969-79), the one issue which surfaced more than any other was the scope of responsibility of the medical staff in relation to Kern View's board of directors and administration, and this issue persistently permeated the entire operation of the center.

Growth and Expansion

The NIMH grant requirements for the development of community mental health services and related requirements for the composition of governing and advisory bodies also continued to influence

Kern View significantly. The board of directors tried to identify new directors as well as to establish advisory councils reflective of the ethnic, racial, sexual, and vocational distribution found in the West Kern Catchment Area. Over a period of years the wide geographical area from which board members came, including the southern California region, was narrowed and limited entirely to Kern County.

Under the leadership of Sigmund Kosewick, the medical director, Ernest M. Solano, then chief of social services, and Larry R. Yoder, administrator, the community mental health center program again moved forward with the center receiving its first accreditation from the Joint Commission on Accreditation of Hospitals in 1972.

Throughout the 1970s there was considerable program development in many areas. The day treatment service was expanded to include adolescents, and through a contract with the Kern County High School District an integrated treatment and educational program was developed. In addition, this grant-funded relationship with the high school district enabled Kern View to establish two group homes for adolescents, one for boys and one for girls. Outpatient services for adults were also expanded during this period with the re-establishment of a Bakersfield clientele, which had been lost when the psychiatrists left, and the opening of satellite clinics in the outlying communities of Delano and Wasco. The latter two projects were made possible through a contract with Kern County Department of Mental Health and a poverty grant from NIMH, respectively, and enabled Kern View to better serve the Mexican-American and underprivileged populations of Kern County.

This period of growth in the 1970s also saw the opening of a methadone treatment program, expanded services to both geriatrics and the chronically mentally ill, the opening of a community home to help formerly institutionalized persons learn to live independently, and expanding outreach efforts through the consultation and education services. Needless to say, these various expansions seriously strained the space capacities of Kern View's facilities. As a result, some additions were made in 1970 (craft room, storage space, and offices) and in 1973 (a classroom, multipurpose room, offices). In 1976, with the assistance of an NIMH construction grant, a major building project was initiated. In the fall of 1977 new outpatient offices, a new administration building, and remodeled inpatient facilities were dedicated for use. For the first time, Kern View's facilities nearly matched its program needs.

As implied already, much of the program and facility growth was only possible through expanded contracts with Kern County Department of Mental Health Services and renewed funding from

NIMH. In fact, in 1974 the board of directors applied for an NIMH continuation staffing grant since the initial grant was expiring and it did not appear that either the state or the county was prepared to fill the financial gap. The continuation grant was awarded and provided Kern View with an additional eight years of NIMH funding.

Another significant development for Kern View in the 1970s was the growth of its public information department, which by late 1970 had become an integral part of the overall operation. In fact, in 1980 Kern View was granted the Public Information Award by the National Council of Community Mental Health Centers for the best public information program of a medium-size community mental health center.

While Rosalyn Carter was campaigning in California on behalf of Jimmy Carter in the fall of 1976, she requested to visit Kern View Mental Health Center, and after touring the facilities, she spoke briefly to the crowd that had assembled. At that time, she announced that if her husband was elected president, he would again authorize a careful analysis of our country's services to the mentally ill. As it turned out, this announcement at Kern View foreshadowed the Mental Health Systems Act of 1980.

— Larry Yoder

Growing Skepticism About Public Funding

After the board experienced the anticipated loss of NIMH funding in 1974, even though it did not occur, the directors began to focus their concerns about future funding bases. The result was the development of a second corporation known as the *Kern View Foundation* for the sole purpose of fund raising on behalf of Kern View. This foundation was incorporated in 1975 and activated with thirty trustees representing the leading citizens of the Bakersfield-Kern County community. Through direct solicitation and a major "Kern View Estate Project" the foundation had raised over $80,000 by 1980. This money was used to begin the Kern View Endowment Fund which continues to grow significantly.

Besides the threatened expiration of the federal grant in 1974, there were other problems related to public monies—specifically, audit exceptions. In the summer of 1975, Kern View was notified by the Kern County Mental Health Department that the state had made audit exceptions for four years (1969-1974) totaling approximately $260,000. In effect the state was saying that funds in that amount, which Kern View received through county contracts, had to be paid back. Much of this was related to the fact that Kern View had

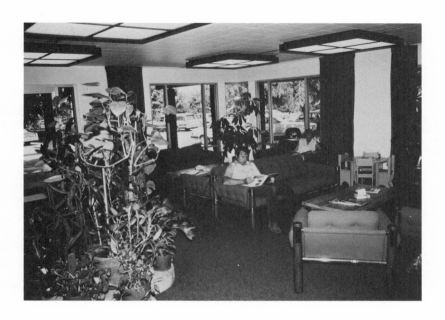

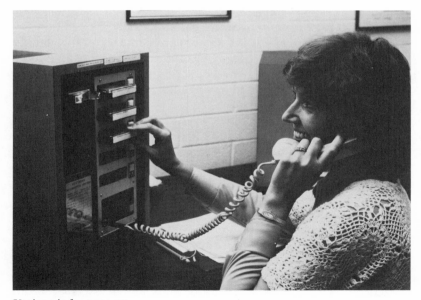

Various indoor scenes .

received a federal staffing grant, an amount by which the state wanted to reduce its obligation to Kern View as a contractor. By engaging a firm with experience in government funding mechanisms, Kern View obtained a significant reduction in the audit exceptions. However, an amount of approximately $180,000, related to the federal grant issue, remained.

After lying dormant a few years, the issue was reactivated late in 1978 when the county of Kern requested payment of this audit exception. The board of directors immediately took action in January 1979 and agreed to file suite against the state and the county, believing that the federal NIMH grant was given to Kern View to develop a community mental health center and that as "seed money" the grant was not intended to reduce the state's obligation. Late in 1979, Kern View received a favorable decision which canceled all audit exceptions that were related to the treatment of the federal grant by the state. Notwithstanding this favorable outcome, the experience with California's Department of Mental Health served to strengthen both the board's and the administrator's growing skepticism of public monies as major funding bases.

Through revenue produced from its inpatient services, Kern View was able to develop a privately funded base of approximately 50 percent, which provided some stability for its services. The directors and administration continued to be concerned about the uncertainty of services which were heavily dependent upon federal and state funding. Developing services and then dropping them when government funding disappeared not only created hardship for Kern View but also had a very negative impact on the community. By the late 1970s the board and administrator were identifying goals for the center which would provide greater stability of services and less dependence upon federal grants.

Changing Medical Leadership

Although Kern View's administration remained stable under Larry Yoder throughout the 1970s, its clinical leadership changed hands frequently. The demand for psychiatric time had become extremely burdensome to Sigmund Kosewick within a short time of his appointment in 1970. It was not until 1972 that the medical director was given some relief by the addition of a second full-time psychiatrist. Also, Antonio Perelli-Minetti, Jr., a Bakersfield psychiatrist, joined the staff part-time, taking time from his private practice to assist with the inpatient load. This appeared to be a step forward in improving Kern View's relationship to the local private-practicing psychiatrists. Even though additional psychiatric time was made available, the load on Kosewick as medical director became too much. He resigned as medical director in the summer of 1973, but continued at Kern View as a staff psychiatrist. Albert Sheff, another psychiatrist, was then recruited for the medical directorship and served in this capacity until the fall of 1974. His specialty was primarily related to quality assurance programs and he was able to offer Kern View guidance and leadership in this area. Perelli-Minetti became medical director on a part-time basis upon the resignation of Sheff. He was assisted by Ernest Solano, who served as associate clinical director.

In 1978, the decision was made to change the title of medical director to clinical director to more clearly define the role and scope of that position at the center; nonetheless, the position continued to be filled by a psychiatrist. Late that same year, Kern View's general and clinical administration agreed that Kern View was of sufficient size that there should be one full-time clinical director as compared to a part-time director and an associate director. In addition, Perelli-Minetti had other interests he wished to pursue and as a result was willing to step out of his clinical director position. Recruitment began but the scene had changed. Legislation had been passed in California which required any private agency contracting for state funds to recruit the best qualified mental health professional for any administrative position from the professions of psychiatry, psychology, and social work. As a contracting agency, Kern View had to announce and recruit from these disciplines for a full-time clinical director.

Summary

During this ten-year period (1969-79) Kern View was able to add services and facilities largely because of its financial support from the National Institute of Mental Health. It became much better known throughout Kern County through the efforts of the Kern View public information service and the Kern View Foundation. Other than having the constituent churches represented on its board, the center's relationship to the local Mennonite churches was minimal. For Kern View, the broad-based Kern View Foundation was a greater support group than the sponsoring church constituency.

Major Period of Transition (1979-1981)

A New Clinical Director

Kerry T. Yamada, a clinical psychologist who had previously held positions at the University of California at Los Angeles and several community mental health centers, was employed as Kern

View's full-time clinical director in November 1979. Yamada was Kern View's first clinical director who was not a psychiatrist. Reaction to the appointment was strong, both from the employed staff, who felt that the board and administration should not have hired from outside the agency, and from the psychiatrists, who believed the clinical directorship should only be filled by a psychiatrist.

Yamada attempted to implement policy to better integrate the professional groups of psychiatry, psychology, and social work, but these were fought and rejected. Changes in medical staff bylaws, which would allow psychologists and social workers the latitude to work within their scope of licensure, were also rejected and became major issues of disagreement between administration and the active medical staff.[21]

Since Kern View was a very small organization, the clinical director established one multidisciplinary meeting of staff rather than having each discipline meet separately. Meetings of such groups as the social workers or psychologists at this time had turned into political action gatherings rather than professional development meetings and there was considerable staff discontent. The multidiscipline approach was seen as a move to erode power bases for the disciplines. Some unhappiness continued about the hiring of an "outside" clinical director. As a result there even was an effort to organize a union at Kern View, but this was successfully defeated in an election held in December 1980.

Old issues with the medical staff, never fully resolved, again surfaced. The board again had to deal with the attitude of the psychiatric community, which included some of the same persons who had expressed their desires in 1963 and who continued on the active medical staff. The new clinical director was unable to implement policies to improve patient care when the recommended changes could be rejected by the active medical staff. Administration found it increasingly difficult to meet accreditation standards as recommended policies were frequently rejected. Since there was more than a ten-year history of various attempts to resolve the issues between the medical staff and the board of directors with only minimal success, the administrator and the clinical director recommended to the board of directors that Kern View actively consider moving toward a closed staff at some point in the future. The board accepted this recommendation in October 1980.

The reaction of the medical staff was severe. Several psychiatrists who were on the medical staff at Kern View were also officers of the Kern County Medical Society, and they chose to use their positions to involve the entire medical society. They announced that Kern View had "closed" its staff, when in fact, the board had agreed only to consider moving in that direction. In the winter of 1980 private-practicing psychiatrists in the community did not admit patients for approximately two months, and this had a significant negative financial impact on the center.

New Opportunities

Out of crisis, however, came opportunity. The West Kern Counseling Center, located in Taft, obtained funding from Kern County Department of Mental Health Service and became an immediately viable service for that underserved community. As positions became available within the center, new professional staff could be hired who were supportive of administrative directions and who wanted to move toward a more private "entrepreneur" agency stance as compared to that of a quasi-public agency. A group home for six girls was opened on the Kern View campus, funded by contracts with the local probation and welfare departments. Many contracts were also made with private industry to promote the sale of employee assistance programs, which eventually led to contracts with Kern View. And most significantly, a program for alcoholism treatment was transferred from a hospital in Delano into the underutilized inpatient facilities.

With all the changes that were brought about in a relatively short period of time in early 1981, Kern View began changing as an organization. The new programs added financial stability which Kern View had never really enjoyed before. Staff members were encouraged with the new developments and worked hard at upgrading programs and services.

Through the experiences of 1980, the board of directors began reviewing how organizational structure and the definition of professional relationships affect the overall operation of the center. Active medical staff was defined as open only to psychiatrists and licensed clinical psychologists who were employed or under contract to Kern View. The relationship of the clinical director to the president of the medical staff was also defined. The active medical staff was to be a policy setting body and the courtesy medical staff privilege was to be available to all private practicing psychiatrists applying for admitting privileges, provided they agreed to abide by the bylaws, rules, and regulations of the medical staff. This was an attempt to solve a long-standing problem at Kern View. Whether it successfully brings about resolution in the long run will have to be judged at a later date, because at the time of this writing these changes are just being implemented.

Patrick C. Barker, a psychologist on the staff of Kern View, was appointed clinical director upon the resignation of Terry Yamada in

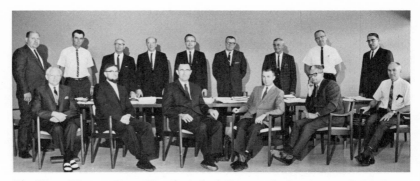

The Kings View — Kern View board of directors before it was divided into separate boards, c. 1966. **Standing** *(l.-r.) Roy Fast, Orland Friesen, John Bartel, Abe Ediger, Edwin Wiens, Arthur Jost (Kings View Administrator), John C. Penner, Clayton Auernheimer, Daniel Horst.* **Seated** *(l.-r.) Henry Brandt, Harvey Dyck, Henry Hooge (Kern View Administrator), Allen Linscheid (Kings View Assistant Administrator), William Klassen (MMHS Director), Victor Janzen.*

1981. Barker was thus the sixth clinical (or medical) director to work with Larry Yoder, administrator, since 1969.

1981 and the Future

At the time of this writing, Kern View is preparing to function without a federal grant. This is a new experience since Kern View has had an NIMH grant for its entire history, 1966 to 1982. Although the grant has been extremely beneficial to Kern View in its development and growth, it also tended to develop a public agency attitude. Kern View is preparing itself for the loss of the federal grant by promoting and marketing revenue-producing services such as alcoholism treatment and employee assistance programs, and by expanding referral sources for its patient treatment programs by communication with nonpsychiatric physicians, nonmedical therapists, clergy and churches, schools, other mental health services, and private industry.

For the first time, the board of directors feels free to establish its own identity outside of the guidelines of NIMH. The board is again evaluating its own identity and its relationship to MMHS. There is greater awareness of the center's historical roots and a renewed interest in maintaining this voluntary fraternal relationship with MMHS and the consortium of mental health centers under the MMHS umbrella.[22]

In Kern View's first fifteen years, more than 10,000 patients have been treated, and Kern View has become well established in the Bakersfield-Kern County community and has been highly successful in its public information efforts. It has been successful in developing community support through the Kern View Foundation. It has attempted, in various ways, to address the original concerns of the private-practicing psychiatrists in Bakersfield. In 1982 Kern View enters a new era. Indications are that there has been sufficient preparation to cope with changing funding patterns and that overall Kern View will be stronger as a private agency, with the board of directors developing a greater sense of identity and determination. Time, professional relationships, economic conditions, community environment, and leadership will all influence Kern View's next chapter.

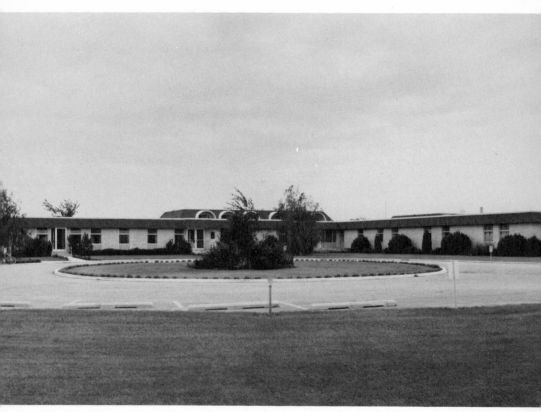

Front view of Eden M. H. Centre.

CHAPTER 10

Eden Mental Health Centre Winkler, Manitoba

Gerhard John Ens*

The motto of Eden Mental Health Centre, "Let us do good unto all men," accurately reflects the central mission of the center throughout the fifteen years of its history. Conceived and born in the Mennonite community of southern Manitoba, with deep roots and a long tradition of caring and serving, Eden has provided a wide range of mental health services for all persons in its service area.

Eden was officially opened and dedicated at its present site in the town of Winkler on June 3, 1967. Six weeks earlier on April 24 the first seven patients had been admitted from Selkirk Hospital of Mental Diseases. Thirty-eight other patients were subsequently admitted that first year, representing in large part Mennonite patients transferred from hospitals in Brandon and Selkirk, and Bethesda Hospital in Vineland, Ontario, as well as new admissions from the Winkler, Altona, and Steinbach area.

A venture between eight Manitoba Mennonite conferences and churches[1] and the government of Manitoba, Eden represented a modern church-oriented mental health facility featuring both inpatient and outpatient treatment. Eden's stated purpose was to serve the community by providing facilities and staff for the comprehensive care of the mentally ill and to work at the prevention of mental illness in the community. As such it was in the forefront of the development of Mennonite mental health services in Canada and in step with the latest policies on the Manitoba government. Operated as a private nonprofit corporation, Eden provided mental health services with an overall Christian emphasis, not only for Mennonites but for other south central area Manitobans as well.

The establishment of Eden Mental Health Centre did not occur suddenly in 1967, but was the result of ten years of arduous work

*Gerhard John Ens is a graduate student in history at the University of Manitoba.

and planning by dedicated Mennonite leaders. It also involved the gradual education of Manitoba Mennonites to the realities of mental health care, and the growing cooperation and coordination with government health services. Eden's history must be seen in the context of the development of mental health services among the Mennonites and the general development of mental health care in Manitoba and Canada.

(J. M. Pauls) came into many homes, I guess they were referred to him by the pastors or ministers, and saw how these people were treated in isolation and lonely... The attitude that Mennonites took to mental health! That when a child was retarded—or here was a mental patient—they were hidden, it was secret... He came into homes and found, yes, somewhere in the attic or in the back room, this family had a person that was mentally ill.

He visited a patient that he knew in the Brandon mental institute and found out there how Mennonite people were treated. Religious materials were taken away, their Bibles were taken away, and he felt that that was unfair for people raised in a Christian setting to be treated that way when they were mentally ill.

—J. F. Pauls[2]

Mennonite Roots

The Eden motto initially might well have included the remainder of Galatians 6:10, that is, "...especially of the household of faith," for the impetus to establish the center came from the Mennonites' concern for their own members. Care for the mentally ill was not a new concern among Mennonites. From its beginnings, the Anabaptist-Mennonite movement had been characterized by the practice of mutual aid. A sharing in the physical needs of others was simply an integral part of genuine Christianity.[3] As early as 1910, the Mennonites had established Bethania Hospital, an institution for the mentally ill, along the Dnieper River in South Russia (see chapter 1).

In Manitoba, however, such concern was slow to develop. The Mennonites who immigrated to Manitoba in the 1870s were generally poor and not familiar with ideas of care for the mentally ill. Furthermore, the group remained in large part isolated from the rest of society in their "line villages," a pattern they brought with them from Russia. Even among themselves, certain colonies maintained separate identities, so communication and cooperation was difficult or lacking altogether.

The Russian Mennonites who came to Manitoba in the 1920s were more familiar with mental health care because of Bethania

Hospital. They also, however, were not well-to-do. The depression that followed in the 1930s made matters worse and the Mennonites found themselves struggling for bare existence, thus postponing any extensive effort at mutual aid. Many of these later immigrants, especially those settling in the villages of the West Reserve, came with the idea of re-establishing a Mennonite commonwealth in southern Manitoba, and gave new vigor to village life in Manitoba, delaying the integration of the Mennonites into the broader society. It was only after World War II that the economic climate of Manitoba improved, allowing new vistas to open for increased Mennonite involvement and service.

During the war approximately one hundred Mennonite conscientious objectors worked in the province's three mental institutions. While this type of service was more prevalent and important in the United States than in Canada, it still had some effect in making Mennonites realize that better care was needed for the mentally ill.[4]

They brought this concern to the leaders of the churches, whether something could not be done to help the mental patients who were in those institutions who were of Mennonite background. Because, obviously, there were quite a few in those institutions, because the Mennonite people are not exempt from mental breakdowns either. So that was actually the impetus that created or started this movement to begin the mental hospital primarily for the Mennonite people.
—Ben Braun[5]

In the United States, the experience in state mental hospitals led more directly to establishing the first Mennonite-sponsored hospitals there, Brook Lane in 1949, Kings View in 1951, Philhaven Hospital in 1952 and Prairie View in 1954 (see previous chapters on each).

The need for better mental health care became more apparent in the 1950s. A number of Mennonites were hospitalized in government institutions which often proved to be an alien, if not hostile, environment. Relatives at times were unhappy with the care provided, especially when these patients showed little improvement.[6] Moreover, there were few satisfactory alternatives. Mennonite nursing homes would not accept mentally ill persons, who often were difficult to manage. The only Mennonite mental institution in Canada at the time was in Vineland, Ontario, too far for many Mennonites to be separated from their family members. This option was made even more difficult when government legislation refused financial aid to Manitoba residents in mental institutions outside the province. Concerned that the spiritual needs of the mental patients must also be met, Mennonite leaders in Manitoba resolved to explore instituting a Mennonite mental hospital.

Ten Years of Planning (1957-66)

Ten years to start a program—why so long? In retrospect one can note a number of obstacles, each requiring considerable time and effort to resolve. Three major tasks were getting the several Mennonite groups together to cooperate in the project, negotiating with the government for its cooperation and support, and agreeing on what kind of institution to establish. Achieving the goal of a mental health facility could not be accomplished overnight. Time was needed for the idea to grow and mature before it could become a reality.

Mennonite Cooperation

The possibility of establishing a mental institution was first formally broached at the annual meeting of the Mennonite Relief Committee on January 19, 1957. Over the next several months Archie Penner, John P. Loewen and P. J. B. Reimer, ministers of the Evangelical Mennonite Conference (EMC), held meetings to discuss and promote the idea of a mental hospital. Convinced that the project was too ambitious for one conference to manage by itself, they appointed a five-man committee to explore inter-Mennonite involvement. Among those contacted was Bishop J. M. Pauls, the spokesman for the Manitoba Bergthaler group. This interview in turn led to a wider forum for discussion when a general meeting was called in the EMC Church at Rosenort on May 11, 1957, for representatives of all Mennonite churches in Manitoba. Sixty-seven persons attended this meeting, representing the Evangelical Mennonite Church, Bergthaler, Blumenorter, Whitewater, Niverville, Lichtenauer, Steinbach, Bethel Mennonite Church in Winnipeg, Arnaud, and Elim congregations. Here the need for a Mennonite mental hospital was affirmed and a study group of five persons, headed by Pauls and Reimer, was elected to make further investigations and do preparatory work.[7] Pauls, having played a large role in getting the various Mennonite churches in the Winkler area to cooperate in building the Salem Home for the Aged, was particularly instrumental in getting the various conferences to work together to establish Eden.

It is perhaps fortunate that this attempt to gain wider Mennonite involvement occurred precisely at the time when greater inter-Mennonite cooperation was being experienced in other areas.[8]

In June of the same year ten members were added to the study

The biggest obstacle was the working together with other churches. That was very new at that time. We hadn't had any prior experience, outside of a little bit of MCC. *That was to convince all the different conferences that, yes, this is what we need. That was a big obstacle. And there my father (J. M. Pauls) pioneered a lot, he laid a lot of ground work.*

—*J. F. Pauls*[9]

committee. The larger group was more formally organized on July 2 with separate committees elected to work on building and financial planning, with an executive committee headed by Pauls as chairman and Reimer as secretary to take overall responsibility. From this point on meetings were held regularly and delegations were sent to the different churches to promote the idea among the membership. Delegations also visited Prairie View Hospital in Kansas and Bethesda Hospital in Ontario to investigate their operations and note possible applicability to the Manitoba situation.

The committee was aware from the first of the distinction between an active treatment clinic and a custodial care home, but favored the latter where the chronic mentally ill Mennonites could be cared for. As already noted, Mennonite experience in government institutions in Manitoba had been such that the leaders were determined to establish an institution where at least their own members could get loving care.[10] There were some in the churches and on the committee who were critical of this limited goal, but in large part it represented the desires of the majority. By 1958 the committee had decided that the new proposed institution would have seventy-five to one hundred beds and would be called the *Mennonite Sanitarium of Manitoba.* (MSM)

Contacts with Government
It was not until the committee of this proposed sanitarium began meeting regularly with representatives of the Manitoba government regarding grants for the building and ongoing operation of the institution that the concept of custodial care began to change. When the Mennonites in the Winkler area built the Salem Home, they had contacted the provincial government regarding grants and subsidies. The favorable hearing they received at that time was in many ways a breakthrough for the leaders in dealing with the government and provided a stepping-stone for negotiations regarding Eden.[11]

So it was natural that J. M. Pauls, who had worked with the Salem project, and members of the committee should meet with

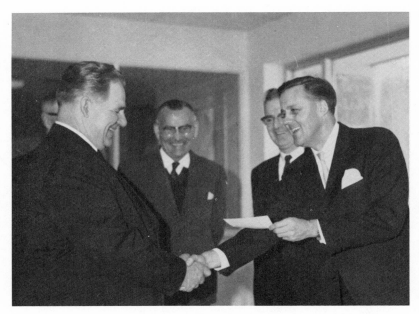

Presentation of Eden M.H. Centre from the federal and provincial governments, December 23, 1966. Standing (l.-r.), I. R. Dyck, Eden board chairman; Dr. E. Johnson, Provincial Director of Psychiatry; Dr. Morrison, Deputy Minister; and the Honourable C. H. Witney, Minister of Health.

Robert Bend, then Minister of Health for Manitoba. This meeting took place on May 23, 1957. They found the government representatives sympathetic and supportive, though unwilling to make any firm commitment for financial assistance. Discussions with T. A. Pincock, the provincial psychiatrist, led the delegates to believe that the most practical type of institution would be in the form of a convalescent home. This advice may have been given because Psychiatric Services was unsure whether Mennonites would have the skills and trained personnel to run an active treatment center, but it also may have represented the provincial policy at that time.

In 1958 the Manitoba government changed hands with the election of the Conservative party led by Duff Roblin. When this new administration re-evaluated its health program, the result was a change in mental health policy. No doubt the revolution in mental health care in North America, with the beginning of the community mental health movement, was having its effect.

Up until 1920 mental health care in Manitoba had consisted of placing patients in institutions at Selkirk and Brandon which accommodated the greatest number of patients possible. The years between the wars was a period of gradual disenchantment with the "asylum." New psychiatric units were established and new treatments were initiated, but this did not stop the burgeoning patient populations in Selkirk and Brandon.[12] The first seeds of a changing policy were sown when after the Second World War the federal government initiated a series of national health grants to extend public health to veterans. At this point, Pincock planned psychiatric services which were not limited to institutional care. Yet the growing disdain for custodial care did not significantly change treatment in Canadian psychiatric hospitals, as most remained largely custodial institutions.

The introduction of new tranquilizer drugs in the late 1950s and early 1960s permitted more effective treatment and symptomatic management of many psychotic patients. Moreover, the adoption of new methods of treatment, which focused on social psychology and group techniques, had enormous effects on mental health policy.[13] These innovations, along with official censure of custodial-care hospitals, led to a policy of de-institutionalization in Manitoba. Chronically ill, long-stay patients were given "remotivation therapy" and returned to the community.[14] From 1960 on Manitoba's resident population in mental hospitals dropped radically, from over three thousand in 1960 to under one thousand in 1978.

A Changing Concept of Care

It was in this context of change that the committee formed to establish a Mennonite sanitarium petitioned the Manitoba government for aid to establish a custodial care hospital. Laregly unaware of contemporary developments in mental health care, the committee was pursuing a course already proved unsatisfactory. As late as 1962, Eden was still slated to become a custodial care home for patients who would not respond to active treatment at other hospitals, even though the government was counseling Eden to keep open the possibility of developing into a mental health clinic.[15] The patient population in Selkirk and Brandon was decreasing rapidly by 1962, so from the province's point of view there was no need for another custodial care facility.

In 1963 the center board seemed to budge a little from its position, and included plans for an outpatient treatment clinic. By September 1963 the government had committed substantial aid, but only on condition that the center become a clinic staffed by a provincial psychiatrist, not be identified as a Mennonite institution, and serve as a regional community mental health center. The name of the proposed institution was subsequently changed to *Eden Mental*

---

*There was a new chief psychiatrist of the province who had to also give
his consent to plans that were being made. And the first time that I
had opportunity to meet with him and his associates, he threw over
our plans completely. In fact when we presented our plan that we had
of building such an institution, it was supposed to be a two-story
building and I think we had rough sketch drawings of it already...
And he looked at us and he said, "Whoever condoned these plans
should be shot!" And of course we were shocked, I guess, we laughed,
but I guess we were a bit disturbed. And then he came out with what
he meant and explained to us that in our day they were not prepared to
support a plan like this...*

—J. K. Klassen[16]

Health Centre from its original designation as *Mennonite Sanitarium of
Manitoba.*

Now the board of Eden was faced with the problem of not only
reorienting its own thinking but also selling this change in concept
to the churches. This was not easy, since many of the older Mennonites felt that this change would only further delay a project already
long overdue.[17] As late as 1964 congregational delegates indicated
that their members still favored a custodial care home over a modern
mental health clinic. This led the board to reconsider its plans, but
the Manitoba government refused to move from its position and to
agree to any reduction in the scope of services.

Another factor in the campaign to establish a Mennonite mental health center in Manitoba, and in changing the attitude toward
treatment of the mentally ill, was the role of Mennonite Mental
Health Services (MMHS), an arm of MCC. Early in the discussions, in
the fall of 1957, Orie Miller, then executive secretary of MCC, was
invited by Mennonite leaders in Manitoba to confer with them
regarding the proposal to build a mental health facility.[18] In 1964 H.
Clair Amstutz, chairman of the MMHS board, spent eleven days in
Manitoba discussing the proposed mental hospital on invitation of
Eden's board and the Canadian Mennonite Relief Committee.[19]
Similarly between 1963 and 1965 William Klassen, also affiliated
with MMHS, visited Winnipeg and southern Manitoba on numerous
occasions speaking to and advising Eden's board on the role of
Christianity and the church in psychiatry, and the benefits of an
active treatment center. Klassen, having been trained at the Men-
ninger Foundation in Topeka, Kansas, was familiar with the latest
developments in the field of mental health. Sponsored by some
Mennonite churches in Winnipeg, Klassen not only informed
Eden's board about the programs administered by Mennonite men-

tal health centers in the United States, but also supported the current plans to make Eden an active treatment center.

Planning and Construction

During this time board members also were trying to choose a site for the center. By May 10, 1958, the MSM Committee was considering several sites with preference given to a farm in the vicinity of Morris. *Peck Farms*, as it was known, was in a central location but proved to be poorly situated to make use of the sewer and water services by the town of Morris. This along with the limited support base of the Mennonite churches in the Morris-Rosenort area led the committee to look elsewhere.[20] The site that was finally chosen was farmland owned by W. C. Enns near the Salem Home for the Aged on the outskirts of Winkler. The main attraction of this location was its reasonable purchase price and its close proximity to a large center of Mennonite population. Other possibilities looked into at that time were the purchase of the Steinbach Hospital and a Morden area farm, and developing a psychiatric ward in conjunction with Concordia Hospital in Winnipeg. For various reasons none of these alternatives proved feasible.[21] Having decided on the Winkler site, the MSM Committee purchased thirty acres for $6,000, half of the actual value of the land.

By 1964 both the site and the nature of the institution had been determined, and all that remained was to make financial arrangements with the government and member congregations. Throughout the late 1950s and early 1960s the government had maintained that no financial assistance would be available for construction before 1968,[22] but as it became clear that Eden would be a community mental health center, federal and provincial funds were made available almost immediately.

On April 16, 1964, the Manitoba legislature passed "An Act to incorporate Eden Mental Health Centre." Legal responsibility was lodged in a seventeen-member board of directors. At a historic meeting on July 25, 250 to 300 delegates representing the different Mennonite conferences and churches in Manitoba accepted the "draft regulations" proposed by the government for the incorporation of Eden, later finalized in a Memorandum of Agreement and duly signed February 15, 1965. In response to the commitment to raise at least 25 percent of the construction funds, the delegates agreed to an annual contribution of $1.50 for each church member for ten years and authorized the board members to canvass conferences and churches who had not yet committed themselves to the project. It was further agreed that Eden was to be a fifty-bed institution providing facilities for "accommodation, psychiatric care and treatment of persons with mental diseases or disorders of the mind," and also "to provide facilities in the institution for a community mental health clinic."[23]

Planning continued and soon construction began. Walter Katelnikoff and Associates was awarded the architect's contract. The building plans were altered at one point to change the proposed building from two stories to one and the plans received government approval. Construction began in May of 1966; the sod-turning ceremony had taken place on April 25. The approved cost of the building project was almost $700,000, with the federal and provincial governments assuming 75 percent of the cost and the participating conferences and churches paying 25 percent or approximately $175,000. The building provided 32,464 square feet of floor space with an inpatient capacity of fifty-four beds and facilities for outpatient services. Built of steel, cement and tyndale stone, the facilities were ready for the first patients in April 1967.

Eden's History (1967-81)

Eden's fifteen years of operation fit into three rather distinct periods. The years 1967 to 71 were years of early growth, coinciding with the appointment of Eden's first medical director, Clarence Labun, and the establishment of Eden's initial policy and program. With the death of Dr. Labun in 1972 and the inability to find a successor, the center lost much of its direction and continuity. This adversely affected the center's effectiveness, and the years 1972 to 75 saw Eden's admissions drop steadily. The last period beginning in 1976 and carrying through 1981 was one of renewed growth and direction, marked by the coming of Henry Guenther as medical director and the creation of the new position of executive director.

Years of Early Growth

By the time Eden opened its doors in 1967, the leadership of the board had undergone considerable change. J. M. Pauls, the leader during the early years of planning, had been replaced by J. K. Klassen in 1961. With the founding of the center assured, Klassen had resigned in 1965 to take a pastorate in Vineland, Ontario. He was replaced by I. R. Dyck who served until June 1967, when Ben Braun was elected chairman for Eden's first year of operation.

The first concern of the board was the recruitment of staff. Arnold Schroeder was hired as administrator in December 1966, before the center opened. John Kroeker was appointed director of social work and Tom Faulkner director of nursing. No full-time psychiatrist could be found to fill the position of medical director, largely because of the center's rural location and remoteness from larger urban centers.[24]

On April 24, 1967, our first patients arrived. They came from Selkirk, Brandon, and Vineland, Ontario. They were the kind of patients who we refer to as chronic mentally ill, meaning that they have been in mental hospitals a long time, one of them since 1933. This type of patient has improved, some considerably more than others. Two have been discharged from the hospital. One of them will be going home to relatives in the near future, others we expect will be placed in foster homes and Old Folks' Homes... The balance of our patients have been, what we call, acute mentally ill. They enter the hospital from four to eight weeks and are discharged.

—Arnold Schroeder[25]

With the admission of the first patients in April, Eden's board of directors became increasingly concerned about the planning and implementation of a comprehensive program without the services of a full-time medical director and psychiatrist. The center was served three half-days per week by psychiatrists provided by the provincial government, among them W. A. Large, Gordon Smith, Henry Guenther and Edward Johnson. Yet the program suffered from a shortage of psychiatric services. As the patient load increased, appointments had to be made four to five weeks in advance and the center's follow-up program was in need of improvement.

During the year and a half without a medical director, the staff of the center nevertheless worked steadily at community education and at providing inpatient and outpatient services. The first admissions to Eden had been chronic long-term patients from other institutions, but over the next few years more and more short-term acute-care patients were admitted and outpatient services were expanded.

One of the other early acts of the board of Eden Mental Health Centre was to affiliate itself with MMHS on the basis of an associate membership. The MMHS board, supervising the five Mennonite mental health centers in the United States founded and sponsored by MCC, offered valuable contacts and advice to Eden. The center was unable to join the organization as a full member because the operation of the center was completely financed by the government of Manitoba, while the United States Mennonite centers were MCC-founded and sponsored. Moreover, while the government was not openly against membership in MMHS, it was certainly not prepared to pay the substantial membership fee.[26] When Eden did affiliate

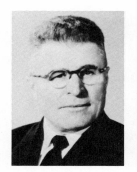

Pauls

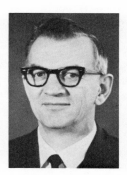

J. Klassen

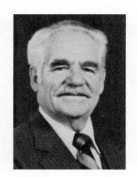

Dyck

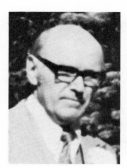

Braun

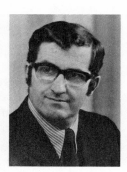

Friesen

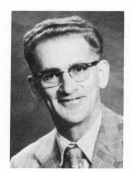

Hamm

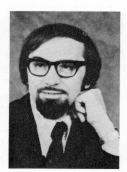

Rempel

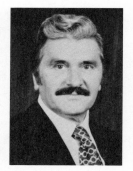

Enns

Board Chairmen: *Bishop J. M. Pauls (1957-61), Rev. Jake K. Klassen (1961-65), Mr. I. R. Dyck (1965-67), Mr. Ben Braun (1967-70), Rev. Henry V. Friesen (1970-71), Mr. Otto Hamm (1971-72), Mr. Ben Braun (1972-74), Mr. Helmut Klassen, no picture (1974-77), Rev. Cornie Rempel (1977-79), and Mr. Ernest Enns (1979-81).*

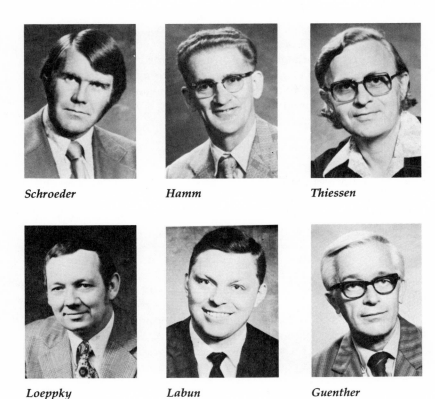

Schroeder   *Hamm*   *Thiessen*

Loeppky   *Labun*   *Guenther*

Executive Directors: *Mr. Arnold Schroeder (1966-72), Mr. Otto Hamm (1972-76), Mr. Ben Thiessen (1976-79), and Mr. Bernie Loeppky (1979-   ).*

Medical Directors: *Dr. Clarence Labun (1969-72) and Dr. Henry Guenther (1976-81).*

itself with MMHS in 1968, it did so with the cooperation and financial help of MCC (Canada).

In 1969 Clarence Labun was appointed medical director of Eden Mental Health Center. Eden's programs were re-evaluated, and an attempt was made to define whom the center served, whom it wanted to serve, and what the role of the church was in its program. Shortly after Labun's appointment a program to teach counseling techniques to ministers in the area was initiated by John White, a psychiatrist. Included in this education program were topics related to psychiatry and religion designed to enable pastors to recognize problems in mental health, to deal with them personally, and to help them refer patients for further treatment.

To provide more time and better service for the acutely ill, many chronically ill inpatients were discharged to nursing homes, foster homes and other facilities on an ongoing basis. The number of admissions to Eden continued to rise, reaching a peak in 1971. By this time, the center also had begun to consider applying for accreditation, both to assure the public and funding bodies of the quality of the institution, and to attract professional staff and teaching affiliations with universities.

Difficult Years

The development of Eden took an abrupt turn after 1971. Clarence Labun fell ill in early 1972 and died of cancer a few months later, leaving the center without a full-time psychiatrist and medical director. His death in June 1972 was followed by the resignation of Arnold Schroeder in November. So the loss of medical leadership was compounded by a change in administration. Otto Hamm, chairman of the Eden board from 1971 to 1972 and administrator of nearby Morden General Hospital, was asked to replace Schroeder as Eden's administrator, but on a half-time basis for a six-month experimental period. Hamm divided his time equally in running the two institutions. This arrangement continued until 1976.

The distress created by Labun's death was intensified by funding problems that arose after 1971. Lack of a medical director hampered the center both financially and in overall direction. Eden's funding from the provincial government was based on a per diem rate for patient days and on outpatient visits to the psychiatrist. By 1971 Eden had discharged many of its first long-term chronically ill patients to personal care homes and this, along with steadily decreasing admissions, helped create a funding problem. Without a full-time psychiatrist to assess and treat potential patients, the center was unable to admit many new patients.[27] While the number of outpatients expanded throughout the 1970s, this did not take up the slack in funding because payment for outpatient sessions was based on visits to the psychiatrist. Since there was no full-time psychiatrist at Eden between 1972 and 1976, many visits were handled by social workers and were therefore not billable.

Eden's problem during these years, however, was not only financial but also the lack of clear purpose and direction. A government study of mental health services in Manitoba in 1973 reported that the development of Eden was hindered by the absence of clearly defined goals and responsibilities. During the center's early development, no one had defined its relation to other government programs and Eden had not been assigned responsibility for any "catchment area." The study went on to recommend the reorganization and regionalization of government mental health services, suggesting that Eden become a regional inpatient facility for the south central region of Manitoba. But responsibility for community mental health services was not delegated.[28]

As these government programs were slowly introduced, Eden began to define a dual catchment area. The immediate area included a population of some thirty to forty thousand. Within this region Eden took on the responsibilites for community mental health. This included hospital care, outpatient clinic services, follow-up and foster home placements. Some 25 to 30 percent of Eden's patients came from this defined area. The secondary area included persons from throughout the province of Manitoba as well as a small percentage from other geographic areas. Follow-up and foster home placement in the secondary catchment area was generally seen as the responsibility of provincial community mental health workers.

Another issue emerged during this period. In its annual report of 1973 the board of Eden expressed concern to the participating churches "for their apparent lack of interest for Eden Mental Health Centre." Without any financial responsibility for maintaining the center, participating churches had lost much of their original interest in Eden.[29] Without input from the church, the center lost some of its sense of direction and by 1975 the board was calling for a restatement of Eden's purpose. At the invitation of the board, Vernon Neufeld of MMHS was asked to help evaluate the Eden program.[30]

Renewed Growth and Direction

It was not until 1976 that matters began to be turned around with the appointment of Henry Guenther as medical director and Ben Thiessen as executive director. Guenther, appointed in September 1975, brought with him a large increase in the number of Mennonite patients from the Winnipeg-Steinbach area, and other areas outside Eden's immediate geographic catchment area. This was in no small part due to Guenther's high standing in the Mennonite community. Before 1976 the Winnipeg-Steinbach area, and other areas outside Eden's region, had represented approximately 30 percent of Eden's patient load. After 1976 this area consistently made up more than 50 percent of Eden's patients. Along with attracting more patients from outside the immediate geographic area, Guenther once more helped bring Eden to a high level of performance in the mental health field.

The creation of the position of executive director in 1976 to replace that of administrator demonstrated that the board was intent on providing new direction for the center. The board realized

*Man, this position is tailor-made for me. I love it. Always have. The
only reason I wasn't here from day one when it opened was because it
was in Winkler and not in Winnipeg... There's no place like it!*
                                                        —Henry Guenther[31]

that the position needed to be expanded in scope of responsibility
and be filled with a full-time executive director. A half-time administrator simply did not have the resources of time and energy to work
as needed with government agencies, strengthen ties with the constituent churches, and lead in long-range planning for the future
growth of the center. Thiessen previously had been associated with
the provincial government, knew many of the government officials
personally, and consequently was able to iron out quickly any financial and administrative problems which may have existed between
Eden and the Provincial Department of Health.[32] Eden's admissions
and discharges rose steadily during this period, drawing both inpatients and outpatients from a variety of backgrounds and places.
While the greatest majority came from the Mennonite population,
ranging from 98 percent in 1967 to 82 percent in 1977, from different
backgrounds, different parts of Manitoba and Canada, and even
some from foreign countries.

Eden's main problem during this period of growth was government fiscal cutbacks initiated in 1977. Despite an increased patient population and an expanding community mental health
program,[33] the center was unable to employ the additional staff
needed. Furthermore, Eden's occupational therapy space was declared unsafe in 1978 by the fire commissioner, but no money was
forthcoming to upgrade this facility until late 1980. Plans for a
community residence[34] and a move toward accreditation likewise
were shelved and delayed due to government cutbacks. Eden kept
functioning, but doubts began to arise whether Eden should be
wholly dependent on government funding.

Another problem which became more critical by 1979 was a
steady increase in the number of chronically ill long-term patients
who required additional staff time. Though Eden kept up its strin-
gent admission requirements, elderly patients once admitted were
difficult to discharge.

At the end of 1978 Ben Thiessen resigned as executive director
and it became clear that Henry Guenther, though remaining medical director, would enter part-time retirement at the end of 1979. The
center was able to employ another psychiatrist, Jeff Ivey, on a
contract basis, thus actually increasing the total psychiatric staff
time. Bernie Loeppky, a former teacher, principal, and pastor from

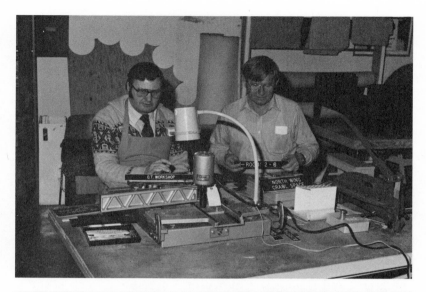

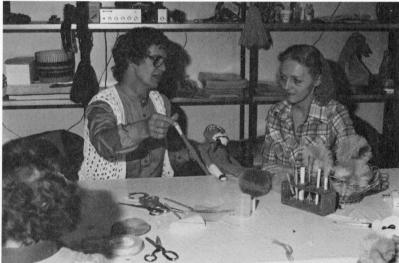

Patient activities.

the Winkler area, was hired as the new executive director in early 1979. This transaction did not create any discontinuity in Eden's development. Loeppky continued the growing and building process which began in 1976. Under his direction the staff of the center began a planning process which resulted in a "five year plan." New bylaws were accepted in 1979 which brought Eden in line with the

We admit a lot of older, sick people, mentally ill people, depressed people, confused people, assess them and treat them. Once they're here, often it is extremely difficult to get them out. Nobody wants old, confused people. It's very hard. Our nursing home beds are all filled up. Often there is a waiting list. Families often can't or do not want the burden of looking after confused old people. Things have changed dramatically... We build beautiful custodial homes or nursing homes, or whatever we might call them; we build more and more of them. I just state this as a fact, not as a criticism, but it's a fact. But maybe we do that partially in order to compensate for our guilt.

—Henry Guenther[35]

requirements of the Manitoba Corporations Act. The five-year plan projected new trends in therapy (occupational, industrial, and music therapy) and the gradual increase of more staff. A full-time volunteer coordinator was hired to organize the large volunteer program, and a program known as *Supervised Pastoral Education* accredited by the University of Manitoba was introduced in 1979. To insure the implementation of these plans it was proposed that a foundation be established to provide funds to supplement government funding. This foundation, incorporated in 1981, represented a radical departure in Eden's funding policy and promised new initiative in program development.

In 1980 the provincial government approved the necessary expenditures ($321,473) to upgrade the center's fire safety standards and also authorized Eden to proceed with its plans for a community residence for persons in transition between hospital and home or community. It was also in this year that Eden increased its medical personnel to three with the appointment of Gary Sloan. These developments demonstrated that Eden was maintaining the government's confidence. The renewed involvement of the Sommerfelder constituent church group in Eden's board of directors, after years of absence, demonstrated that Eden also had earned the trust of the Mennonite community.

Conclusion

Having provided professional mental health care in the context of the Christian church for the last fifteen years, Eden Mental Health Centre continues to develop its services and outreach. The early problems of the center, most excruciating in the difficulty to find a full-time medical director, seem to be in the past. Henry Guenther's tenure as medical director and practicing psychiatrist has brought continuity to Eden's psychiatric staff and treatment program. The executive director position, filled by Ben Thiessen and Bernie Loeppky, has facilitated a program of planning and development which keeps Eden at the growing edge of mental health care in Manitoba. Eden offers a first-rate physical plant with a creative staff that is both qualified and dedicated. Working with the churches as well as with the community and government health services, Eden plays a unique role in the mental health care of Manitoba.

What We Learned

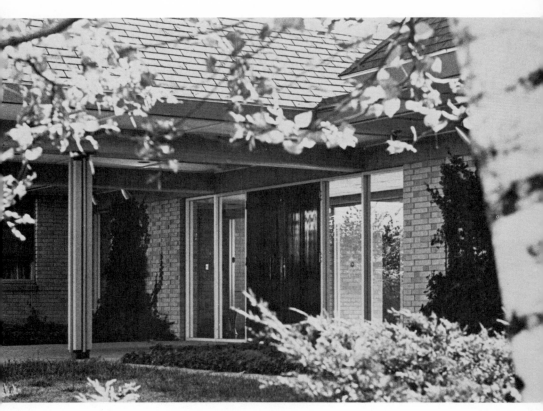

Prairie View, Newton, Kansas.

CHAPTER 11

Center Organization, Leadership and Governance

Larry W. Nikkel*

From the broad and varied experience of eight different mental health centers, there is much to share about how they have been governed, organized, and administered. Three themes emerge above others which seem particularly interesting, important, and perhaps unique. These themes are the subject of this paper. This chapter treats, in order, what the MMHS centers have learned about organizational wholeness, the dual leadership model of administration, and the evolution of the lay governing boards.

Organizational Wholeness

The story of Mennonite mental health is in a sense an expanding concept of what is involved in health and wholeness. The initial focus was largely on the wholeness of individual patients. As the hospital staff began to apply the concepts of the therapeutic community to help the patient, it became evident that they themselves would have to incorporate the same principles of openness and responsibility with each other that they espoused for the patients. After these concepts were applied to the staff, they began to emerge as ideals both for the organization and for the community.

Professional skills in consultation and organization development began to evolve. It was necessary to learn the practice of organizational development from the experience of the local centers and the theory from the behavioral sciences.

Although none of the centers would claim to have achieved organizational wholeness, some principles which contribute toward that goal seem to have been identified.

One principle is the realization that there will always be ten-

---

*Larry W. Nikkel is administrator of Prairie View, Newton, Kansas.

sion within organizations. Of ultimate importance, however, is that there is a commitment to the creative management of conflict as contrasted to the natural tendency toward denial or avoidance.

Some of these tensions are of an interpersonal nature. Some are the result of service needs being greater than the resources available to meet those needs. These issues cause programs to compete for highest priority even to the point of survival. In such situations it must be recognized that organizations are like people in that a part of their task is to learn coping skills. The error of organizations is not in having problems or conflicts but in the failure to acknowledge and deal appropriately with the problems and tensions encountered.

Furthermore, the maturing organization realizes that not only is conflict inevitable but within the solutions for today's conflict are the seeds for the conflicts of tomorrow. For example, a crisis of today may center around the problems of autocratic leadership. The solution may be in the delegation of responsibility. But even as one delegates responsibility and authority, one can expect that within this very solution are contained seeds of the next crisis—the inevitable need for more coordination, as Larry Greiner has pointed out ("Evolution and Revolution as Organizations Grow," *Harvard Business Review*, July-Aug. 1972).

A second principle related to organizational wholeness is the extent to which there is a "conscience" with regard to patients and staff. This conscience manifests itself in various ways. In Prairie View's early history, there was a growing conviction that the hospital doors should not be locked. It was felt an unlocked hospital would say a great deal to both patients and staff about responsibility, mutual trust, and openness. The Prairie View doors were unlocked on an experimental basis and were not again locked as a matter of official policy.

This conscience generally assures that there is a sense of joint responsibility which takes into account the needs of the organization, of the staff, and of the patients. It is primarily through the efforts of people that the effectiveness of an organization can be assured. Therefore, people should not be considered objects to be manipulated solely for the organization's advantage.

Another aspect of organizational wholeness is commitment to building trust. As is the case in any relationship, trust does not evolve unintentionally or automatically. Many efforts to understand and to be understood result in misunderstanding and damaged relationships. This is also true in organizations. Therefore, conscious attempts must be made to build trust. As one strategy for trust building, Prairie View has engaged an external consultant who has worked with the organization over a fifteen-year period. Sometimes the consultant meets with individuals and sometimes with departments and teams to assure open communication. The focus may be on the broader organization goals or on more personal issues. In building trusting relationships, each participant must be assured that his or her own interests and needs will be taken into consideration.

A fourth element of organizational wholeness is the sense of mission. The organization must know explicitly or implicitly why it exists. The mission of an organization may be stated very simply, as was the case in the early years of the Mennonite Mental Health Service (MMHS) centers. The centers were to serve the mentally ill in a large geographical area and function within the financial limits of what fees and contracts would support.

One of the early goals for the MMHS centers was, in the words of Robert Kreider, "to care for their own." Kings View Hospital at Reedley, California, was to take responsibility for the area west of the Rocky Mountains; Prairie View Hospital at Newton, Kansas, was to respond to needs in that area between the Rocky Mountains and the Mississippi River; and Brook Lane Hospital at Hagerstown, Maryland, was responsible for the area east of the Mississippi River. Although the churches and the Mennonite Central Committee (MCC) agreed to assist in the development of the physical facilities, the centers/hospitals were to "make it on their own" from that time forward.

As the centers developed and as new staff and board members were added, the mission of each of the centers needed to be reviewed, clarified, and expanded. This process is essential to organizational wholeness. The mission of an organization must be understood and agreed upon by staff, board, and the public served by the organization.

The ultimate test of "wholeness" is not, however, whether the mission of an organization is clearly defined but the degree to which the organization is getting the job done.

The fifth principle is the courage to risk, to venture, and the freedom to fail—as individuals and as units of the organization. Entrance into the contractual relationship of MMHS centers with the federal government for financial grants represented such a venture. There were fears of governmental control, loss of constituency support, and altering of mission. In retrospect these fears have not been realized. The relationship has not had these damaging effects upon the centers but has helped to create a partnership which enabled the dramatic expansion of services.

A final element of organizational wholeness is the development of capacity and process for self-renewal. This implies that there is a willingness to let some things drop and to take on new things. For individuals this may be done through reassignment of responsibilities, through sabbatical leaves, or through continuing professional or personal development. Organizationally, renewal is enhanced through the updating of one's mission and through an ongoing evaluation process which provides information on how services or management areas are performing. Wholeness is not indicated by perfection but by the organization's willingness to consider changes that may be necessary and by its capacity to change.

The Administrator and Medical Director Dual Leadership Model

Because of inherent values, MMHS centers developed for their purposes a near-dual leadership pattern represented by the administrator and medical director. The model of a nonclinical administrator was borrowed from the general hospital. This was done despite the fact that the state psychiatric hospitals and many private psychiatric hospitals had the model of a medical director-superintendent as the chief executive officer. The administrator model seemed natural because it was in keeping with the pattern of other MCC programs. The administrator was selected as the one who embodied the churchly and the managerial aspects of the program. Furthermore, churchman-administrators were available while medical director-superintendents were not.

The churchman-administrator as chief executive was continued as the predominant characteristic in the MMHS centers with, however, some modifications.

Even though the chief executive function has been assigned to the administrators, there has been an acknowledged need for strong clinical leadership in the centers. In their early experience this need for dual leadership was often demonstrated by both positions being shown at the same level in organization charts and in some cases even showing both positions in the same box. This model was totally unacceptable in academic and professional management circles as having too much room for ambiguity related to authority and ultimate responsibility. But the dual leadership model clearly had a high degree of compatibility with the mission of the centers and the values of decision making in a brotherly way.

The dual leadership model assumed that responsibility for decisions could be conceptualized as two separate but overlapping circles. Some issues were clearly of a clinical nature and the medical director would take primary responsibility; for example, the qualifications of the professional staff, the contents of the medical record, the philosophy and quality of treatment services. Other issues were clearly administrative in nature for which the administrator was responsible; for example, maintenance of buildings and grounds, administration of the fringe benefit program, the procurement of resources, and policies and procedures related to personnel. In areas where the issues were not clearly defined, they would have to consult and come to agreement. It is here that the professional management critics would press their point of ultimate responsibility and authority.

At a special conference on the interrelationship of these two positions held in Newton, Kansas, in 1971, several observations were made by Robert Hartzler, administrator of Oaklawn Center in Elkhart, Indiana, and Elmer Ediger, the administrator of Prairie View at Newton. A central thread in the presentation was the obvious commitment to a concept of shared leadership in the MMHS centers. This included not only the medical director and the administrator model but also other members of the professional staff. This participative management value should not, however, be construed to imply that critical decisions were necessarily arrived at through a democratic process or by consensus of all staff. Such key decisions were made primarily by top management staff and needed approval by both the administrator and the medical director.

Another element in the success of the dual-leadership model is the continuity of leadership provided by the longevity of the administrators and medical directors. Administrators in most of the current MMHS centers have had amazingly long periods of service — eleven, thirteen, seventeen, twenty-five, thirty-five years. The tenure of medical directors in these centers is almost as impressive. The demonstrated ability of these individuals to work together over such a period of time has surely been a central ingredient in their success.

An additional value of the model is the belief that "good administration is a part of good treatment." This required a close working relationship between the administrator and the medical director. This realization led to more focus on what it takes to provide good patient care than on issues related to authority and control.

Over the years there has been an increasing external emphasis on specificity and accountability. These forces, together with the increasing complexities encountered as the MMHS centers have moved from being primarily small psychiatric hospitals to large organizations, have pushed the centers to be more explicit about the person who is ultimately responsible to the board.

It is possible that in the future there may be further evolution of this process in the direction of professional administrative training and in the use of mental health clinicians as administrators. At its heart, the MMHS centers are a combination of that which the church and the mental health disciplines can provide. This requires not only a board which has a strong element of the church in it but also a person at the top level of administration who is a strong representative of the church's values.

The Evolution of the Local Board

The local boards have evolved to have the primary responsibility to carry out the Mennonite mental health mission. MCC, with headquarters in Akron, Pennsylvania, received the mandate from the constituency to initiate the program. Like all other programs of MCC, it was assumed that this one also would be administered through a director responsible to the executive secretary. Locally there were to be advisory committees representative of the various Mennonite groups in the area.

From 1947 to 1957 this was the pattern. Budgets and all personnel selections were controlled from the Akron office. This approach seemed to work quite well for the establishment of the new programs but became increasingly difficult as experience and expertise began to build at the local level. The local professional staff and administrators were not employed on a short-term basis as were most MCC relief personnel. Local professional and management staff were the ones who had to take the immediate consequence for staffing and other decisions.

Over a period of years local representatives challenged the MMHS board to rethink the arrangement so that authority on the local level would be commensurate with their responsibility. There was considerable resistance, but eventually the decentralization described elsewhere in this book was made in 1957 (see chapter 2).

In the second stage of evolution the locally incorporated boards gradually learned how to assume and carry out their responsibility for the church-sponsored professional mental hospital program. The MMHS program was an alliance in effect between representatives of the church board and mental health professionals. The board was the church side of the equation. The administrator was their church-administrator inside the center. The church board represented a variety of vocations, including professionals, but generally not "mental health professionals" and, therefore, the church board members in the context of mental health were clearly "lay boards." The task of learning the nature of the "mental health business" was a big one for each board member.

How to relate to the medical director and the professional program in general was a problem for the boards. Fortunately in the selection and self-selection process there was a high degree of compatibility with the medical directors.

In order for the boards to be responsible, they had to learn to be more willing to challenge professional opinion. The gradual learning to know each other and becoming more knowledgeable in the field made for amazing growth and understanding and a sense of compatibility. Even though medical directors were frequently not inclined toward administration or public speaking, they had been trained to be understanding and warm in their relationships to small groups and these were strengths in building the type of public trust that evolved in most situations. Board evaluations of proposals initially were largely from the viewpoint of finances or the needs and desires of local constituents represented by the board. Over a period of time the board criteria for evaluating programs from the mental health point of view grew tremendously.

The boards of Brook Lane, Kings View, Prairie View, and others in their turn, sometime in their history, came to the point where they felt they really had to take responsibility in a new way. Often this was precipitated by some crisis, such as, finances, or the loss of a medical director or administrator. Such experiences tended to give boards self-confidence which had its impact long afterward in how they carried out their responsibility. At such points board members learned to say, "It has to make sense to us," and to act accordingly. It was through these situations that the board began assuming the responsibility which legally had been theirs all along.

New board members frequently remarked that it took them two or three years before they felt they could understand and really help shape decisions. The boards still face the question of how they can hasten this process.

Another stage of evolvement for many of the centers was in the matter of composition of the board membership. Most of the local boards have changed their bylaws so that approximately 50 percent represent the community-at-large while the other 50 percent represent the church constituency. A sense of need to change in this direction generally stemmed from the need to get community involvement and ownership in order to more effectively carry out a community program.

The change toward more equal representation began to take place in the early 1960s. During the time of this transition, the primary concern was that members-at-large also share the Christian ideals of the center. A "fifty-one percent" type of balance of power was briefly discussed, but the spirit was not that of retaining ultimate control by such arbitrary means. Centers had learned that there were many people in the community with whom they could have a high sense of compatibility. Community members-at-large frequently became the strongest advocates for the Christian heritage and spirit of the center and for a strong relationship between the local center and MMHS.

MCC constituents, however, only vaguely aware of the fact that changes had been made with regard to the board composition and involvement with the community, sometimes assumed that the center was "no longer MCC." With some interpretation, however, such misunderstandings were generally overcome. None of the boards have gone below the 50 percent church representation.

In what might be another stage is the various efforts to help the board work more effectively in fulfilling its purpose. The MMHS board has become increasingly concerned and effective in cooperating with the local boards in carrying out the MMHS appointment function of board members. All board members, Mennonite and members-at-large, are screened by the MMHS executive and appointed by that board.

As a whole, MMHS and the local center boards and administrators are in accord that the decentralization toward local board responsibility was the right decision. At the same time the local boards and administrators have become increasingly appreciative of the importance of MMHS in accomplishing their mission as church-sponsored psychiatric centers.

From the experience of developing healing communities in our hospitals, we have learned principles and processes which can also lead to more organizational health and wholeness, trust, supportive relationships, openness, and personal responsibility for conflict within an organization as well as in our homes and communities.

The dual leadership model of administrator and medical director as the primary leadership team has served a useful purpose. It became the model which facilitated a successful marriage between psychiatry and the church. Although the model has been modified in most of the centers, the concept of shared leadership has continued.

The local boards have evolved from being advisory to full authority governing boards, from inexperience and insecurity to much more self-confidence and backbone, and from total church constituency representation to a blend of church and community representation. Often the community representatives have been the most vocal advocates of maintaining a strong tie with the church constituency. The evolution of the boards has contributed greatly to the strength of the center.

Through an overarching sense of church purpose, through the evolution of organizational philosophy and structures, and through carefully nurtured relationships, there has been a working together of church, mental health, and community representatives to fulfill a mission of serving those in need.

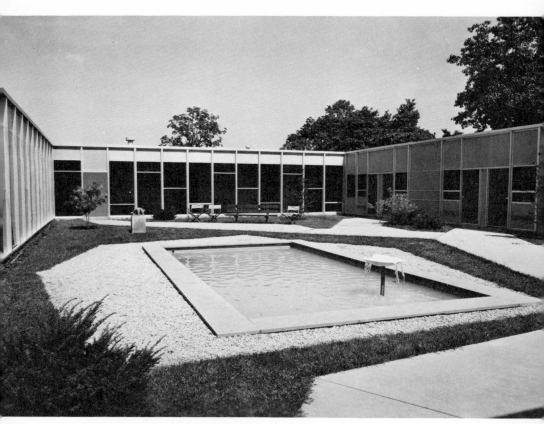

Oaklawn Center, Elkhart, Indiana.

CHAPTER 12

Providing Clinical and Other Programs
Vernon H. Neufeld*

The MMHS Center Experience

Goals for the Earliest Centers

The purposes and goals of the first Mennonite mental health centers—Brook Lane, Kings View, Philhaven and Prairie View—were uncomplicated; some would say "simplistic." All four were conceived in the aftermath of World War II, and their beginning should be viewed against the backdrop of a church interest stimulated by the Civilian Public Service (CPS) experience and the state of the mental health care at that time. All were planned beginning in the late 1940s and were opened within a span of a little over five years (1949-54).

The institutions were seen as alternatives to the vast, crowded state hospitals into which conscientious objectors had been thrust. There had to be a better way. The planners for the Mennonite Central Committee (MCC) mental health program first visualized a centrally located institution, but later conceived the idea of three smaller homes to solve the geographical problem and provide the opportunity for different models. In the words of Orie Miller, these were to be "experimental, to see what we could do."

The programs were to serve the "mentally ill," at first loosely defined. Beginning with the state hospital experience, the initial thought was to serve the needs of chronically ill, long-term patients. Consultations with numerous mental health professionals and visits to many institutions led to active treatment programs for acutely mentally ill persons. The centers started out to serve their own, for

---

*Vernon H. Neufeld was director of Mennonite Mental Health Services from 1967 to 1982. Much of the material in this chapter is derived from a survey taken by Chester Raber in 1981 and from interviews in February 1982 at Oaklawn and Prairie View.

example, the Mennonites. But in each case, by the time the first patients were admitted, the doors were open to everyone who needed help.

Though each began as a hospital, unlike the state hospitals, the emphasis was upon a home-like atmosphere. Patients were seen as persons and treated with dignity and respect. The total environment, twenty-four hours a day, was important and vital for the patients' welfare. The mental health services were to be the best possible. Though initiated, administered, and mostly staffed by nonprofessionals, the hospitals very soon began employing the best professional staff available. The initiation of the mental health programs was a ministry of the church, a service "in the name of Christ." (This topic is treated more fully in chapter 13.)

Significant Changes and Trends

The thirty-plus years since the first MMHS institution began have seen many changes. The evolution from the first "homes" to the more complex and diverse centers has been rapid and dramatic. In considering some of the more obvious and spectacular changes, one should note that these do not apply equally to all centers, since each developed in its own setting. Moreover, the MMHS centers of more recent origin may not have experienced the transformation in the same way as the first ones. They came along at various points in the changing scene. The major changes or trends included the following:

1. *The change from hospitals to centers.* The first three MCC hospitals dropped the hospital title (Philhaven retained it) as the concept changed and services multiplied. The next two institutions to begin, Penn Foundation and Oaklawn, did not have any beds and were started primarily as day treatment and outpatient care programs. The last two, Kern View and Eden, were started as centers, although both provided inpatient services.
2. *The change from treating sick persons to serving also those with other needs.* The focus on patients—inpatients, outpatients, day patients—shifted to others at home, school, work, who may have experienced problems or who simply wanted to enrich their lives. This expansion did not diminish patient services, however.
3. *The change from the individual to society.* The patient or the person with a problem could not be treated in isolation. He or she was part of one or more social groupings—family, school, church, community. So treatment of the individual shifted to an emphasis which included education, consultation, and prevention.

4. *The change from limited treatment methods to more expansive ones.* This was due in part to changing modalities (e.g., from electroshock to drug therapy) as well as expanding services and diversified staff which led to a variety of therapies, activities, and educational and training programs.
5. *The change from limited to multi-disciplinary professional staff.* As programs were added and diversified, specialized staff also was added. This change included the loss or diminished role of volunteers.
6. *The change from a medical-psychiatric focus to a broader behavioral-psychological-social-educational dimension.* This change paralleled several of those named above. The medical directorship in one center (Kern View) became a clinical director position open to other disciplines and is currently filled by a psychologist. The more frequent use of *client* or *consumer* rather than *patient* is a further indication of this change.
7. *The change from a limited accountability to a much more complex one.* The original accountability which was mainly to the church has been compounded by the need to answer also, in varying degrees and ways, to "consumers," the community, the mental health professions, funding sources, regulatory and licensing bodies, and accrediting agencies.

What the Centers Have Learned

With such a rich and varying experience, the task of identifying major lessons learned is not a simple one. Several general observations can be made, however, about what the MMHS centers have learned in providing clinical and other programs, while also noting areas of weakness and areas where the centers may have made distinctive contributions. What follows is based on the observations of staff members from several MMHS centers.

The Nature of Sickness and Wellness

Like other issues of a theoretical-philosophical nature, (for example, psychiatry-religion), the MMHS centers have not spent much time making clear written definitions of *mental illness* and *mental health*. They have devoted their energies to relieving problems of mental illness as they occur. The approach has been to act upon basic assumptions and think about it "on the run."

Yet one can say that a broadly perceived view of mental illness has to do with "(a) problems of living and feeling, (b) disability of living in harmony with self and others in the environment, and (c) emotionally disadvantaged" (Chester Raber). The spectrum of illness is broad and complex, from incapacity and dysfunction at one end to limited emotional problems related to life stages or periods of stress at the other.

Mental health, on the other hand, has to do with the ability to care about oneself and others, to "love your neighbor as yourself," and to work or be productively active (Mervin Bontrager and Orval Shoemaker). It is more than the absence of illness or emotional stress, but the energy which promotes wholeness (health = wholeness), "sense of emotional robustness" (Eli Bowers; referred to by Merrill Raber). Nor is mental health to be defined as adjustment to one's circumstances where normality means fitting into the system. The nonconformist may be the healthy one, and rather than adjusting, there may be a need to change the system (Vernon Yoder). Wellness includes a "spiritual" dimension of being at peace with oneself, with the world, and with one's Creator.

Interrelatedness of Personhood

The mental health centers have come to see the individual—sick or well—as a whole person, "combining the interrelated biological social, emotional, intellectual, and spiritual needs" (Oaklawn Philosophy Statement). One's place in society and in the natural environment also are vital in shaping or affecting personality. These qualities of life are not separate "compartments" of the personality; they are aspects of a single, whole person.

This view of humanness probably is not a new or unique discovery, but it has been recognized more openly in recent years. While helpful in working with persons, this view does not simplify dealing with personal problems. The "spiritual" problem may be an indicator of a deeper personality disorder or a physical problem may indicate spiritual confusion. The migraine headache is a painful physical affliction, but something else is triggering it. While alcoholism can be placed in remission, the causes remain somewhat unclear, whether genetic, environmental, or psychological. Clinicians have discovered that the "symptoms" which cry for attention often are "different wrappings of the same problem" (Sanford Kauffman). While specialists still deal with aspects of a problem in their area of expertise and training, there has been increasing recognition of and respect for colleagues who approach the problem from another angle.

The holistic view also has helped wipe away older views and debates. The nature-nuture argument—whether heredity or environment is at fault—is no longer significant since usually both are seen as factors. The organic, genetic, physical aspects, for example, the somatic, have taken on greater meaning in mental health. The use of biofeedback illustrates this.

A result has been a greater emphasis upon teamwork, the integration of services, and the development of a "system" approach, not only within the center but with other providers in the community. So the task becomes even more difficult and complex.

Treating the Mentally Ill

It would be interesting to take a look at the various ways in which patients have been treated, to evaluate what has worked and what hasn't. If one development in the mental health centers stands out it is the number of therapies and approaches which have multiplied through the years—among them verbal therapies, milieu therapies, activities, and drug therapy. Some modalities are more effective than others. But it probably is true that "most everything works if it's applied sincerely by a well-motivated therapist and a well-motivated patient, in good faith and within reason" (Vernon Yoder). So rather than look at individual approaches, several factors in treating patients might be lifted up as significant.

From the beginning of the centers the total milieu was considered important to the recovery of the patient. This belief has not changed. The actual therapy—individual, group, activity, or whatever—is important, but so is all the time in between: the contacts with other patients, as well as ward and housekeeping staff on the ward, in the hallways, on the grounds, and in the dining room. The whole experience is treatment.

The other factor is the emphasis upon the patient to take responsibility for him- or herself. This, too, while a part of the MMHS philosophy from the beginning, has continued to be an important ingredient in treatment. This focus upon patient responsibility shows itself in different ways. Oaklawn reports how charts are shared with clients, based on the notion that "I have a right to know whatever there is to know about me, and which puts me in charge of my health in some way" (Sanford Kauffman). In recognizing the dignity of the individual, Prairie View has found "to focus on the strengths of the client...makes a lot more things possible than if we think only of the patient's weaknesses" (Cindy Martin).

Rehabilitation

One of the significant developments, in many ways successful, has been the attempt to work with chronically ill patients. Once doomed to state institutions, in the 1960s these long-term care patients were being returned to the community in an effort to empty the hospitals, although unfortunately this did not always mean a better alternative.

The five-year aftercare project of Prairie View demonstrated that former hospitalized patients could be cared for in the community, with appropriate residential facilities, follow-up with medications, and home visitations. Other centers had similar experiences with the chronically ill. With rehabilitative services and continuing care programs the needs of chronically mentally ill persons can be served. It is not that they are "cured," but the best that the centers can do is to maintain and support the chronically ill and control them "to some degree in a manageable level" (Harold Loewen).

The centers have discovered that not only is continuous hospitalization unnecessary, but some persons in nursing homes also can live in less restrictive and limiting residential alternatives (semi-independent living apartments, for example). Through periodic contact, in person or by phone, the centers are often able to prevent recurring psychotic episodes. Not all regression can be prevented, but admitting patients into a local hospital for a short period of time, even an "elective short-term hospitalization" (Vernon Yoder), helps prevent long-term hospitalization and, in some instances, develops a level of acceptance by the patient and his family of the problem. After such an intervention there are ways of supporting them. Another lesson coming out of efforts to rehabilitate is the need for "pursuit of the chronically ill who are not motivated to maintain their treatment program" (Vernon Yoder). The center needs to go to the patient.

Another significant development of the centers' programs has been progress in treating alcoholism. A number of the centers have found that through a combination of intensive counseling, collaboration with self-help groups, medication and hospitalization, persons suffering from alcoholism, once all but written off as "incurable," can be rehabilitated.

Preventing Mental Illness and Promoting Mental Health

From the beginning of the Mennonite mental health programs there were those who urged that the prevention of mental illness should not be neglected (for example, P. E. Schellenberg). The earliest efforts to "educate" the churches were in part intended to do this. The developing education and consultation programs, and later "growth" services, made prevention and promotion an integral part of the centers' programs.

Preventing illness and promoting health have presented problems. Funding has always been difficult; it is easier to pay for patient services than a vaguely defined education program. "Money is for illness, it is not for wellness" (Melvin Funk). While almost everyone agrees that it makes more sense to "turn off the faucet" than to continually "empty the bucket," it is difficult to document that prevention pays off. "Academics and theoreticians tend to point to the lack of evidence that any mental illness is prevented..., pointing to the vast lack of research data available" (Merrill Raber). The centers believe prevention is "going on right and left... We can hypothesize it and I think it is a fair hypothesis, but we can't prove it" (Walter Drudge).

Yet the centers have contributed to both prevention and promotion. Staff members, functioning in settings away from work, influence the wider community indirectly with attitudes and insights, by rubbing elbows in the community. Similarly, clients take their experiences to home, work, church, or other settings and indirectly contribute to prevention. There is an overall impact of the center upon the community which is preventive and promotes sound mental health.

The centers also have contributed directly to prevention. These are the specifically planned efforts, such as parent-training classes, marriage enrichment workshops, pastor's seminars—the list is long. Another approach is by linking up with other community agencies which also work at prevention—the schools, churches, courts, probation, police, welfare, and so forth—so it becomes "a systems kind of thing" where the center is only one part of a complex network (Sanford Kauffman).

Another way to prevent illness is to maintain persons with disabilities at a high functioning level. The success in working with the chronically ill, already referred to, is an example of "preventing regression and maintaining relatively optimal status of health" (Vernon Yoder).

The holistic emphasis also has broadened the concept of promoting mental health. "People that are able to take care of their bodies can usually take care of their minds. There is a relationship between the two" (Sanford Kauffman). Proper diet and exercise, and refraining from the use of alcohol and tobacco become efforts in promoting health, both physical and mental.

Priorities

What have the centers learned about priorities? The job has always been too large to manage comprehensively. What each center has done was often determined more by available funds than any other factor. The centers that moved in the community mental health center direction, funded by federal, state, and local governments, were able to provide all kinds of new services not possible otherwise. As some of this funding diminished, a few of these programs had to be dropped.

In the continuum of needs—extending from psychiatric hospitalization on the left to promotion of mental health on the right—the centers place greatest priority to the left. Short-term hospitalization, preventing long-term institutionalization, crisis intervention, and providing outpatient and day patient services all take priority over programs which move over toward education, consultation, and growth events. This is dictated in part by funding sources— government as well as third-party payers—but also by the urgency from within and insistence from without to meet the obvious needs, the crises, the catastrophes in life, before giving attention to needs which take much longer and are not openly crying for attention.

New Approaches

The MMHS centers on balance have stayed pretty much in the middle of the road as new methods, approaches, trends, and experiments have come along in the mental health field. There are those who would consider the hospital aspect conservative. "In our inpatient program we represent conservative, mainstream psychiatry and have been very reluctant to shift with the fads" (Robert Carlson). The centers have avoided extreme experiments, in part on a common sense basis, in part because of their church orientation. Yet programs which at one time were controversial have found their way into the centers, for example, mind control (biofeedback), sex education, holistic health, physical approaches, behavior modification, and transactional analysis.

The "techniquey" approaches to therapy (Donald Munn) have never dominated or detracted, but when adopted have complemented or supplemented mainstream approaches. The "pendulum swings from one theoretical stance to another or one methodology to another" have been avoided. The center (Oaklawn) "has retained what it set out to do but it has added new approaches" (Walter Drudge).

Are There Any Weaknesses?

It would be easier for someone outside the MMHS center orbit to identify the weaknesses. Yet the centers themselves recognize some.

Whether a weakness or not, there are endeavors which the centers by and large did not undertake, by choice or default. Center staffs are not known for writing, for sharing with others what has been experienced and learned in the center programs. Nor has there been much research to evaluate the effectiveness of particular methods of treatment. Centers have not spent much time trying to untangle knotty philosophical or ethical issues in any direct, conscious way. The center staff members have not been theorists and academicians, but rather doers and activists.

There is some dissatisfaction that the centers have not related as they might to the churches. "...Everytime we try to list what we've done with the churches we end up being surprised at the length of the list. . .; but it always feels like we haven't begun yet" (Robert Carlson). "...We have got a lot of work left to do in relating to the churches" (Harold Loewen). "...We feel more comfortable working with physicians than we do with clergy" (Sanford Kauffman). Similar self-criticism is leveled at almost everything the centers attempt to do.

On the other hand, some wonder if the centers have tried to do too much. "We want to treat the whole person...and we like to work in an interdisciplinary setting, but finally we can get so caught up in trying to get all the pieces in that we end up weighing down the process incredibly to where we can't make a decision" (Sanford Kauffman).

"Sometimes I feel like we're trying to do it all. We try to do too much. We spread ourselves too thin" (Julie Neufeld).

Are There Any Distinctives?

It is difficult to claim, even if one believes it, that the MMHS centers are distinctive or unique in any way. In most ways, perhaps, the MMHS centers are more similar to other mental health programs than they are different. They have offered services and programs which others also provide; they have similar staffs in training and experience; they have similar goals in meeting human need. But at the risk of seeming parochial, one still might suggest certain qualities or characteristics which, though also found in other programs, stand out more prominently in the MMHS centers and so in some sense might be called "distinctive."

One such emphasis is the way patients or clients are viewed with "a deep kind of sensitivity and caring about human values-...the humaneness" (Melvin Funk). Instead of being treated with the "custodial mechanisms that dehumanize the individual" (Robert Carlson), the person is treated with dignity and respect. People can get well—there is optimism and hope. Persons have responsibility for their own health—this shows confidence and respect. This emphasis may be a heritage from the Quakers and the "moral treatment" tradition (Elmer Ediger).

There is a distinctive ethical framework or value system which underlies the work of the centers. "We do have a kind of core of values... There is a values system that permeates the program" (George Smucker). How patients or clients are perceived and treated is one way the values are expressed. How staff relate to one another and others also reveals the values underlying the system.

The centers exhibit evidence of hard work, productivity and industriousness. "...Our ethic got engraven in stone back there. We dare not break the tablets! (Melvin Funk). There is a no-nonsense kind of approach. Staff work hard and produce; the pencil-pushers, gad-abouts or clock-watchers are not found. And this emphasis upon work transfers to clients, who also are expected to work and produce in their own behalf.

A team approach also characterizes the MMHS centers. "We moved from a doctor-patient treatment setting, of a patient in milieu, to establishing a 'professional team' in which there was a partnership in the healing process" (Robert Carlson). The lines drawn between the different professions, often important in other settings, are all but erased, with "various members in the team...having an equal footing in the program..." (Elmer Ediger).

The partnership idea also finds expression in the community. In referrals, in collaboration, in prevention, the centers increasingly see themselves as one community resource among others; each is important, and links and lines of communication are vital. What works best is the person-to-person contact, not institution-to-institution. "I think that the personalized touch that we believe in giving our clients is also a personalized touch we are still learning to give to our referral sources... As an institution we need that relatedness to the community, otherwise we would be fostering again a kind of impersonal organizational system that would lack the personal touch" (Walter Drudge).

One still must confess there is little that is unique clinically. There may be some difference in how the whole is put together. "We borrowed a great deal but the way we put it together has been somewhat different." A particular staff, "with a sense of purpose along with a history of stability," provides "a kind of quality control that raises it above the ordinary kind of treatment setting where the individual parts may be very much the same" (George Dyck). To this another adds, "I think it is a common philosophy and the common commitment to make it work for the sake of the patient" (Elmer Ediger).

This, then, leads to the common denominator. It is the origin of the centers as part of the church's mission, the roots of that beginning, and the continuing influence and guidance provided by the larger church constituency and by staff and board personnel that contributes most to the difference. The church through staff provides the salt which gives the distinct flavor, the leaven which raises the whole lump.

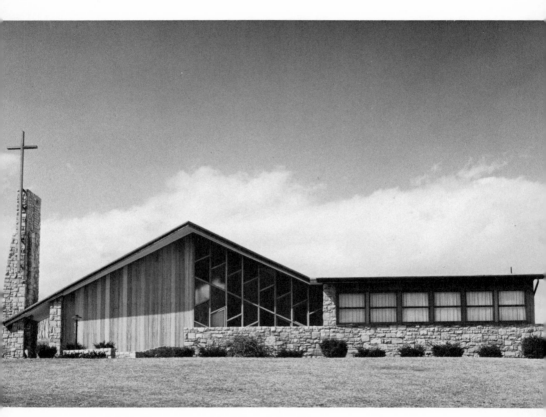

Brook Lane Chapel, Hagerstown, Maryland.

CHAPTER 13

The Church and the Centers

Vernon H. Neufeld and Donald M. Wert*

The Mennonite and Brethren in Christ churches, working together through MCC, were responsible for giving birth to the first mental health programs. The church built the centers.

This chapter discusses the experience of the Mennonite Mental Health Services (MMHS) centers in relating to the church. ("Church" here refers first of all to the church constituency responsible for founding the centers and functioning at each center location, but also to other denominational groups which became involved locally.)

Rather than evaluating the MMHS centers as a single group, the chapter presents two broad, and somewhat distinct, approaches to the church-center relationship question, one represented by the five centers founded by the Mennonite Central Committee (MCC) and the other by Philhaven Hospital. These are similar and yet varied methods which evolved or were adopted by the centers as each considered and worked out its mission as a church-related program. In addition to sections dealing with the MCC centers and Philhaven Hospital, a middle section briefly discusses the other two MMHS centers, Eden Mental Health Centre and the Penn Foundation.

The Experience of the MCC Centers

The Church Built the Centers

At the outset, and roughly for the first decade following the 1947 MCC decision, the first three centers were clearly identified as church-sponsored programs. The church provided the religious soil, the tradition, and experience from which the centers took root and grew. The church had the vision to serve its own members and

*Vernon H. Neufeld, director of MMHS (1967-82), prepared the first and second sections of the chapter as well as editing the whole. Donald M. Wert, director of education at Philhaven Hospital, prepared the section on Philhaven.

others. The church provided the leadership—members of boards, committees, and most staff—which planned, implemented and operated the programs. The church gave its money, material aid, and volunteers to construct the centers. The church gave the broad purpose and values which guided the beginning and the development of the programs. Within the brief span of a little more than five years (1949-54), Brook Lane, Kings View and Prairie View were completed and operating.

The Centers Develop

As the first MCC centers began to develop their own individual identity, MCC granted them greater autonomy. Decentralizing administrative responsibility from MCC headquarters was in process when Oaklawn was being established in the late 1950s and 1960s and the transition was already complete when Kern View opened in 1966. Local boards composed of church representatives, at first only from the Mennonite constituency and later from other church groups, replaced MCC in having primary responsibility to operate the local programs.

The MCC centers, though church-sponsored, were also committed to provide competent professional care and to work in and with the local community. This multiple commitment led the centers to work at combining the vision and care of the church with the best of the mental health professions in collaboration with the larger community. This was no simple task for the centers, and the degree of success varied considerably from center to center. Moreover, the local center development created some difficulties regarding church relationship for MCC-MMHS and the local church constituency.

MCC-MMHS Struggles with Change

As we have already seen, MCC delegated responsibility to the local level with considerable apprehension and fear that the centers would slip away from the church. There were trends and developments which seemed to support these fears: The need to employ nonconstituent staff members, often in key positions, created uncertainty about the centers' ability to provide a Christian ministry. The growth of strong professional staffs led to doubt that the lay leadership of the church (MCC, administrators, and boards) could control the direction of the centers. A strong professional approach caused concern that the spiritual aspect would lose out. Then came greater involvement in the community, leading to the appointment of nonconstituent church members to the board. Also, by accepting public money, as some did, the centers gave further indication that they were less dependent upon the church.

MCC and MMHS in various ways tried to deal with these trends and perceived problems. After 1958 MCC gave supervisory responsibility to the MMHS board and markedly strengthened its membership to deal more effectively with the growing centers. The roster of the MMHS board in the late 1950s and early 1960s reads like a "Who's Who Among the Mennonites." Some control—at first retained by MCC and then passed on to MMHS—was exercised in appointing all local board members, approving the appointment of the administrator, the medical director, and the chaplain, and ratifying bylaw changes. Much of this practice continues.

.MMHS tried to deal with issues of psychiatry and faith. A series of Mental Health Study Conferences were sponsored in various sections of the country to deal with philosophical and theological questions. The subject was frequently raised in MMHS meetings; for example, a whole day was set aside at the October 1959 meeting to discuss "the Christian faith and mental health programming," with outside participants including Paul Pruyser of the Menninger Foundation. Representatives of MMHS attended and participated in the Academy of Religion and Mental Health to find answers. Delmar Stahly, the MMHS staff person, in April 1961 expressed his frustration over criticisms from "our theological schools" and church leaders that "MMHS does not offer answers to questions of relationships between psychology and Christianity." That same year MCC encouraged MMHS "to make the religious aspect of our Mennonite health service effective in line with the concern which the church had—and still has—in establishing our mental hospitals." There were other efforts to resolve the issue, when for example a 1965 MMHS study group produced a statement on "The Role of the Church in the Field of Mental Health."

So the response of MCC and its subsidiary MMHS to what was happening at the local level was to balance the strong professional staffs with strong boards locally and at the MMHS level, to influence the appointment of key personnel and changes in bylaws, to work at finding answers to the faith-science dichotomy, and, as is described later, to encourage a strong chaplaincy program. Even so, there were suggestions, at least from some MCC leaders, that perhaps some of the centers should be turned over to the local communities—a model followed by MCC in some of its overseas service programs.

Local Center-Church Relationships

Many of the developments which troubled MCC-MMHS also troubled the local churches. The sense of local church ownership greatly diminished after the early planning and building stage. The

major lines of growth and development—strengthening professional staff, involving the community, securing public funding—
contributed to the local congregations' perception that they no
longer were needed by the center. Some church leaders felt "left
out" when they were not included in the treatment team; at times
there seemed to be a chasm between the local minister and the
center therapist. The fact that some centers with public funding at
times "played down" the Mennonite church identity also contributed to some of the rejection felt by the churches.

Yet throughout their history all five of the MMHS centers, in
varying degrees of success, worked at maintaining and strengthening church relations. There were, after all, significant church ties in
each center, with a churchman-administrator, a board composed of
constituent and other local church representatives, and a core of
concerned Christian staff. So there were contacts and visits,
speeches given in churches. In some centers church members continued to provide significant financial support. The centers worked
with area pastors and members to help them with their tasks,
bringing them to the center, providing workshops and study
groups.

The Chaplaincy Question

One answer to the church-center relationship question at both
the MCC-MMHS and the local levels was a chaplaincy service. This
possibility became an issue in the late 1950s and early 1960s. The
1956 MCC study which led to greater autonomy for the centers
recognized the problem. This committee observed the "uncertainty
and lack of broad clarity in the program as to the role of the spiritual
ministry in the total treatment program of the hospital unit... A full-
or part-time chaplain is frequently recommended, but...there is a
difference of opinion here... ."

H. Clair Amstutz in his April 1960 chairman's report to MMHS
delineated the questions as he saw them at that time: "Does a
chaplain do spiritual therapy by virtue of personal relations or by
virtue of office? Does he bring healing through his discussions with
patients or by bringing hope and courage through sacraments,
liturgy and other symbols? Does a chaplain minister to the personal
needs of the staff? Is he a general 'trouble-shooter?' Is he the public
relations man, especially relating the hospital to the church constituency?"

Originally the hospitals felt little need for a "pastor" on their
staff. The earliest staff members, including volunteers, aides and
nurses on the ward, provided a Christian milieu and helped meet
the personal spiritual needs of patients. Key professional staff, for

example at Oaklawn which had several clergymen as therapists, were particularly able to deal with religious matters themselves, and there was no obvious reason to add a chaplain. The spiritual ministry was often perceived as indirect rather than direct.

While there was pressure from the constituent churches for concrete evidence of a Christian ministry, other internal and external factors moved all the centers eventually to add a chaplain or director of pastoral care to their staffs. Among mental health professionals generally there was increasing acceptance of the validity of a religious dimension in providing services. The chaplaincy as a distinct mental health profession was developing, and persons like Chester Raber and Robert Carlson were instrumental in bringing new concepts and practices into the MMHS centers.

What We Have Learned

1. *The church centers have learned to lead in community mental health development*. The MMHS centers have learned that treating mentally ill persons needs to be extended to preventing mental illness and promoting mental health. This means utilizing local resources and cultivating local responsibility, that is, a community mental health development approach. Some of the MMHS centers have come to see this effort as the church being the salt in the community by "losing itself" in a collaborative community development program.

2. *The centers have come to see the local churches as partners in a common cause*. Local pastors are front-line workers dealing with a variety of personal and emotional problems. The local congregation at best is itself a therapeutic community which provides stability, meaning, care, and healing. The linkage between center and church is vital for each to better fulfill its mission and purpose. The interest which at first was directed mostly to constituent churches has expanded to include all Christian groups and other religious communities within the local areas.

3. *The role of the chaplain or director of pastoral care has emerged as a vital one*. The function has become varied, not necessarily filled equally in all the centers. Four major tasks emerged: (1) to serve as pastor to patients, providing or planning group activities, doing individual counseling, serving as liaison with the patient's own pastor, (2) to serve as a resource to other professional staff members, particularly in dealing with religious and spiritual matters, (3) to provide training for pastors, most often in a Clinical Pastoral Education program, and (4) to serve as a pastor in the community, a pastor to pastors, using various methods as group sessions, work-

shops, training events, one-to-one contacts, to help pastors do their job.

The chaplain must be, and has been, accepted by center staff as a vital skilled member of the team, and yet needs to remain a member of the clergy with links to his or her own pastoral peer group. He or she must avoid becoming a "therapist" at the expense of giving up the pastoral role and at the same time avoid becoming a "preacher" only to be boxed in by colleagues.

4. *Church sponsorship and relationship continues to influence the centers.* The church continues to affect and influence their functioning in providing purpose and vision, a set of values, and such qualities as integrity, productivity, and "common sense." As part of its legacy, the church provides a Judeo-Christian view of humanity. Clients and patients are seen in a more holistic way, as persons with differing needs, and there is greater recognition of the interrelatedness of the physical, mental, spiritual, and social aspects of life.

5. *Combining church and mental health has been validated by experience.* Theoretical questions concerned with relating or integrating the Christian faith and mental health disciplines have been better dealt with in practice in the center than in philosophical discourse or debate. Within the institution, the goal has been to combine the best of the church and the best of the mental health professions under the leadership of the church (MCC-MMHS, local board, administration). The center program is not of the church alone nor of psychiatry alone; each utilizes the other, each learns from the other, each is accountable to the other. The balance between the two has varied considerably from center to center and from time to time, but the centers remain committed to the "marriage" of the church and psychiatry. The combination has been validated by experience.

6. *The church has become more accepting of mental health.* The Civilian Public Service (CPS) experience taught Mennonite churches something about the need to utilize the best wisdom and skill available from the mental health world. Mennonites gradually allowed themselves to learn that the mental health professions had something to offer. Uncertainty and suspicion have given way to greater trust and receptivity. The stigma associated with mental illness also has been greatly reduced as church people learned to make use of mental health services. Church agencies, some of them still fearful and cautious, are increasingly accepting the MMHS center programs.

7. *Mental health professionals have come to accept the church administration of mental health programs.* The boldness and audacity of the church (MCC) to start and operate professional programs has

proved not only to be accepted but at times to be lauded by the mental health world. Fortunately there were those who gave MMHS and its church administrators a chance to develop this church role. The acceptance by mental health professionals has probably been one of the happy surprises of the MMHS experiment. The centers have found a number of well-qualified professionals—Mennonites, as well as Christians from other denominations and some non-church persons—who feel a kinship with the values of MMHS-administered programs.

8. *The centers value and desire to strengthen linkages with the church.* The value of the larger church as represented in MMHS has been reaffirmed by the centers. At one and the same time, in MMHS, the centers join together to learn from one another in their common purpose; and they find the vision, the sense of mission, the guidance, and the discipline which the larger Mennonite and Brethren in Christ constituency offers.

The Other MMHS Centers

Eden Mental Health Centre

The beginning of Eden was quite similar to that of the five MCC centers in that the impetus came from the several Mennonite conferences of the province. However, there was no inter-Mennonite organization like MCC to take responsibility, so one needed to be created. But the rationale and the energy came from the churches.

Largely because Eden was completely financed by the province, the tendency after Eden opened was for the churches to lose interest. The board, made up of representatives from the conferences, and the staff worked hard to make the tie with the churches meaningful. Conference representatives made an effort to serve as a link in reporting to their respective groups and bringing back concerns. An annual meeting was held for church constituents.

The chaplaincy developed at Eden much as it had in the MCC centers, with a multiple role within the center and in the community, including a Supervised Pastoral Education program.

Milieu has been important at Eden. Partly because Eden is located in a region with a heavy concentration of Mennonites, the center staff is composed mostly of members of the constituent churches. But there is also a conscious effort to maintain a Christian staff that is concerned about Eden's function as a ministry of the church. For a center that is totally dependent upon the government for financial support, Eden has been remarkably successful in retaining a strong sense of church identity.

Penn Foundation

The Penn Foundation is quite different in its origin and development, in that it was not sponsored by any organized church group. However, the board of directors, the medical director, and other staff members had strong personal ties to the churches of the area, mostly Mennonite, and a religious interest and sense of mission persisted through the years. In more recent years, the center is working more deliberately both to serve the churches and to represent the churches in its program. The new administrator-medical director leadership team, with board endorsement, is determined to move in this direction. Consequently, the first chaplain for the Penn Foundation has been employed and the center has affiliated with MMHS.

The Philhaven Hospital Experience

The story of Philhaven Hospital's founding by the Lancaster Conference of the Mennonite Church is told elsewhere (Chapter 5). Like the MCC centers and Eden the initial conception and energy came from church interests, vision, and purpose. There was a basic organizational difference between Philhaven and the MCC centers in that Philhaven was sponsored by one fairly local church conference (Lancaster), to which it remains structurally related and whose congregations constitute the local church constituency. Yet Philhaven Hospital eventually needed to develop its own understanding of itself as the church's mental health ministry, to clarify its vision and philosophy, and to develop its programs.

The Need for Self-Definition

Philhaven Hospital has clearly and consistently identified itself as a ministry of the church and this, more than any other factor, has maintained the whole fabric combining church and center. Though connected to the organizational structure of the church, the tradition of the hospital has been articulated and interpreted by the institution. When Philhaven faced a crisis of purpose and definition in the years 1969-71, the renewal of the hospital's mission did not come from the bishops or the constituency except as reflected in the institution. Rather, resolution was furthered by staff members and board members who were concerned to preserve the tradition of the hospital and to cooperate in the ministry of the broader church even when the conference was not demanding this of the center.

The importance of personnel policies is, perhaps, the most important working-out of the hospital's self-definition. Philhaven demonstrates the continuity of its tradition because the hospital is committed to hiring persons who uphold and reflect the values of the institution. The commitment of Philhaven to the vision of the center as a ministry of the church is what distinguishes its integration of faith and practice.

The Pastoral Nature of Health Care

In the Catholic and early Reformed traditions, the role and responsibility of priests and other members of the clergy was indicated as *cura animarum*, "the cure of souls." In the Anabaptist tradition, however, responsibility for the "cure of souls" is collective and cooperative. Every member of the "priesthood of all believers" assumes a personal responsibility for ministry through the fellowship of the church. This is not to suggest that there is no need for an ordained pastorate, but rather to emphasize the responsibility of every believer and to affirm the importance of the Christian community. Erland Waltner has said that an authenic Anabaptist perspective is the "emphasis on Christian community as the appropriate context for pastoral care to persons in crisis." From the Philhaven perspective, the church exercises her "cure of souls" through the Christian community within and around the mental health center.

From the beginning, Philhaven was intended to be the means whereby the church expended her gifts on behalf of the ill, the distressed, and the deprived. The staff of the hospital was expected to employ native talents, spiritual gifts, and acquired skills in professional disciplines which were clearly acknowledged as forms of ministry. Certainly, the ministry of the church is not limited to the practices of professional "helpers," but our theological tradition affirms the potential incarnation of the gospel in every Christian occupation, including the mental health disciplines. It is in bearing the gospel that our professional lives are transformed, because the gospel is not addressed to any component or part of an individual but to the whole person. The ministry of Philhaven is to the "whole person," to the emotional, physical, intellectual, and spiritual dimension of personhood. As our professional labor reflects this dedication to wholeness, it remains true to the inspired vision of our foundation.

In his MMHS paper, "The Church and the Mental Health Community: Why We Need One Another," Harlan Ratmeyer identifies the primary pastoral functions within the Judeo-Christian community and suggests that these functions are shared by the Mennonite mental health centers. Citing Clebsch and Jeckle (*Pastoral Care in Historical Perspective*), Ratmeyer mentions "healing, sustaining, guiding, and reconciling" as "pastoral" functions that are "goals which are at the heart of the mental health community as well." As mental health professionals, we strive with our colleagues throughout the mental health community for the attainment of these goals.

But, as Christians we also recognize that our concerns are broader and higher than those of any professional discipline. We are concerned for the whole person, and we know that healing, guidance, sustenance, and reconciliation are not achieved without a tender regard for the "cure of souls." If Ratmeyer is correct, then mental health professionals must learn about pastoral ministry. If pastors care in ways that are different from other mental health professionals, then Christian professionals need to learn these "ways" if they will achieve their own therapeutic goals. The achievement of our professional goals necessitates our dedication to spiritual care; we are called in our several disciplines to be pastors. Furthermore, we understand that spiritual care cannot be provided alone by a single person or department; sensitivity to spiritual needs must distinguish every department and every provider of service.

Care Is Not Given in Secular Settings

We recognize that in our work as well as in our worship, we are the church. Our ministry to persons in crisis still depends upon the vision, guidance, and support of the whole "household of faith" of which we are a unit. The gratifying growth of Philhaven during the past thirty years is a reflection of continuing growth throughout the church community. The broader church, in turn, has been blessed through this venture of service as the church is enriched by every aspect of her ministry. We are not hired laborers set to work in strange fields; we are taking our places in the "family business," doing the work closest to our heart. If a "gap" develops between the professional practice of health care and the "pastoral" care of persons in a broken world, then we have lost the splendid vision that inspired our foundation. The relegation of pastoral care to a specialized and subordinate role in mental health care is not a sign of maturity, but of negligence. To minimize the spiritual dimension of all our work is to undermine the peculiar strength of our center, our dedication to healing and wholeness, in every dimension of personality.

The practice of health care in secular settings can aspire to compassion and high regard for people, as Ratmeyer assures us it does. But we are enabled to aim even higher. We can bear witness to the transformation of persons by the power of Christ. The characteristic "peacemaking" of Anabaptists is founded upon the "peace that passes understanding." The newness and freshness of approach to mental health was inspired by the One who "makes all things new." We do not pretend that we can no longer learn from our colleagues throughout the broad mental health community. Nor

do we wish to exaggerate our differences with "secular" professionals, but we recognize that our work is inspired and upheld by
the "Shepherd and Bishop of souls," Jesus Christ.

The Role of Pastor in the Hospital

Although we are all called to be "pastors," we all need the
comfort and guidance of a pastor. Here we discern some important
elements of the pastor's unique role. Like other mental health professionals, the director of pastoral services ministers to the needs of
the whole person in his professional practice. But, unlike, most
professionals, the skill of this pastor is extended both to the patients
within the hospital and to the staff that cares for them. The whole
Christian community of the center comprises the parish. This pastor
offers guidance, healing, reconciliation, and sustenance to those
who are striving to offer the same. As pastor of pastors, the director
of pastoral services gives to those who give, provides for those who
provide, and serves those who are serving.

Whether through the structure of the treatment team, in
classes and training groups, or in conversation with individuals, the
director of pastoral services assists other mental health professionals to perform pastoral functions. This person teaches staff
members to assume leadership in worship, offers guidance to therapists who are challenged by the spiritual needs of their clients, and
encourages every member of the community to participate more
fully in the spiritual life of the institution. As enabler, the chaplain
helps the community to express its faith in worship and prayer. As
coordinator, the chaplain insures continuation of the chapel services, Bible studies, and inspirational groups. As catalyst, the chaplain facilitates the growth of mental health professionals so that they
might undertake more completely their pastoral responsibilities.
Whether enabler, coordinator, or catalyst, the director serves the
entire Christian community of the mental health center.

The Hospital as the Church

Throughout the hospital, the faith of the community is displayed in subtle ways. Team meetings begin with prayer as do
professional meetings and the sessions of the administrative council. In the dining room, individuals observe the ancient custom of
"saying grace" before eating. The literature in the patient library and
the reading material in the public areas reflect the hospital's commitment to spiritual growth of staff and residents. An intimate medita-
tion room is available for patients who wish to study or reflect
quietly by themselves. Persons who are being introduced to

Philhaven soon discover an understated but pervasive atmosphere of spiritual encouragement.

Formal programs of spiritual care are focused upon the chapel. The director of pastoral services arranges the schedule for daily chapel; members of the staff volunteer to lead worship. Because their participation is scheduled, chapel leaders are often able to involve patients with the planning and the execution of the program. Sometimes patients work with music therapists in preparing vocal or instrumental musical offerings. With clinical pastoral interns studying at the hospital, the daily chapel services are evaluated and discussed. This promotes continuing emphasis upon the importance of these programs and enhances quality standards in providing spiritual care.

On Wednesday evenings, inpatients and visiting family members or friends are invited to participate in a chapel program that most often is conducted by church groups or speakers from the communities near Philhaven. The program has become less formally structured and includes concerts of sacred music, movies of a religious nature, or celebrations organized around a theme and presented by inpatients. These programs are also evaluated by the evening duty staff and then reviewed by the director of pastoral services.

A special celebration of worship involving the whole hospital community takes place each week on Thursday mornings. A significant portion of the inpatient population is joined by members of every hospital department including professional staff persons, patient care personnel, and members of the support services. In addition to mealtimes, this is one event in which the whole community at Philhaven can share together. The worship service is very well attended and often involves groups of staff members in choruses, dramatic productions, choric readings, or instrumental ensembles. The coziness of the crowded chapel powerfully affirms the spiritual foundation of the community and the importance of prayer and fellowship.

Although they represent more than twenty denominations of Christian belief, the staff easily finds common ground for worship. The service is nonsectarian, incorporating elements of many Christian traditions. The residents of the hospital, some of whom profess no religious faith or non-Christian beliefs, are moved often to deeper understanding and appreciation of Christian faith. Occasionally, former patients communicate that their Philhaven experience marks a new awakening of their spiritual life.

Small group activities, often initiated by patients, also offer spiritual guidance and support. Bible studies, songfests, and inspirational groups for prayer and sharing are well attended—especially in the evening hours. For some inpatients, attending chapel is fraught with emotional distress or conflict. The informal groups, meeting in the living rooms or activity areas, are more accessible physically and emotionally.

Philhaven has developed a staff that is comfortable in discussing questions of religious faith or practice. In the innumerable interactions between staff members and the persons whom they serve, confidential personal relationships develop and are nurtured. In these friendships, client and therapist share convictions and experiences that include spiritual concerns. Where desired, counselor and client can share in prayer which reinforces for both parties the transcendental meanings of suffering and of healing.

Staff members also seek fellowship in small group activities. A biweekly Bible study meets during the lunch hour on Fridays. Discussions in this meeting are moderated by various volunteers from many parts of the hospital. Periodically, this noon meeting is devoted to prayer for the community at Philhaven and for the work of the hospital. Twice a month, the "Integration Luncheons," which attempt to integrate Christian faith and professional practice, are consistently well attended and widely supported. The formal presentation of an issue is usually made in a half-hour by any staff person interested in that subject. The second half-hour is then used to discuss the issue. The richness of the dialogue among the staff has been provocative and helpful.

Conclusion

The MMHS centers have used basically two approaches in finding and fulfilling their role as church-related institutions. One course, followed by the MCC-founded centers as a group, is a "development" model not unlike the practice of MCC in its overseas relief programs. The church sponsors and administers the program and provides at least a core of Christian staff to provide services, but in the local setting uses other resources and personnel, cultivates local responsibility, and collaborates with other groups, Christian and non-Christian, in achieving its goal.

The other approach, used by Philhaven Hospital, is to make the entire enterprise, staff and program, consciously and purposefully Christian. The hospital, in its work and in its worship, is the church. Clinical staff provide a combined professional and spiritual ministry. The director of pastoral services is the hospital pastor, primarily ministering to the members of that Christian community. The milieu is openly Christian.

To suggest two models means that there are at least two broadly defined approaches to becoming a church-related mental health center. It does not mean one is superior for all situations. In MMHS all eight centers have found a common church base from which to develop their individual programs. And from that base each desires in its own way to fulfill its mission as a church-sponsored service agency in its own setting.

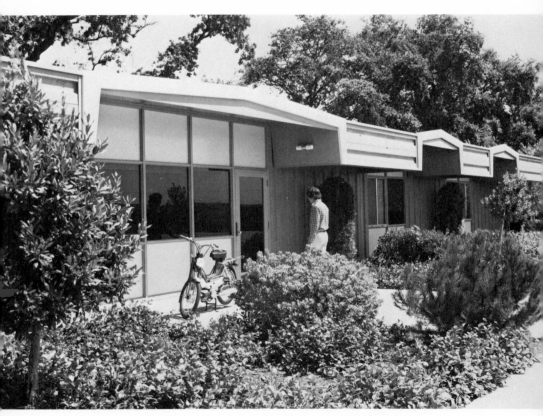

Kings View Rio Vista Transitional Facility, Reedley, California.

CHAPTER 14

Private Centers and Public Funding
Arthur Jost*

"What have the MMHS centers and hospitals learned from their experience with public funding?" This is the question addressed in this chapter. All eight mental health centers or hospitals, now part of the Mennonite Mental Health Services (MMHS) organization, have been touched by local, state, provincial, and/or federal funds. But there is a wide range of experience, from minimum public support at Philhaven Hospital and Brook Lane Psychiatric Center to practically total support at Eden Mental Health Centre.

This chapter treats first of all the historical context of church sponsorship out of which the first centers developed, and thus deals with the period before any public funding was accepted, about 1947 to 1957. Secondly, the chapter records the Kings View experience, somewhat as a case history, because of its extensive use of federal, state, and county funds. Finally, after comparing how the experience of the other MMHS centers is similar to or different from Kings View's, the chapter concludes with an overall evaluation of the total experience.

Before Public Funding (1947-1957)
The Mennonite Central Committee (MCC) mental hospitals which were planned, built, and opened during the first decade (1947-1957) — Brook Lane, Kings View, and Prairie View — gave little thought to receiving government funds either for construction or for operation prior to 1957. Of course, there was not much available to them. Moreover, the continuing debate over the issue of separation of church and state may have been a prohibiting factor, for the issue has continued to be a concern in Mennonite circles as well as in other

*Arthur Jost is president of the Kings View Corporation. He was assisted by the editor in the preparation of this chapter, particularly the first and last sections.

267

religious groups and on the United States political scene generally. But the first hospitals clearly were private, church-sponsored, and church-related institutions. They were born and grew up during their early years in a church environment, and government funds were not in the picture.

A Dual Emphasis

In the church environment of the time there was a dual emphasis or mission. One idea, expressed earlier in the Mennonite experience with Bethania Hospital and Bethesda Hospital, was to care for the needs of one's own group, to serve "the household of faith." The other, coming from MCC and the Civilian Public Service (CPS) experience, was to meet a need in society, to serve persons who are suffering, regardless of who they may be. These two threads of concern are brought together in one of the earliest MCC policy statements concerning the mental health program, "that the concept of services to be rendered be approached by MCC here also in the same spirit as in its other services, having due regard to the needs of *all men* but especially of *the household of faith*" (May 3, 1947).

Serving Mennonites

The "household of faith" interest at first dominated. Mennonite churches, in the earliest discussions of caring for the mentally ill, were concerned mostly about serving their own. Church members told of their relatives whom they visited in the large state institutions, where the patients were strangers in semiabandonment. CPS workers in state hospitals looked for familiar names of Mennonite origin among the patients, and felt a kinship with them as they together contemplated their geneology. Surveys and studies were conducted among Mennonite congregations, and the results were used as arguments to support initiating mental health programs.

From the beginning there was a mandate from MCC, expressed clearly by Orie Miller, the executive secretary, that (1) the mental health facilities would be built with church funds but (2) the program itself would be self-supporting. Once built and operating, the hospitals could not expect the churches to continue providing regular support for the operating budget. There apparently was some fear among the Mennonite groups that the new MCC mental health program would be a drain on contributed dollars otherwise earmarked for mission and other projects. So the stated policy concerning operations, also delineated in May 1947, was "that the cost be borne where possible by the patients or their families or, if necessary, by the congregations or conferences of which the patients are members." This was the Bethesda Hospital model, which was wholly church supported at that time, patient fees being guaranteed by the supporting churches.

What actually happened with the anticipated church support? As planned, the original facilities were built largely from funds and labor contributed by the churches, with only peripheral support provided by the local, nonconstituent community. Contributions from the churches for general operations continued for some time, but subsidizing patient fees did not have substantial support. In order to keep costs down and make fees more affordable, the first hospitals made significant use of volunteers and attempted to keep salaries down, near the level paid by other church institutions.

Patient fees in fact became troublesome to some in the churches. They had paid for the building so to pay fees for services, or to help with them, or to contribute to operations, seemed like double taxation. At various times attempts were made to bridge the gap by giving Mennonites special rates, providing a sliding fee schedule, setting up a "patient assistance fund," establishing a "membership benefit association," or exploring other forms of assisting patients. But in the end, the patient and his or her family who had difficulty paying the cost of treatment were not satisfactorily provided for. This created a serious problem for the hospitals and a cause for deteriorating relations with the churches.

Serving Others

And what of the second emphasis, to serve "all men"? The doors of the hospitals, once opened, were open to all—certainly all who could pay. In the earliest period of development very limited thought was given to the poor, who now are found in the mainstream of community mental health care of some MMHS centers. Curiously, the twenty-year MCC tradition of serving the needs of persons "out there" had taken second place to the early preoccupation with the "household of faith." Patients whose families could afford the treatment found a comfortable and welcome alternative to the state institutions in the Mennonite hospitals, but for the Mennonite and non-Mennonite residents in the community who were poor, an alternative form of paying the fees would have to be found.

Two other developments at the local hospital level should be mentioned as factors which opened up the hospitals to consider public funding. One was the increasing move of the institutions to serve the local community. Early support for constructing the mental health facilities was sought from Mennonite churches, but, by the time programs and buildings were ready, the projected services were no longer limited to Mennonite churches. Those who presented the programs already anticipated some community involvement and participation, and acknowledged that these mental hospitals would be demonstration programs located in areas of dense Mennonite populations to serve anyone needing help.

The other development was the financial difficulty encountered by the hospitals. Kings View Hospital closed its inpatient services for almost six months in 1957 and '58; Prairie View came close to closing its doors a little later; and Brook Lane too experienced financial problems. So the desire to operate on a fiscally sound basis, indeed, to survive, made the hospitals receptive, if not vulnerable, to public money when this became available.

So the three main reasons that the Mennonite institutions — those that did — began to receive public funds were the desire to serve everyone in need of services, including the poor; the objective to serve the local community, which then would be expected to help pay for those services; and the need to survive.

The Kings View Experience (1957-1981)
Of all the MMHS centers and hospitals, Kings View has been the most heavily involved in public funding in terms of dollars received. It has worked with and received funds from three levels of government — county, state, and federal. What has been Kings View's experience and how shall this be evaluated?

Construction Grants
The first opportunity to receive public funds came to Kings View in the late 1950s. Even while its inpatient services were temporarily suspended in 1957 and '58, Kings View was granted federal funds to add bed space to its hospital, the first government grant received by any MMHS institution. The Hill-Burton Hospital Construction Act was a federal program which provided matching grants mostly for general hospitals. In California, the state legislature made provisions to match Hill-Burton money with one-third state funds so that a federal match of one-third left a balance of one-third for the private agency. Kings View Hospital received two major building grants during its history.

Hill-Burton grants placed few restrictions on the recipients, but did include building standards and timelines, and a prohibition of discrimination against race, creed, or religion. A requirement to provide a certain amount of free care lay dormant for almost twenty years. When the requirement was revitalized nation-wide, Kings View Hospital was already providing care to the poor through its contract programs, but Kings View also adopted a formula to give free care at the hospital.

Community Mental Health Programs

A second government program affecting Kings View provided the opportunity for collaboration and funding at the local county level. In 1954, California officials borrowed plans from New York to fashion its own Community Mental Health Act, which was adopted by the legislature in 1957. Kings View influenced the development of legislative language which permitted Kings View Hospital's participation in the program. While the legislation was being debated in California, Kings View officials saw an opportunity to resolve the problem of treating the poor, because the law mandated care at a cost affordable to the patient or his family, or at no cost at all.

From 1957 to 1964, Kings View officials negotiated with two rural counties to contract for the provision of mental health services using the available public funds. During this time it became clear that rural counties especially had very little interest in exercising their option to develop and operate county mental health programs. It soon became apparent that to obtain such a contract Kings View would be expected to provide for the program planning and operation of county-wide programs, involving large sums of money. Kings View would be an agent for the county, yet would have basic freedoms as a contractor. Kings View would select and hire its administrators, professional staff, and support staff; set fees for patients on the basis of predetermined guidelines; and provide the services to the community. Mandates from the state included admission policies requiring Kings View to accept patients without regard to creed, race, or religion. Kings View would also be required to treat court-committed patients who needed to be held involuntarily.

During the course of its history, Kings View at the peak of its experience contracted with nine counties under the state mental health program.

Federal CMHC

The federal Community Mental Health Centers (CMHC)Act (1963), at first providing funds for construction, in 1965 made staffing grants available to existing or new mental health centers. A nonprofit corporation needed to make application to the National Institute of Mental Health (NIMH) for approval in order to serve a defined geographical region called a *catchment area*. Staffing grants provided funds to compensate staff employed in agencies serving designated catchment areas. Kings View applied and in 1966 was designated a CMHC for the northern half of Tulare County and all of Kings County.

The CMHC Act permitted freedom to serve patients within broad guidelines. Center patients were required to reside within the defined catchment area in order to be eligible to receive services rendered with grant funds. Certain reports and monitoring arrangements were mandated. A governing board from the community was an important requirement. Since the state program already required advisory committees, the federal requirements caused duplication. This duplication caused a diminished role for the federally-mandated boards because contracts with California counties demanded some degree of sharing of authority with the county-appointed committee. The situation was complicated even more by the fact that the federal catchment area did not coincide with county boundaries (in Tulare County).

The 1975 amendments to the CMHC Act generally tightened the regulations to correct weaknesses of the previous act. This affected Kings View most critically at the governing board level in that the community policy board, heretofore essentially advisory, would need to be given greater authority. To satisfy this requirement, the Kings View board delegated responsibility to the CMHC policy board to determine the local program and employ the program director. The reorganized policy board raised the issue of control more clearly than any previous issue. The other requirements, which meant more active monitoring through frequent and extensive site visits, more referrals to the regional federal office to resolve issues, did not have a major negative impact upon Kings View operations.

Patient Assistance Programs

In the mid-1960s a number of federal programs were enacted which provided direct assistance for the patient, and therefore only indirectly affected the institution. The Social Security Title XVIII and Title XIX entitlement programs authorized Medicare and Medicaid. These acts of Congress revolutionized payment for general medical care for the poor and the aged. In mental health, the laws were discriminatory and limits were placed on both programs. Another federal act, Civilian Health and Medical Program of the Uniformed Services (CHAMPUS), providing care for the dependents of military personnel, was more liberal, as was also an act providing insurance for federal employees and their dependents (Federal Employees Health Benefits Program).

The California Medicaid Program (Medi-Cal) was liberally applied in state-funded mental health programs. With the application of Medi-Cal billings, Kings View was paid for day treatment and other nonhospital programs, and for the services of nonmedical personnel working under the direction of psychiatrists.

Central Valley Regional Center

In 1971, Kings View initiated a significant new contract with the state of California for Central Valley Regional Center (CVRC). The local Fresno Association for Retarded Citizens previously had contracted for one year to provide a program of diagnostic, placement, and other services for the mentally retarded and certain other neurologically handicapped persons. This program covered six rural counties with the hub situated in the large and central county of Fresno, with a total population of over one million. CVRC is one of twenty-two centers in California operated by nonprofit agencies.

With state funds, Kings View served as a conduit for the purchase of essential services, and significant funds also were available to employ caseworkers and specialists. The program began with a modest staff and budget, but has grown until the records currently indicate 8,000 active cases. The categories of clients treated fit the federal definitions for developmental disabilities, and the purchase of essential services range from eyeglasses to workshop fees. This program has given Kings View much satisfaction.

The regional center system opened numerous opportunities to serve the poor and the handicapped in every community of the six-county area. Developmentally disabled persons were neglected prior to 1971 when such publicly funded services were provided mainly to state hospital patients. This created extremely long waiting lists for state hospitals. CVRC has been a program that fit well into the objectives of the Kings View mission statement.

The Effects Upon Kings View

Rapid Growth

One of the obvious results of public funding was the rapid growth of Kings View over a relatively short period of time. As a small private hospital with thirty beds in 1958, Kings View by the mid-1970s was responsible for all the mental health services in nine counties, for a federal community mental health center with a catchment area covering 1½ counties, and for services to developmentally disabled persons in six counties, all funded by government money.

Rapid growth and the resulting size of the total program, as in any similar situation, created problems. There was difficulty in procuring adequate, qualified staff. The corporation outgrew staff capabilities in some positions of top management, and changes needed to be made to keep up. The increasing size and perceived authority of the central offices led to problems of a "we-they" relationship at the local program level, and it was difficult to maintain a spirit of unity within the corporation. The contracting government entities viewed with some questioning, if not suspicion, the high costs of maintaining a relatively large central staff, the cost of which each was expected to share. So size alone created problems, though in themselves the difficulties were not specifically caused by public funding.

Quasi-Public Image

But there were problems arising more directly from the ties with government. One of the early effects upon Kings View, resulting from government collaboration and funding, was a developing quasi-public image and the problems inherent in that role. Even with the initial Hill-Burton construction grant in 1957, members of the constituent churches and other community residents perceived that the hospital had been "taken over" by government. The earlier sense of pride in owning a facility which local members built and furnished seemed betrayed. No amount of public information and personal efforts could erase that sense of disappointment. Internally, however, Kings View was not unduly affected by serious government intervention.

In the publicly funded mental health and mental retardation programs the identification problems were more serious and persistent. Staff members themselves seemed unsure about whether they worked for the private Kings View corporation or for the county or state which provided the funds. Contracts, which were considered and renewed annually, existed at the pleasure of the county or state, so there was a constant uncertainty about the future. In several instances, where counties canceled contracts with Kings View, staff showed some relief in the final determination that they would "serve only one master," albeit the less desirable one of the two.

A similar uncertainty existed within the community. The county and state programs, in that Kings View provided all the services within a specified area, were seen by the community for the most part as public services. All the pressures, the scrutiny, and criticism which any public service experiences, were encountered by Kings View in operating the programs for government. The fact that Kings View, a private, nonprofit corporation, was contracting with government was not obvious to most persons in the community, and those who were aware of the relationship often were critical: Kings View was "taking over," Kings View was too expensive, Kings View was making a profit from contracts, and so forth.

Governance

One specific area of confusion and difficulty involved the Kings View governing board and the public policy/advisory boards. The quasi-public image emerged and was influenced by government mandated public policy board structures as they interfaced with one another in Kings View programs. The mental health advisory boards appointed by each county, the policy boards appointed by Kings View for CVRC, and for the federally designated community mental health center, all shared government designated authority and view for impact on the programs. In two counties, for example, the Kings View board, the county advisory board, and the CMHC policy board all had some responsibility or authority for the mental health program.

Financial

Financial problems seemed inevitable. One cause was the cost reimbursement financing model used in the county community mental health programs. The idea was that Kings View's costs of providing services were to be reimbursed by a given county. The catch was that Kings View would be reimbursed for *audited* disbursements. With government guidelines often vague, there were not only misunderstandings and arbitration, but costly audit disallowances as well. In other words, it was a no-win arrangement. At best it was break-even, and Kings View never broke even.

How then could Kings View manage financially? Largely because one of its programs, Kings View Hospital, consistently operated with a high patient census and was able to maintain reserves sufficient to offset the losses incurred in the public programs. While the Kings View board never adopted a policy stating that the hospital reserves would be available for corporate-wide subsidy, this in fact was the unwritten policy and practice. It is not unlike the practice of private patients and insurance companies subsidizing publicly funded patients in general hospitals.

As a result of the problems arising from the cost reimbursement system, Kings View sought ways to remedy the situation. In the early 1970s attempts were made to alter the contracts to a negotiated form that would both allow surpluses to accumulate and remove postaudit disallowances. It became apparent that new state legislation would be required, so with Kings View sponsorship, new provisions were adopted by the legislature to make possible new contracts to replace current cost reimbursement contracts. In 1981 the Kings View board summarily adopted two policies to guide future operations: not to contract with government unless there is assurance of adequate funding to cover costs and to restrict the use of hospital surpluses.

Summary

One can draw several conclusions about Kings View's experience with government funding:

1. The construction grants (Hill-Burton) by and large contributed to the needed expansion of the hospital and did not have a negative impact upon the Kings View organization, although, as already noted, there was some adverse reaction from the church and community.

2. The fee-for-service programs aimed to assist patients (for example, Social Security), though not very significant or extensive, have worked satisfactorily with little or no negative influence felt.

3. The federal staffing grants enabled Kings View to provide a wide spectrum of programs, including consultation and other community services, and to that extent was a positive experience; the difficulty with the policy board, already mentioned, and the gradual phasing out of the funding became negative aspects.

4. Public funds from state and county sources have been a mixed blessing. These funds enabled Kings View to formulate extensive programs and services in keeping with its mission to serve all persons in need, including the poor. Yet, these contracts proved the most troublesome of all forms of public funding, with unclear bureaucratic regulations, undesirable program priorities, some waste in spending funds merely to conform to regulations, and disallowances and liabilities for Kings View.

The Experience of Other MMHS Institutions

Brook Lane, Philhaven, and Penn Foundation

Of the first three hospitals to be established by MCC, Brook Lane (1949) has maintained most consistently the private psychiatric hospital stance. Two times during its history Brook Lane considered applying for federal construction grants (Hill-Burton), but finally decided against it. More than once, Brook Lane also considered moving aggressively in the direction of becoming a community health center, but never became a mental health center in the state or federal sense and was not funded as such. Brook Lane has, however, provided numerous services on an individual, contract basis for various public entities, for example the schools.

Philhaven Hospital (1954), which was born in the same period as the first three MCC hospitals, has also remained free of government ties. Like Brook Lane, Philhaven has provided various services for government agencies, but has avoided the role of a CMHC which utilizes federal and state funds. It has been careful to function as a private psychiatric hospital under the direct sponsorship of the Lancaster Conference of the Mennonite Church.

As we saw in a previous chapter (Chapter 7), initially, Penn Foundation applied for a Hill-Burton construction grant and was assured of funding, but ultimately turned down the grant when the center learned it had to include beds in the facility in order to comply. Penn Foundation cooperated with and received funds from the state in providing certain services on a fee-for-service basis, but not as a community mental health center.

Eden

Eden Mental Health Centre (1967), located in Manitoba, Canada, has received the most public funding of all the MMHS member institutions, in effect 100 percent funding. The cost of operating is established on the basis of an annual budget and paid by the province. The Eden arrangement needs to be understood in the Canadian context, where collaboration of church organizations with government is more liberal and flexible than in the United States, where universal access to medical care is an established reality, and where the relationship with government is much simpler (for example, at the single, provincial level rather than at a multiple level as in the United States). Approximately 75 percent of Eden's initial construction costs came from federal or provincial funds, but both channeled through the province. Patients receive care as part of the provincial health plan and do not pay fees to Eden for services rendered.

Prairie View, Oaklawn, and Kern View

The other three MMHS centers—Prairie View (1954), Oaklawn (1962), and Kern View (1966)—like Kings View have had considerable experience with government funding at all three levels: federal, state, and local (county).

Under 1961 Kansas legislation, Prairie View in 1962 arranged to sell mental health services to three local counties on a fee-for-service basis. A middleman, tri-county corporation was set up to receive county funds and purchase Prairie View services. Under the 1963 CMHC Act, Prairie View in 1966 received a construction grant to help finance a building program. A staffing grant under the same program was received the same year, and succeeding years on a decreasing basis, as a stimulus to expand the range of services within the three-county catchment area. In 1964 the state began providing subsidies to the counties on a matching basis, and these funds when available were channeled through the tri-county corporation, not directly to Prairie View. More recently the middleman corporation has been dissolved and Prairie View now contracts directly with each county.

Oaklawn Psychiatric Center in the early 1960s helped finance the construction of its original facilities with a federal grant (Hill-Burton), made possible with the support of Elkhart General Hospital. Elkhart County, in which Oaklawn is located, in 1964 began making annual grants to Oaklawn in exchange for making available mental health services to residents according to their ability to pay. Similar arrangements were made with four other counties until they as a group established a separate community mental health center. In 1973 Oaklawn was designated a CMHC for Elkhart County by NIMH, and was awarded federal funds accordingly. Most of the slack in funding caused by decreasing grants has been picked up by the state, which makes annual grants directly to Oaklawn.

Kern View Hospital at its beginning also received a Hill-Burton construction grant, matched by the state on a one-third basis. Within months after opening in 1966, Kern View received a staffing grant as a federally designated CMHC. Unfortunately, the specified catchment area was roughly the western half of Kern County, the eastern half being assigned to the county itself, with the boundary running through the heart of Bakersfield in which both Kern View and Kern County Department of Mental Health services were located. Under the state Community Mental Health Act, Kern View contracted with the county for certain services on an annual basis, but never for all services, even within the federally designated catchment area.

Comparison with Kings View

When one compares the experiences of Prairie View, Oaklawn, and Kern View with Kings View's there are similarities as well as differences. All four programs have had an overall positive experience with federal construction grants, whether CMHC or Hill-Burton. These funds assisted with building programs without serious impact from government regulations or controls. All report that the federal staffing or stimulus grants assisted in the development of new services which were not possible otherwise, and this funding had overall positive results. An exception was the "withdrawal pains" caused by decreasing funds and the need to secure additional funding or phase-out programs. Experiences with public programs to assist patients (Medicare, Medicaid) were similar to all four and posed no problems of regulation or control.

There were differences in how the four institutions handled

the CMHC governance issue. While Kings View delegated certain responsibilities to the CMHC policy board, Kern View attempted to make its own governing board comply with federal guidelines regarding residence and other demographic considerations in the catchment area. Oaklawn set up a CMHC corporation, the board of which was composed of the Oaklawn governing board members residing in the catchment area; and Prairie View enlarged its governing board to make possible better representation from the three-county catchment area.

Prairie View and Oaklawn seemed to have had better experiences with local community mental health center programs, financed by both county and state funds, than Kings View did. Some of the difference was due to California conditions, for Kern View encountered some problems similar to Kings View's, for example with audit disallowances. Prairie View had problems in one of the contracting counties, but this apparently was caused more by local conditions than by the system used in contracting. Kern View's problems with the county and state, in addition to audit disallowances, were caused largely by the situation in the local county where contracting was made very difficult in the hands of local government.

What Have We Learned?

Our experience with government via funding mechanisms has not been uniform. Of the eight institutions, five chose to become involved significantly and three chose to be relatively free. Even among the five and among the three, there are variations in philosophy and experience. So there is no single experience; there are eight different experiences. Consequently any conclusions made are general and will require qualifiers and exceptions.

1. Relationship to the churches has not been directly and adversely affected by public funding. We have noted that leaning on government for funds coincided with a diminishing sense of responsibility on the part of the churches, that in some centers there seemed to be a tendency to downplay the Christian/Mennonite identity, that there was some drifting of the constituency from the centers (or vice versa) over a period of time. But it would be difficult to demonstrate a direct tie between these developments and receiving government funding. Of two centers attempting to maintain a strong and open Christian identity, one is almost wholly funded by government (Eden) and one is almost free of public funding (Philhaven).

2. Public funding has made possible expansion of services in areas difficult if not impossible to fund on a private basis. Joining

with government made services available to everyone in a given area, especially including those who could not afford to pay. Public funding increased the opportunity to serve special groups, for example the elderly, those addicted to drugs and alcohol, and those released from state institutions. Government grants expanded the opportunities to serve the larger community with education, consultation, and growth events, which are seen as prevention programs.

3. Risk is involved in accepting public funds, for example to serve the poor, but it is a calculated one. The choice, at extreme ends, is between maintaining a private practice position and serving those who can pay or collaborating with government in order to serve everyone, especially the poor. There is some "trade-off" in collaboration, depending somewhat upon the purposes of the institution.

4. Some services can be provided more readily than others on a private basis. The overall experience has been that inpatient, and increasingly outpatient, services can be given without public support, but services of a public health nature cannot. Treatment costs are more easily recovered than costs of education and prevention, individual care than community-wide services. The earlier problem of some patients being unable to pay the cost of treatment has been alleviated, though not completely resolved, by increasing third-party payers (Social Security and insurance).

5. Public funding makes it possible for private institutions to provide services in behalf of government qualitatively superior to and more efficiently than services provided by government itself. This is difficult to document, but center administration and staff, as well as persons in the community and in government, generally agree on this.

6. Public funding inevitably means some government influence and regulation. The truism, "He who pays the piper calls the tune," has meaning and relevance. While no center felt that government was oppressive or overly regulatory, each grant carried with it specific conditions and requirements. Grant applications, reporting, and site visits at times were more troublesome and exhausting than the regulations themselves. The severity of the control generally varied according to the type of grant. There was less restriction with construction grants, greater regulations with grants for services and programs; less for fee-for-service, greater with operational subsidies.

7. Collaborating with government has complicated and may have adversely affected staff development. It was difficult if not impossible because of regulations against discrimination, to be up

front about desirable though forbidden stipulations (for example, religious) in recruiting personnel. Staff positions needed to be open to all, so screening and selection became more subtle and indirect. The rapid growth of staff resulting from public funding also made a difference in the quality of staff.

8. Public funding can be seductive, and there is a point beyond which the centers do not go. Where the line was drawn varied greatly. The increased cost and required use of union labor was enough for Brook Lane to say no to a Hill-Burton grant. The stipulation to add beds to a planned outpatient and day treatment facility was enough for the Penn Foundation to refuse a construction grant. The severe requirement concerning the governing board in the 1975 CMHC Act caused all four centers receiving funds to ask, Do we pull out? Kings View said, No more, to the cost reimbursement funding mechanism. The key question concerned the degree of control: when the tail wags the dog, it needs to be amputated.

9. Public funding does lead to some waste, some excesses, some irrationalities. This is illustrated by the increased cost of construction caused by federal guidelines (Hill-Burton). Penn Foundation concluded that by refusing the grant their cost was less than their share would have been with the matching grant. Another example is the arbitrary, impractical boundaries drawn for catchment areas (Kings View and Kern View).

10. A collaborative relationship with government moves the private center into the political arena. At various times centers found themselves negotiating contracts, influencing legislation, dealing with union activity, arbitrating disagreements, and filing a lawsuit—activities which developed from a quasi-public position assumed as a result of receiving public funding.

11. Working with various levels of government has been a learning experience, and centers are much wiser because of this experience. Especially those who received considerable government funding have rediscovered the value of both the private stance and the church connection. The uncertainty of public funding and increased regulation make for an uncertain future. Long-term, meaningful survival depends upon an appropriate role as private, church-related institutions.

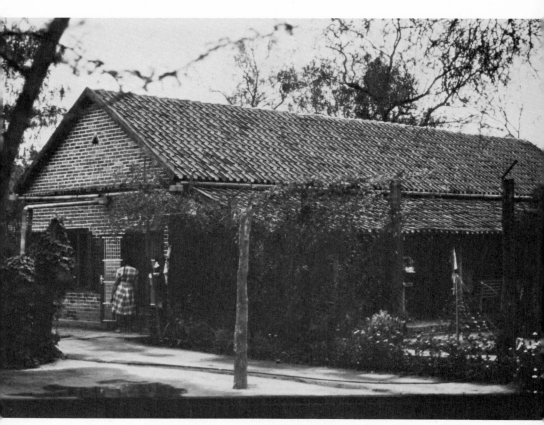

One of several patient cottages at Hoffnungsheim Sanatorium, Filadelfia, Paraguay.

CHAPTER 15

MMHS in Perspective
Aldred H. Neufeldt*

By any yardstick the Mennonite Mental Health Services (MMHS) story is unique. MMHS was born in the aftermath to World War II out of a conviction that people who are deeply troubled with psychiatric problems deserve a better fate than to be locked away in the large, faceless wards of state institutions. Brought into being as the administrative arm of the Mennonite Central Committee (MCC) and responsible to guide the establishment and development of the mental health centers, MMHS has evolved into an amalgam of the church which gave birth to the mental health program and the centers themselves.

If it were possible to consider simply the mental health service story, apart from both the involvement of the church throughout and the precise origin of MMHS as a nonresistant response to militarism, one might find some rough parallels in the development of community mental health systems in the United Kingdom in the 1950s and a province like Saskatchewan or states such as New York and California in the 1960s. There was some similar motivation of a professional and humanitarian nature in all these settings. Yet there is an essential difference that makes such comparison inappropriate.

If one focuses only on the individual mental health center part of MMHS, one would be in danger of missing the overall theme of what MMHS is all about. MMHS is more than a collection of individual centers, significant as these may be. In the overall assessment of MMHS one can come to a number of conclusions: (1) MMHS has become a forum where the church at large and the professional

---

*Aldred H. Neufeldt was a member of the MMHS board 1969-78 and its chairman the last three of those years. Currently he is senior partner in Applied Research Consulting House, Mississauga, Ontario.

community can wrestle with issues as common today as thirty years ago. (2) MMHS provides a common set of beliefs and values for centers scattered through a number of widely diverse jurisdictions. (3) MMHS has served as a means of uniting the centers in a system which serves as a safeguard to their vitality. (4) In the process of giving up responsibility for administering these centers and becoming a cooperative venture between the individual centers and the churches of the MCC constituency, MMHS also evolved from being inward oriented to being concerned about reaching out beyond itself.

An assessment of MMHS, then, needs to take these and other factors into account. Comparison with an external norm has some uses with respect to individual parts of MMHS activity, but not to the whole. A more useful frame of reference is to examine the MMHS experience from the point of view of what has been learned. What follows, then, is derived from a conceptual analysis of various events in the MMHS history.

MMHS *as a Forum for Continuous Learning*

There is a body of evidence in literature that human organizations of all kinds, whether business and industry or the service professions, have a life cycle not dissimilar to that of the people who comprise them. There is a period of infancy in which growth is slow and tentative, followed by exciting periods of rapid growth. Most organizations then move into a mature phase characterized by relatively minor adjustments, and essentially aimed at maintaining the *status quo*. Donald Schon has called this a state of "dynamic conservatism"—working hard at keeping things the same. This is followed by a period of slow decline of its vibrancy and relevance, ultimately leading to a situation where it is largely out of step with its original purposes. This process seems almost inevitable unless ways are found of ensuring that the organization regularly comes face-to-face with its own irrelevancies and learns from them. Few organizations seem capable of learning until they are faced with death. (Consider, for example, the North American auto industry which waited a disastrously long period of time before developing fuel efficient vehicles.) Mental health centers generally are no different than other organizations in this regard.

As in other domains the mental health field has had its informal and formal means of promoting learning, with informal means often being most important. One of the reasons MMHS centers have continued to have a vibrancy is that some have deliberately and continuously sought out the best available information relevant to providing services. When the first MMHS centers were begun there were no patterns to follow. The small center approach was an idea borne out of a concern that there must be a better way. The initiators were both naive enough not to be intimidated by the immensity of the task of preparing new directions and wise enough to ask for advice from wherever it was available. The National Institute of Mental Health (NIMH) programs such as those provided by the Menningers and others provided valuable early assistance. This pattern of seeking new and improved ways of doing things has remained with most centers to the present. As a result, there grew an informal means of information exchange that has had a continuity to it with long run implications.

External sources of learning, though, often are hard to maintain and by themselves tend to be insufficient. When times are good it is easy to look elsewhere for ideas. When times are difficult, it is much less easy to learn—whether the difficulties stem from internal tensions and mistakes or external factors. It is in this latter kind of context that the MMHS structure has been most helpful.

The forum where issues involving the centers are exchanged and debated is in the context of the MMHS board. Although composition of the board has changed a number of times since its inception, it has continued to have the following general characteristics. With rare exception, all members have had a close identity with the Mennonite and Brethren churches. As a result, there is a prevailing common sense of purpose for meetings which for the most part is quite unspoken. Membership of the board usually involves a cross section of human service professionals, educators, theologians, center representatives, people from the business community, as well as representation from various church constituencies and MCC. As a result, when issues of importance are discussed they have the benefit of a broad range of experience. Indeed, it has been said many times that it would be impossible to purchase better consultation.

The fact that there is a great deal of continuity of membership also helps the learning process. Since the board meets only twice a year, it takes several meetings before a new member is really effective. However, with terms that are three years long, and each term being renewable up to three times, the learning that is gained in one generation can and is passed on to succeeding generations. The common judgment of board members past and present is that serving on this board is an enriching experience—both personally and professionally. With this kind of prevailing atmosphere it becomes understandable why continuous learning is as much a "way of life" as a deliberate act.

The MMHS learning forum does not end with the board meetings. Associated with every board meeting is a gathering of administrative heads from the centers. Usually scheduled for the day before the board meeting begins, this meeting provides a forum to share problems, examine ways of solving them and, in general, provide helpful advice and common support to each other. Because the number of people in a given community who can fully understand the problems and complexities faced by a chief executive officer are few, these meetings have become highly valued by the people involved.

Once a year, again associated with board meetings, one day is devoted to learning about current issues that have a bearing on human services. The MMHS center hosting that particular board meeting organizes the program either to highlight a given set of broad issues (for example, values implied in clinical decision making, the role of the church in psychiatric service, and so forth), or to highlight effective approaches to difficult clincial problems (for example, alcohol or drug abuse, adolescent behavior issues). Personnel and board members from all centers are invited to join together on such occasions. Again, an opportunity is afforded to exchange ideas between clinical and program leadership of the various centers, as well as for all persons present to reflect on a common set of issues as presented through the formal program.

A significant vehicle of learning is the role played by the MMHS director. At least twice yearly the director has attempted to visit each center. Such occasions are used to review with the chief executive officer of the center, the chairman of the local center board and other persons what current issues and problems are being faced by the center. The director is not only immediately helpful in terms of providing advice based on this experience, but he is also able to identify commonalities between the issue as presented and problems faced previously by other centers. It then becomes easier to identify resource people who might help resolve the issue of the moment.

MMHS as a Continuing and Guiding Value Base

A growing secular literature is beginning to recognize that one's fundamental values are critical to determining the direction any individual or organization will move. This has not always been so. In western culture generally we have placed great stock on the role that empirical knowledge plays in determining the answers to problems or goals to be pursued. The prevailing "beliefs" have been that knowledge will lead to insight and technology which, in time, will solve our problems. These beliefs exist for some good reasons. There has been a technological revolution which in fact has dramatically improved our quality of life as measured by how much of our time is spent on putting food on the table, traveling from place to place, and even in coping with various diseases and pestilence. The net result has been that society generally has placed more value on "information" and "technology" than on other values.

There is growing recognition, though, that despite our vast store of knowledge the fundamental problems facing us—war, poverty, and disturbed personal relationships—are not solved through technology. In other words, the message of the church that fundamental values are important is beginning to be recognized in corporate and social circles. In decision theory terms, it is not only a matter of the information one has at one's disposal, it also matters what "criterion" is used to judge that information.

This suggests that one of the most unique and important dimensions of MMHS in relation to its centers is that it provides a continuing, guiding value base against which the inevitable pulls and pushes of emerging technologies and secular professional values can be tested. Conversely, MMHS can interpret professional concerns to the church constituency. It has become a forum where professionals can voice criticism over too narrowly defined church practices, and have these tested and reflected upon.

The issue of "professional" view versus "church" view was a point of tension particularly in the early MMHS history (from the mid '50s through the early '60s). Even professionals who had been reared in the church found it difficult to reconcile the belief system learned as part of becoming a professional (for example, that the clinical knowledge one has should solve the problems one confronts) with broader values related to faith. The net result was that a period of relative estrangement existed between the sponsoring churches and the individual centers. Indeed, questions were raised by MCC as to whether the centers should be encouraged to go their own way. These tensions began to resolve themselves when the church constituency became less suspicious of new technologies, new funding mechanisms, and new ways of organizing, and when the professional community became more appreciative of how values interrelate with knowledge.

As this tension diminished, another set of conflicting values emerged. The MMHS centers had been some of the very first community mental health programs in North America. As such, their early work was often unappreciated and unrecognized. In the early to mid 1960s the "community mental health movement" was exploding across the continent. Some of the MMHS centers, as a result, became very visible. Given that public funding was now available, should these centers "buy in," became a question. Over time a number have, but not without considerable debate locally and at

MMHS meetings. (See Chapter 14.) Some were pressed, both by state governments and some of their own professionals, to become regional community mental health centers. This led to a tension of whether the centers should cut their ties with MMHS to assume a strictly local/regional and secular identity.

On each occasion the idea has been examined and, after careful deliberation, discarded. MMHS provided a continuity of principles and values against which such conflicting societal values could be tested. If one examines the histories of individual centers and MMHS minutes it is interesting to note how individuals associated with given centers assumed different roles at different times — at one point in time struggling with whether or not a local center should become independent, at another arguing persuasively that the centers must continue to band together with the church through MMHS so that these very contentious issues could be dealt with in a forum that was not conflicted with local monetary, political, or professional jealousies and issues.

These conflicts have not been without a positive side effect. While the early centers were directly under the administration of the MMHS board, over time individual centers became largely independent with local boards of directors. MMHS evolved into a fraternal organization with equal representation from the centers and the churches. The only residual controls remaining with MMHS for the five original centers were the authority to appoint local board members and approve the chief executive officer and the chief clinical officer, and the final authority with respect to bylaw changes. As a result, issues of local autonomy have largely subsided, although the professional personnel in various centers occasionally raise the question of more local autonomy. Usually these questions are raised by personnel who have not been appreciative of center origins and the Anabaptist traditions. Each time such a debate emerges, however, it is renewing in another way. It causes not only the MMHS board but also local board members and leading personnel to examine the reasons for their continued existence. Such an examination of purpose, aspirations, and ideals always becomes a renewing experience. It is highly likely that without MMHS, several of these centers would have departed from their original purposes. The existence of MMHS, as a means of keeping original purposes and underlying values before the centers in order to test their continuing relevance, is unique.

MMHS as a "Safeguard to Center Vitality"
One of the reasons many organizations fall into disarray and either die or become irrelevant is that in times of stress no outside

force is available to either counsel the organization in how to avoid doing itself harm or to help it become revitalized. Few organizations (as few people) are prepared to be very forthright when they are either in organizational difficulty or when they wish to cut their ties with original intents and purposes. In these circumstances most organizations become withdrawn and self-centered—usually a step toward demise. From previous chapters it will have become apparent that the MMHS centers have been subject to the same stresses and strains as other organizations. It also has been said that MMHS has provided both a values-based frame of reference against which ideas and concerns could be tested, and a forum to promote continuous learning. Neither of these would have been possible to maintain, however, without a structure that did not allow centers simply to withdraw and wither when the going got tough.

We noted earlier that the MMHS had certain legal responsibilities with respect to its five original centers: to appoint board members and to ratify senior personnel and center bylaw changes. (These provisions do not apply to the three centers which were begun independently of MCC and later affiliated themselves with MMHS.) While for the most part the appointment and bylaw approval process is straightforward, consuming little time at board meetings, these actions have three important effects.

First, the approval process symbolizes that there are, in fact, tangible and obligatory ties between MMHS and the centers. For the most part these ties are perceived in a positive way by both centers and MMHS—one that is of particular benefit to the centers since it helps centers (and their boards) avoid becoming entrapped in local and parochial issues.

Once in a while, however, a given center will propose a change in bylaws or an appointment that is of questionable benefit. On occasions such as this a second effect becomes apparent; namely, that the MMHS board can indeed provide a very real "check and balance" to local or state initiatives. There have been occasions, for example, when a bylaw change is proposed prompted by some new state government requirement and which the center found difficult to avoid. While MMHS in all likelihood would have approved such a bylaw change if pressed to do so, the testing of such a proposed change by personnel from other jurisdictions on more than one occasion has caused the submitting center to withdraw the proposed change in favor of some additional consideration at home. Similarly, there have been occasions in at least two centers when its professionals have virtually persuaded the center to turn into a secular or private program. Again, it is doubtful whether MMHS would have turned the proposal down in the final analysis. However, because the issue had to come up for discussion at MMHS, the opportunity presented itself to question the underlying issues, intents, and motives. On each occasion matters were raised that had not been considered and which caused the centers in question to review their organizational goals and internal processes. Similar observations could be made of occasional nominations for board members or senior personnel being presented for approval.

The third effect of the approval process is that it creates an agenda for the MMHS director to visit each center. Again, there is no need for an agenda when things go well. The director is more than welcome to visit each center. However, when a center is in a period of internal conflict, the need for the MMHS director to review local board membership and functioning with the center head and the local board chairman creates a welcome agenda for a visit which otherwise might be difficult to arrange. Such occasions allow the director to meet with center leadership, exchange ideas, and serve in a facilitating and supportive manner as in a way that is easily justified to all concerned.

There has been questioning from time to time as to whether these residual responsibilities of MMHS toward its centers are important. The argument put forward is that MMHS and its director could continue these various functions without the present formal structural link. While goodwill is an important and very present ingredient in MMHS, the experience with other systems and organizations suggests that inevitably forces arise which tend to cause such an organization to disintegrate. To prevent such disintegration one needs some constraining force that binds the organization together in a way that is more difficult to sever than by means of a "Mexican divorce." One of the very real uniquenesses of MMHS has been that the five original centers have had a continuing structural relationship which at one and the same time is both elastic and yet very real.

MMHS as a Means of Reaching Beyond Oneself

One final dimension contributing to the ongoing vitality of MMHS has been its sense of mission. Just as individual centers have been outward oriented, seeking to benefit from experiences elsewhere so as to improve their service at home, so too has been MMHS itself. In its early history MMHS almost foundered when it focused only on center development and administration. One might well surmise that after the centers were developed, and all that remained was the administrative function, MMHS board members would have become increasingly removed from the day-to-day sorrows and joys of center operations. No wonder, then that there was a move toward greater local autonomy in the 1950s and 1960s.

Once MMHS became a fraternal organization with conjoint membership of the centers and church, new agendas for joint action started appearing. Some early interests were expressed in developing outreach work in the Appalachian region of the United States and in Hong Kong. These never really got off the ground. However, one initiative that did was the MMHS work in Paraguay. This experience, described elsewhere in this book, developed a sense of purpose within MMHS. It gave visible proof that it was possible for the centers and the larger church to work together toward a greater purpose of serving humanity as well as to maintain a high quality program at home. The work in Paraguay has contributed a number of other learning experiences. For North Americans, often used to rapid service growth and change, work in Paraguay has taught patience. Development of new services in a country that had few meant that time and more time was needed. True development takes place in a time frame which considers the cycle of awareness that people have, and not by time frames that are technically feasible. MMHS also learned to respond to locally requested and articulated needs rather than to external perceptions of need.

The second major outreach of centers and church together through MMHS has been the work on the developmental disabilities (DD). In this case, the intent has been to raise the consciousness of North American church constituents to the special needs that mentally retarded and other developmentally disabled persons in their midst have. Over the past eight years a tremendous change has occurred. Where once few mentally retarded youngsters or adults were found in church, today a sizable number can be found. Where once diagnosed retardation was considered as sufficient reason to prevent baptism and participation in congregational activities, today there is a sizable degree of acceptance. Where in the early '70s there was only one summer family camping and retreat program for families with retarded members, there now are a sizable number. We are seeing church school materials that encourage integration of disabled persons into their congregations and many other signs that this initiative has paid handsome dividends for the efforts that have been expended.

In both the above examples MMHS has served as a vehicle which allowed centers and MMHS board members at large to reach beyond themselves. Being asked to think about work under way with Paraguayan leaders (or other countries such as Mexico and Brazil) causes one to think in much more global terms, and to see mental health programs at home in their proper context. Being asked to think about the needs of a stigmatized, neglected, and under-served population at home, such as those with mental retardation, has had a tendency to reduce any feelings of complacency which may have emerged.

Summary: Once More the Question of Evaluation

By any yardstick MMHS is a unique entity. When one asks whether MMHS is a service organization, the answer is ambiguous. While the center members are very much in the direct service delivery business, MMHS itself is not. Is MMHS then a church program of some kind? Again, the answer is elusive. MMHS is very much part of the broader Mennonite family tree (although not always very visible in the past). Yet, it isn't the typical church program as one tends to think of it. Structural ties are loose and the operating mandate has been such that its activities have not often been the center of pulpit presentations.

For all of these seemingly "will-o-the-wisp" characteristics, MMHS itself has made a profound impact. Board members from throughout its history commonly observe that their period of service was one of the most worthwhile experiences in their lives. Center administrative heads say that this organization has played a significant part in their ability to continue exercising responsible and responsive leadership at home so as to continue building excellence in mental health service. The people receiving help from individual centers by-and-large have been the very direct recipients of such pride in the providing of quality care.

The larger world too has been positively affected. From the very beginning, when MMHS centers were the pioneers in providing mental health services in a more personal and humane way, individual MMHS centers have served as a model to countless other programs. The relationship with Paraguay has been of mutual benefit—to both North Americans and Paraguayans. The Developmentally Disabled program in the past decade has launched a new awareness within the church community contributing to the opening of doors for disabled people that heretofore had been shut. In many respects this program parallels the original mental health experience which began opening doors for people with psychiatric or emotional problems.

These and other elements have created an organization with a continuing sense of purpose and vitality that is rare in the annals of human service organizations.

What Others Say

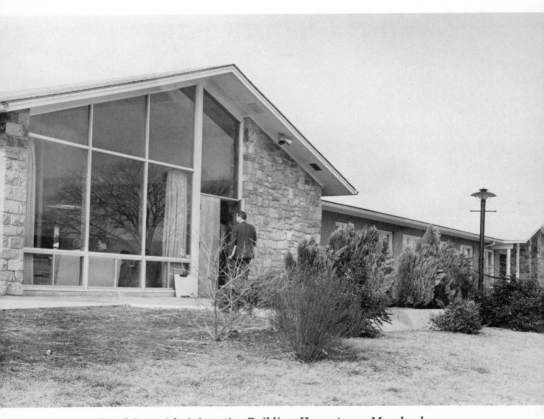

Brook Lane Administration Building, Hagerstown, Maryland.

CHAPTER 16

"From the Inside Out"

Richard C. Hunter*
A Mental Health Association Executive

In my early upbringing, I had not experienced groups with self-imposed sharply defined boundaries which clearly defined me to be on the outside. That is not to say that I had been acceptable everywhere or to everyone. Nor that there weren't groups for which I would have been unqualified. However, I was not aware of groups which would consciously identify me to be an "outsider." This kind of naivete proved valuable when my notice to report for Civilian Public Service on June 23, 1941, specified Camp #5 in Colorado Springs, Colorado.

I knew in advance that the camp to which I was reporting was operated by the Mennonite Central Committee (MCC), but the significance of that was not clear nor of much concern compared to separation from career, friends, and family. It wasn't until my environment and my daily activity became circumscribed by the camp itself that I gave much thought to the people with whom I first expected to spend one year, and then, on December 7, 1941, realized I would spend an indefinite period of time.

Though Camp #5 was totally Mennonite when our contingent of non-Mennonites arrived from the Twin Cities in Minnesota, it was some time before I realized that I was an "outsider." And then it wasn't because I was excluded or treated in some special fashion. There was no discrimination and, so far as I know, the non-Mennonites were treated fairly. Probably the most conspicuous difference, at least so far as I was concerned, was that stemming from urban versus rural cultures. Yet even these differences did not constitute barriers. On the afternoon of the first day in camp, this city dweller/office worker found himself in fresh, brand-new work

*Richard C. Hunter is deputy executive director of the National Mental Health Association.

clothes digging a diversion ditch to prevent erosion. As I recall, it was Jake Hofer, accustomed to hard labor, who worked silently beside me. After a period of observation, he reached out without a word to take my heavier shovel and replace it with his, which proved to be much more manageable. It was experience such as this which helped me to accept graciously the role of "outsider," when I finally realized that that was what I was.

As time went on, I began to hear names like Orie Miller, P. C. Hiebert, and Harold Bender. Then Henry Fast came to the camp for one of his many visits which took place during my twenty-eight months in Colorado Springs. I wasn't sure how I felt about this man of quiet firmness. He had a smile and a twinkle, but he also had what seemed to be a resolute assurance about how things were going to be. I began to recognize that Camp #5 was not just a camp for a collection of unrelated conscientious objectors operated by the Mennonite Central Committee, but that it was a Mennonite community, within which non-Mennonites were permitted to reside. I began to see that *Mennonite* was not just a name of a church denomination, but was a church-centered culture which commanded far greater loyalty and allegiance among its constituents than I had ever experienced as a member of the Methodist church. Although I could tell the difference between Kansas, Nebraska, and Oklahoma Mennonites, and even the difference between those from North Newton and those from Pretty Prairie, Kansas, there were some well-defined and encompassing boundaries which brought together those who were on the inside and established for me my place on the outside.

Initially, I had little knowledge of the oppression experienced by the forebears of my campmates, so I didn't understand the closed nature of the community. However, as I came to know more about the moves from country to country in search of conditions favorable to their peaceful way of life, I began to understand and appreciate the sense of need for protective boundaries and for attention directed primarily to the needs of those who were members of the "household of faith." The MCC faced a major challenge in setting up camps to serve not only those coming out of its common heritage, but also to include strangers who, while opposed to war, came from that outside world which had in so many instances, constituted a threat to all the Mennonite community stood for. In the process, however, the kind of siege mentality long justified by the history of oppression began to give way to a realization that the boundaries established around the Mennonite community might need to be used less as a defensive barrier and more as the simple definition of the group whose members could be free to cross the lines back and forth to minister not only to those within but also to those without.

While I was developing a great deal of respect for the leadership of the church as I had an opportunity to observe it in people like Albert Gaeddert, our first camp director and fellow campers such as Robert Kreider, Ray Schlicting, and Elmer Ediger, I had questions about whether the rank and file among the campers who had grown up in a tightly-controlled culture were objectors on the basis of their own conscience or that of the community from which they came. Pacifism was not actively discussed as it might have been in a college dorm. It was difficult to comprehend the depth of a conviction that was never verbalized. I tended to question the personal commitment of people who seemed to be able to go on day after day patiently putting up with the discomforts of camp and the disruption of their lives. It was then a revelation when, one day, an Amish crew leader out in the field on an assignment, proceeded without any discussion, to load his crew into the trucks at midday, and bring them back to camp when he and others in the crew realized that they were involved in the initial stages of preparing for what later became Fort Carson. There wasn't a lot of talk and debate, nor was the action dramatized for public consumption. When conviction called for action, it was taken quietly and effectively.

There was another gratifying surprise for me as an observing outsider, when service in mental hospitals first became an option offered to campers. Curiosity ran high when word was received at camp that Dr. Arthur Noyes, superintendent of Norristown State Hospital in Pennsylvania, was going to visit the camp in search of persons willing to replace hospital personnel who had left their positions for war service. There was good attendance the night Dr. Noyes spoke, which I attributed largely to a need for a break in the monotony of camp life. I was not at all prepared for the substantial number of young men from a rural background in the Midwest who volunteered to go to work with mental patients in custodial instituions on the East Coast. Their ministry was not to be to troubled members of their own community, but to anyone who was in need of their help.

It wasn't until Congressman Starns effectively prevented overseas assignments of conscientious objectors, lest the rest of the world mistakenly believe that the United States was all pacifist, that I concluded that I, too, should accept a hospital assignment. For a year, I served in the Methodist-operated unit at Highland Hospital in Asheville, North Carolina, as a ward attendant. Working conditions were reasonably good. Living conditions were certainly better than barracks. The members of the unit and the hospital staff were congenial and intellectually stimulating, but it was a situation in which I was neither an insider nor an outsider, for there was no group standard or expectation. I was one of several individuals, each having his own personal convictions. It was a group lacking in the strength and character of an organized culture. Consequently, when, after ten months in Asheville, I received an inquiry from MCC about my possible interest in a position in the Marlboro, New Jersey State Hospital, I accepted without hesitation to return again to the happy role of "outsider" in a Mennonite unit.

As the end of the war approached, talk centered on what to do following discharge. Many of those in the Marlboro unit, as in other Mennonite units, were headed home to the work and life of the communities from which they had come. It was apparent, however, that they would take with them a concern about what would happen to the patients being left behind. They retained a sense of mission which undoubtedly encouraged and supported MCC and the development of Mennonite Mental Health Services (MMHS).

Even before the final discharge of all campers, there was talk in Akron, Pennsylvania, and other places where leaders of the church assembled, about the creation of havens to assure that the mentally and emotionally disturbed members of the Mennonite community would not be subjected to the unacceptable conditions of public mental hospitals. In this planning, there were still the voices of those from the past, with a sense of obligation to "our own" and anxiety about outside, corrupting influences. The desire to preserve the traditions of the Mennonite church was appropriate, but contemporary experience was producing a growing recognition that the time for living behind protective walls was beginning to pass.

I was not a participant in the active discussions of what the church would do, since, following my discharge, I moved off in a different direction. I had, while at Marlboro, become actively associated with the Mental Health Program of Civilian Public Service, which was located at Philadelphia State Hospital. I joined the staff of that organization, which, in mid 1946, became independently incorporated as the National Mental Health Foundation, and later the National Mental Health Association, devoted to building public support for better care of the mentally ill, the prevention of mental illness, and the promotion of mental health.

Again, I found myself in that world where I was neither inside nor out. I missed the family to which I felt I beonged—strangely as an outsider. Thus it was an exciting day, late in 1946, when Norman Loux, Titus Books, and Delmar Stahly came to visit at the National Mental Health Foundation to talk about plans for Brook Lane Farm, which was to be the first in a series of small mental hospitals located near to Mennonite settlements but to be available to serve others as needed. While those of us on the staff of the Foundation were focused on the needs of thousands of patients crowded into public institutions, it was inspiring to know that at least a small part of the total task was going to be taken on by people who would do it well. It is still inspiring to realize that the long- range plan developed in the 1940s was so sound in its fundamentals that it has proceeded essentially on course from then until now.

I have not had an opportunity to follow the development of MMHS closely, but I have listened with pride and pleasure to each report of progress which has come to my attention. Not only has the national recognition given to services such as Prairie View and Kings View been a tribute to the Mennonite community, but it has been a testimony to the positive contributions of Civilian Public Service as an alternative to military service in World War II.

There are two specific situations which have special meaning for me. While Brook Lane Farm was being brought to reality, the Lancaster County Mennonites in Pennsylvania took independent action to create Philhaven for their own people who needed help. A facility to serve "insiders" was a wholly natural development in a county as densely populated with Mennonites as Lancaster County. Even there, however, there was a readiness to look outside for guidance. The National Mental Health Foundation was invited to consult. Kenneth Appel from the Pennsylvania Hospital in Philadelphia, and later to be president of the American Psychiatric Association, was also associated with that service in its initial operation and spoke proudly of the quality of service rendered in this small hospital, operated by devoted people in no way associated with the professional realms in which he was accustomed to move.

I think, too, of another service developed somewhat later, but not identified as a part of the Mennonite family of services. Penn Foundation in Sellersville, Pennsylvania, was without question the fruit of Mennonite concern and influence. However, it was so committed to the service of its community that it avoided any identification that might separate it from all of those who would be able to benefit from its program. The character of the Foundation, taken from those who gave it its start and have remained in its leadership, makes it an extension of what Mennonite Mental Health Services have stood for and indicates the influence of the Mennonite church beyond those services specifically identified with it.

When construction was imposed in 1940, and when Civilian Public Service was instituted in 1941, MCC prepared itself for the isolation which it had known before in resisting the demand of governments to bear arms. By 1946, its defensive posture had been modified by an outward directed mission to serve the suffering mentally ill. Now, thirty-five years later, Mennonite Mental Health

Services are among the best in the country, reflecting the Christian concern of their founders and deserving of the highest praise and recognition which they have received from the renowned leaders in the field.

Now as I conclude, I have a concern that those of the Mennonite heritage, with their defenses down, may become so blended in with all others, that there will cease to be an inside and an outside — there will be no outsiders. Boundaries need not be barriers but they can and should define a unique people who need, for the benefit of the rest of us, to preserve their uniqueness, not to stand against the forces of the outside world, but to inspire those on the outside to something higher than they would otherwise know.

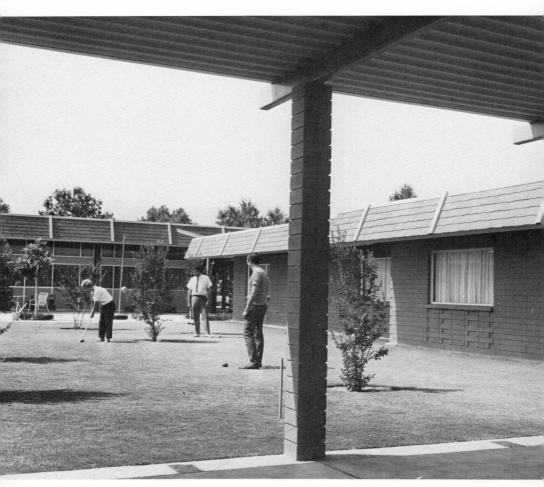

Kern View, Bakersfield, California.

CHAPTER 17

"Past Recollections and Future Concerns"

Lucy D. Ozarin*
A National Institute of Mental Health Veteran

I had not known of the Mennonite Mental Health Services until one day in the early '60s when Elmer Ediger appeared at the Public Health Service Regional Office in Kansas City where I was chief of the Mental Health Unit. The Prairie View staff saw a need to provide follow-up psychiatric care to people in their area who were returning from the Topeka State Hospital 125 miles distant. In due course, Prairie View submitted an application for a grant from NIMH to provide aftercare services. The five-year demonstration grant was approved and became operational in 1964.

Meanwhile, the Community Mental Health Centers Act (CMHC) had become law in 1963, and Prairie View, becoming interested in providing comprehensive mental health services to its surrounding three counties, began a process to meet the federal grant requirements. It was no easy task. Thus began a long and fruitful association of the federal government with a private non-profit agency which became a sponsor of a center. As one of the early operational centers, Prairie View became a demonstration site for NIMH to recommend to national and international visitors as a model center.

Probably the most unique part of the program is the spin-off called the Growth Associates Program which received NIMH staffing and training grants. This educational undertaking is a true venture into extending mental health services through use of nonmental health professionals. But, equally important, its courses aimed at the general public are a thrust to prevention of mental dysfunction by helping people understand the role of stress and how to cope with it.

*Lucy D. Ozarin, M.D., recently retired from the National Institute of Mental Health where she served for many years.

While Prairie View is the MMHS facility I know best, I have also visited and watched other MMHS affiliated programs. I visited the Penn Foundation in Sellersville, Pennsylvania, program in 1964 as a member of a team from the Joint Information Service (JIS) (American Psychiatric Association and National Association for Mental Health). When the CMHC Act was in process of being passed, I had been given the task to find out "What is a mental health center?" The Penn Foundation was unique among the group of MMHS facilities I knew in being closely tied to a general hospital instead of operating a mental hospital and, therefore, selected for a site visit.

The Foundation activities were located in a large attractive residential type building across the street from the general hospital. The proximity of psychiatric staff to general hospital staff was a major factor in providing comprehensive medical care. The fact that the medical staff were in large part responsible for the establishment of the psychiatric service erased the separation so often found between psychiatric and nonpsychiatric physicians. The relationship also smoothed the way to introduce other mental health workers—psychiatric nurses, social workers, and psychologists— and to allow medical and other hospital staff to become acquainted with these disciplines and learn how to use these skills. In the early 1960s, this was an innovation.

Penn Foundation has never utilized federal assistance. Their activities have been supported by individual and group contributors and through state and local funding for services rendered. The willingness of private citizens to support the Foundation, their willingness to provide for the needs of their neighbors, their caring for their community is evidence of the altruistic spirit that seems to pervade the Foundation activities.

I also visited the Kings View Hospital in the mid-1960s prior to their application for federal funding to establish a mental health center. I saw there a pleasant small mental hospital located in the midst of fields. Arthur Jost was hospital administrator and also president of the California Hospital Association. His connections were extremely helpful in those days in bringing respectability and support to the field of mental health which at that time was still viewed with some suspicion by both medical profession and citizenry.

Kings View became another model multi-service center. I recall especially its well-organized emergency service. Emergency service is a vital part of center operations because its provision is crucial to immediate evaluation and treatment of a patient and equally important is that management of the emergency often determines the future treatment career of the patient. It is at this point that action may avert hospitalization which is disruptive to patient and family and also expensive. Because of the rural setting, with patients as far away as twenty-five miles, the emergency team was mobile. The staff went to the crisis or emergency site often in "hot pursuit" as they said of patients previously known to them to defuse the crisis before it reached proportions requiring hospitalization.

Another center I have visited was Kern View. This center as I recall had some difficulty in its early days, but when I joined a site visit team during the early '70s, Kern View seemed to be firmly rooted under Larry Yoder's administration. The small hospital is attractive and pleasant and staff were serving their catchment area with a full array of mental health services. Kern View differs from the other MMHS affiliated centers in being located on general hospital grounds and in the heart of a city though it serves an outlying rural area. The other hospitals are located in rural settings and often provide the only mental health service available. Service delivery in rural areas differs in some ways from services in urban areas.

One of my tasks at National Institute of Mental Health (NIMH) since 1976 is to serve as coordinator of Rural Mental Health. I have become conversant with the special problems of providing mental health services in such areas. Poverty is in higher proportion, distance creates problems, helping resources are in short supply. Staff, especially psychiatrists, are hard to recruit and keep. I do not know why the MMHS chose to establish mental hospitals in rural areas. But whether it was planned or by chance, they have rendered a great service to the people of those areas. The facilities have located highly trained and qualified staff in all the mental health disciplines and have been successful in keeping them for a period of years, no doubt because of the high standards of patient care and the professional opportunities offered.

An outstanding characteristic of the MMHS facilities I have known is the thrust toward change and growth, a willingness to enter new activities and places if people need help. Yet this growth has been carefully planned and carried out in a way to assure a high degree of success. It is no accident that Prairie View and Kings View were selected by the American Psychiatric Association to receive Gold Medal Awards for achievement. They have brought honor to the MMHS and also to the NIMH which helped support them.

Yet despite the religious underpinnings of activities of the MMHS, a religious bias has not been evident. True, work with community clergy has been a prominent activity, but the role of clergy in mental health has been long supported by the federal government through NIMH grants, and the Saint Elizabeths Hospital, a federal mental hospital in Washington, D.C., has had a pastoral training program for years, I see the religious context of the MMHS emerging in the spirit and attitude of staffs of the mental health centers and the support of the members of the parent organization. To help others who are in need of help seems to be the guiding principle and somehow ways are found to do so.

But now, what of the future?

The care of the mentally ill and troubled has always reflected the social and political ethos of the times. For mental health the political and economic situation of the '80s poses problems. Financial support from the federal level is to be diminished, and it will remain to states and localities to support services as possible and to enlist private support. With the escalating costs of medical care, more effort will need to be made to do more with less and, equally important, to find new ways to reach the desired goals.

MMHS made an early decision not to establish facilities for chronic patients, but now the problem must be posed again. The care of chronic psychiatric patients, those people who have lived in mental hospitals for years and those people who have relapsing mental episodes, is a major problem in this country. We have learned by experiment and experience the needs of these long hospitalized people and useful ways to care for them given the financial and staff resources. But a new type of chronic patient has emerged during the last decade and our efforts thus far have not been every effective in helping them.[1] The new chronic patient is described as usually a young adult, who may or may not be psychotic or have time-limited psychotic episodes, impulsive, often involved with drugs, often with a history of behavioral problems in adolescence, at times a wanderer or in trouble with the law, alienated from family and friends.

Residential and supportive services have been suggested as a means to help these young people many of whom seem to have good potential to achieve useful and productive lives. We need to find new ways that are practical and economically feasible to help these new young chronics in spite of the difficulties and frustrations encountered in trying to do so. Somehow, the social context of their lives seems important.

Another problem area is the future role of the public mental hospital. We have seen over the past twenty years that the state hospital is a major treatment resource for poor people or people with drug and alcohol problems and sometimes for the aged. Its role is closely related to the availability of community resources. With funding for community mental health facilities becoming more scarce, it is likely that state hospitals will again become a major treatment resource. But how should they be structured? It is unthinkable that the state hospital can return to the isolated custodial role it played in the past. What kind of new patterns of care can be introduced? How can the problems of the past be avoided? Somehow the state hospital must be brought close to the community. What links need to be developed? The MMHS facilities have good experience in providing a high level of care to psychiatric patients. Their staffs may have ideas that can be put to test. There are still some funds to support research and perhaps demonstration from public and foundation sources.

Still another area to be developed further is the relationship between primary medical care and mental health. The family doctor or general practitioner is usually the first professional to see patients with mental dysfunction, often shown as anxiety, depression, or excessive alcohol intake. These and other symptoms may accompany physical conditions. Currently over half of the patients with diagnosable mental conditions are being seen by nonpsychiatric physicians who refer only 20 percent of these patients to mental health resources. In view of the shrinking financial support for mental health, general physicians will, therefore, have to treat the psychiatric symptoms of their patients. The mental health center staffs can provide assistance through education and consultation and in assisting general physicians to use the skills of all mental health disciplines appropriately.

The MMHS can take pride in its accomplishments on a national scale. Its few centers have had limited input but their performance has served as a demonstration land model to the entire country and has charted the pathways for a nation to follow in providing psychiatric care where and when people need such help.

In his chapter, Vernon Neufeld described the early MMHS philosophy in terms of "service, volunteerism, frugality, and witness." The Judeo-Christian tradition stresses the duty of each person to help a fellow human being. The MMHS seems to have found a way to do so.

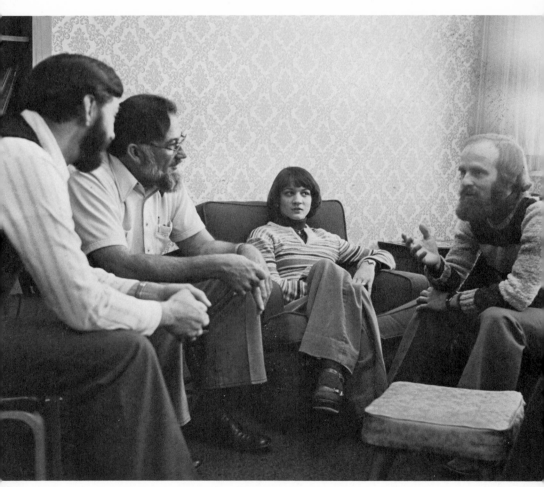

Staff Conference at Prairie View.

CHAPTER 18

"The Words Were The Same, The Music Was Slightly Different"
Jack F. Wilder*
A New York Psychiatrist-Educator

I became acquainted with the Mennonite Mental Health Services in the late 1960s when I had developed and directed the Sound View-Throgs Neck Community Mental Health Center in the Bronx, New York. Our center was the largest urban mental health center at the time, and was located in the poorest county in New York State. The center was a major affiliate of the Albert Einstein College of Medicine and had no problem in attracting highly qualified professionals. We had significant financial and physical resources and an impressive organizational chart. We had a great opening. I quickly found, however, that there was a huge gap between appearances and reality. We disagreed on what we should be doing, the quality of work was uneven, productivity was low, and intra-staff rivalries compromised our performance. There was one saving grace, however, — I attended many area and regional meetings with other center directors and was pleased to learn that our situation was not unique. The relief I would experience from attending those conferences would only be short-lived. There remained the gnawing belief that I could do better.

My awakening came at a national meeting at which I met Elmer Ediger. I heard Elmer discuss his program at Prairie View and we found time to chat informally. He was different from other directors. Where they appeared to be in a constant state of panic, Elmer was calm. Where others were certain that they had hired the "wrong staff," Elmer said he was working with "good people." Above all, Elmer seemed to know what he was doing. He talked intelligently about management principles and practices. He was humble and did not claim to have all the answers. But he appeared

*Jack F. Wilder, M.D., is professor of Psychiatry and associate dean for Planning and Operations, Albert Einstein College of Medicine of Yeshiva University in New York.

to have mounted a reasonable, comprehensive, clinical program that met the needs of patients and yet was engaged in creative efforts in consultation and education. I was a little skeptical. How could someone from a mental health center called "Prairie View," located in a small town in Kansas, have developed a program that had eluded the academicians from the major teaching institutions in Boston, New York, and Philadelphia? I had to see it to believe it. I also wanted to see Elmer again. He had visited with my family and we immediately felt that we were family.

I remember my first visit to Prairie View. I was startled by the setting. In the Bronx, our buildings were surrounded by dirty streets and graffiti. Prairie View was surrounded by green grass and sheep! The buildings were beautifully designed. I later learned that residents of the community had participated in its construction. But what are buildings? I knew that once I went inside, I would feel like I was back in the Bronx. To my amazement, I didn't. The interior was warm and in excellent taste. I was greeted by a lovely receptionist who asked how she could be of help. Staff members were not in committee meetings arguing over how to remove the director of the center, but in their own offices actually seeing patients. The inpatient and day hospital services were alive with activity. Staff were working efficiently, too—I had an opportunity to observe an accountability system that was actually in practice. And the service programs were being carried out in an academic ambience. Studies were being conducted, papers were being written, and training and educational courses were being provided to the center staff, to professionals in the area, and to community residents. Elmer had told the truth. It could be done. A mental health center could deliver comprehensive, high-quality mental health services to a community.

I talked to many of the staff members individually, and, above all, I was privileged to meet with the Prairie View board. It quickly became apparent to me that there were two major reasons why Prairie View worked. First, there was an overriding historic commitment by the Mennonite community to heal the sick. And second, they had hired first-rate management to achieve this noble purpose. It was not easy for me to leave Prairie View after that first visit. I had learned so much and I had made so many good friends. I won't mention names other than Elmer's for fear that I would leave someone out. It was a moving experience. I returned to the Bronx renewed and wiser.

I visited Prairie View and attended conferences in Kansas on other occasions. At times I gave a talk, and when I did I always learned more than I gave. I met directors and professionals who worked in other Mennonite community mental health centers. I sensed that they, too, were working in successful programs. I had the pleasure of actually visiting one other mental health program associated with Mennonite Mental Health Services, the Penn Foundation in Sellersville. My experience with Norman Loux and his staff was similar to the one I had found at Prairie View. They were doing a first-rate job. I especially remember a wonderful evening I spent in Norman's home with his family and staff. We sat around in a circle and chatted. Many of the issues that were raised that night were similar to the problems we were facing in New York. But although the words were the same, the music was slightly different. The staff at the Penn Foundation—whether they were Mennonite or not—were approaching their jobs with a commitment and dedication which I have found to be unique to the programs of the Mennonite Mental Health Services.

Are there any weaknesses in the Mennonite centers? No doubt—no one is perfect. If there is any obvious weakness, it is the failure of the centers to recognize how much they have accomplished. Their standards are so high and the tasks so difficult that they tend to overemphasize how far they still have to go. As such, they have been too cautious about sharing with others what they have experienced and attained. I urge them to write more, to develop more audio/visual material, and to provide more training experiences so that other workers in the mental health field can benefit from their work.

The mental health center movement has come under considerable criticism during the past few years. Like most new programs, it promised too much. The resources of any one program are finite and the mental health needs of any community are infinite. Even if resources were limitless, the know-how to meet the needs of a community is currently limited, especially in the areas of primary and secondary prevention. Many centers, in their search for doing something new, also avoided treating the very ill, the very group they were set up to care for. Above all, many mental health centers suffered from inadequate management.

I long ago took odds with the stated objectives of the National Institute of Mental Health to establish 2,000 mental health centers in ten years. They haven't reached that number yet, and many of the centers that are in existence are not of the quality such programs deserve. I advocated that several centers be established across the country, that we see how they can be made to work well, and if they do a good job, we use them as the training grounds for the prospective directors of new centers. It is not an original idea—MacDonalds and Kentucky Fried Chicken had it long before I did! Actually, it could have been so simple. All the government had to do was to fund the Mennonite centers and use them as the core of an expanding, national community mental health center movement. We certainly would have been much better off today had we proceeded in that way.

This is not to suggest, however, that the quality of all mental health centers across the country would have been equally high. You can teach management skills, copy programmatic models, and duplicate sound accountability systems, but the commitment to do the hard job of caring for those in need is not easily transferable. Had we gone the route I suggested, the Mennonite centers would remain singular, shining examples of what the human spirit can accomplish.

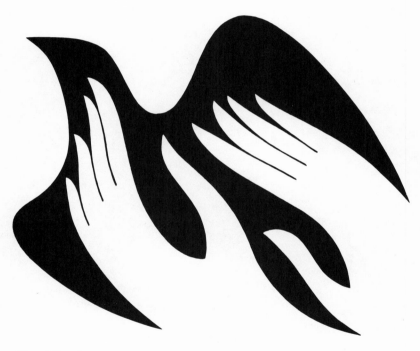

Kings View logo.

CHAPTER 19

"Church Sponsored Hospitals and Church Aims"
Paul W. Pruyser*
A Menninger Psychologist-Theologian

As chance would have it, in my upper teenage years I worked in a small bank in Amsterdam, one of whose managers was also financial secretary of the Dutch Mennonite churches (*Algemeene Doopsgezinde Societeit*). He was an able, dedicated, hard working man who shouldered his tasks with zest. My view of Mennonites at that time was conditioned by the public features of the Dutch group which consisted by-and-large of well-to-do, socially respected, and quite enterprising persons who lived dispersed throughout the country in cities and villages, with notable concentrations (but no compact settlements) in the provinces of Friesland and North Holland. Their family names were Dutch and not Swiss or Rhineland German. They were known to be pacifists and had for centuries been accepted as such. After the Anabaptist uprisings during the Reformation era had calmed down, their ancestors were not under any pressure to emigrate. Over the centuries, those Mennonites had quietly made their mark in all kinds of occupations, from farming to finance and industry. In dress, living arrangements, and demeanors, nothing set them apart from other Dutchmen.

After my immigration to the United States in 1948, and especially when I had become director of professional education at the Menninger Foundation, I came into contact with a different variety of Mennonites, most of whose ancestors had been subjected to persecution, forced to migrate from one European country to another, and in the end had made a kind of tribal immigration to the United States or Canada, where they had commonly started a new life in rural settlements which were spiritually, morally, and socially centered in their church. They plied their agricultural skills and their

*Paul W. Pruyser, Ph.D., is Henry March Pfeiffer Professor, Department of Education, The Menninger Foundation.

trades, and were often conspicuously different from the prevailing mores in dress, habits, language, and family patterns, and sometimes in their selective aversion to certain cultural conveniences. In the '50s and later, some of the offspring of these immigrant groups sought training in the mental health professions at the Menninger Foundation.

In comparison with most other applicants to our education programs their views of their careers and their life plans appeared to be less individualistic, and their motivation seemed to have an aspect of a communal, if not divine, calling. They performed as if they were living up to a pledge—not just to become personally fulfilled but to be socially useful and morally mindful. It was clear that they lived by principles and that their vocations were rooted in their belief system. Indeed, their principles sometimes made them a bit hesitant in endorsing the modern psychodynamic lore we taught, and I was not infrequently enlisted by my colleagues or these students to assist in overcoming some ideological impasse. Despite their individual differences they appeared to share a heritage and outlook that were very important to their career development and career goals. I discovered that many were indeed earmarked for a communal task that needed their individual talents, energies, and dedication.

In conversations with these men and women I began to form my own scenario of what Elmer Ediger has elsewhere in this book described more objectively as the origins, history, and development of the Mennonite Mental Health Services. These idealistic students, who were otherwise rather self-contained and not prone to great effervescence, had been fired up by other Mennonites who, during World War II, had done alternate service duty by manning the staff-depleted state mental hospitals, and in the course of their work had made some interesting discoveries which they felt should be shared with elders and church officials. Among other things, these young men had found that in their own and other people's eyes they were singularly suited for work with the mentally ill and retarded. Their centuries-old peace tradition had given them a degree of serenity as well as a measure of tender respect for the downtrodden that are hard to come by in ordinary employment agencies and institutional personnel departments. Theirs had not been just temporary "jobs" to be quickly discarded for something better after they had fulfilled their government obligations. On the contrary, many of these young men had felt that they were mentally and spiritually thriving on this hospital work, and that some of the patients were equally thriving on the affectionate relations they established. These assigned "aides" acted indeed as "helpers" and not just as assistants in some bureaucratic system.

Upon returning home from their stateside "fronts," as they pondered what had made them so good at helping the deranged, the outcast, the vulnerable, the ridiculed, the deviant, without prior training in mental health work, they naturally sought the cause in their upbringing and its impact on their personalities, including their value system. They had several special things going for them: an abhorrence of violence and cruelty, an acquired sense of responsibility for the welfare of others, a cordial team spirit, a modest self-appraisal, and a sober lifestyle that stimulated community feeling rather than personal fulfillment of brilliance. Being neither angels nor beasts, their quiet manners elicited trust and conveyed compassion; their capacity for sustained work including menial ministrations demonstrated the health-fostering quality of all work well done. They had fulfilled their service obligation as a mission—a peace mission, a mission of compassion, a human betterment mission, rather than an evangelistic outreach campaign. And after the war was over, they felt that it should be one of the contemporary missions of their church to care for the mentally ill, to establish hospitals and clinics, and to enlist the talents of the church's youth in rendering the best professional services required to staff the bold enterprise they advocated.

In 1972 I had the honor of being invited to give an address on the occasion of the twenty-fifth anniversary of the Mennonite Mental Health Services. In that speech (later published in the *Mennonite Brethren Herald* of February 25, 1972) I cited the gold medals that several Mennonite hospitals and centers had been given for the high quality of their work and the inventiveness of their programs. But while it is nice to bask in national recognition, Mennonites are not known for resting on their laurels; they want to go on working harder, improving themselves and the lot of their fellow human beings. What might the future hold for the Mennonite Mental Health Services now that they have amply proven their worth?

I would anticipate that the socio-cultural situation of North American Mennonites is bound to undergo fairly rapid changes in directions that have already become clear. Tribal settlements will decline further as the younger generations will disperse themselves in search of nontraditional, nonagricultural job opportunities. The extended family pattern will decline; proximity will no longer be a major factor in maintaining family ties. Along with these demographic changes the ethnic dimension of Mennonite church affiliation is likely to diminish in favor of voluntary association by individuals who are attracted to the church's programs, worship patterns, pastoral leadership styles, and theological outlook. As the ethnic traditions weaken, the church will have to define its uniqueness by emphasizing its Anabaptist principles and its peace tradition, especially the latter with great vigor in a world that is arming itself to the teeth.

One result of these changes is that the present and next generation of Mennonites will no longer have been shaped by the family patterns and community feelings that molded the preceding generations. Like other North Americans, some young Mennonites today come from broken homes; they have been exposed at close range to alcoholism, marital infidelity, sexual aberrations, deviousness, and a host of other forms of moral erosion or character defects. They will no longer be able to see themselves and their families of origin automatically as models, gratefully to be emulated, as I am sure many old-time Mennonites did with some justification. Thus, with an increasing variety of Mennonite individuals with increasingly mixed backgrounds and increasingly diverse lifestyles it will increasingly fall to the church to compensate for educational processes once entrusted to the families. If its principles are to be vouchsafed and transmitted, the church will have to be conspicuously a teaching church rather than a center for the celebration of old kinship traditions. It should be known for its dynamic missionary spirit that spawns idealistic and constructive undertakings whose tenor is to correct prevalent social and moral evils, lifting up a just peace as superior to aggression, exploitation, and oppression. The same missionary spirit should be evident in the church's concern with individuals through what used to be called "character building": instilling in its members and others a dedication to high principles, willingness to make personal sacrifices if needed, peaceful modes of problem solving, and melioristic zeal.

In other words, Mennonite Mental Health Services will see changes in the youthful pool from which its future personnel is going to be recruited. And it will see changes in its leadership pool. An historically exemplified danger now lies ahead. As the inspired leaders and the first generation of enthusiastic mental health workers will approach retirement, one could witness a repeat of what happened at the end of the so-called "Moral Treatment" era in the middle of the nineteenth century. The Quaker spirit that had produced the first psychiatric revolution sagged, skepticism overtook the idealism of the founders, malcontent rose among the practitioners, and a vast bureaucratization took over under the pressure of unforeseen external circumstances. The once humane and effective hospitals became pauper homes and snakepits. Lest this happen again, great vigilance is needed. And that is why this book is an important document that should not merely celebrate past achievements but also warn of future dangers.

For another grave danger is already at hand: with increasing dominance of medical economics and third-party payment arrangements, hospitals are bound to become more and more beholden to statistical or actuarial norms of "good service" set by strangers to the healing ethos. They are already falling into a commercial and managerial parlance that smacks of the marketplace. Such terms as "health delivery system" do not fit the humanistic tradition of medicine and definitely fly in the face of the religious spirit that started the original hospices from which hospitals in the modern sense eventually developed. Hospices of old were a *Gemeinde* mission; modern hospitals are a *Gesellschafts* arrangement. It seems to me that the church-sponsored hospital or clinic or community mental health center has its *raison detre* precisely in offering to the sick a *Gemeinde* oasis in a desert of impersonal and rather bleak *Gesellschafts* "conveniences."

The religious or church-sponsored hospital, if it is to be true to its principles and mission, will thus have to justify itself (and the high mental and fiscal cost of its existence) by its *differences* from secular alternatives. In what follows I have no intention of minimizing the often splendid services rendered by secular medical institutions, nor of underrating the work of their staff members. But we all know that many patients are not content with the ministrations they receive and that in many quarters of our society a critical spirit toward the "health system" has come into being. This otherwise deplorable situation may be an opportunity for church-sponsored hospitals to take stock of their aims and concentrate on the unique contributions they can make.

In addition to living up to high professional, scientific, and ethical canons, I think that the church-sponsored hospital should live up to church aims. What these aims are may be difficult to define in operational terms. But I will venture to describe them in attitudinal terms, in a language that is both religious and psychological. In the church-sponsored hospital there should be an awareness of the sacred—whether the sacredness of its ultimate auspices or of the persons cared for and treated. There should be some cognizance of Providence—the idea that the care given by the staff is ultimately a derived providential care mediated by men and women. There should be an attitude of faith—not necessarily in creedal terms and liturgical forms, but as a basic disposition expressed by an engaged, hearty, life-affirming approach to the patients that imbues them with hope and courage. There should be an atmosphere of graciousness and gratefulness, in which the idea of merit is suspended by an emphasis on acceptance and forgiveness. In the church-sponsored hospital there should be opportunity for repentance—not as an imposed duty or a mandated ritual, but as a self-initiated beginning of a process of personal change. If remorse and regret are voiced, the doors of conscience are thrown open for inspection of its values. And as Mennonites especially have long known, the church-sponsored hospital should have an almost infectious atmosphere of communion—one in which patients and staff members alike sense that they are gathered by a transcendent power to acknowledge their creatureliness by practicing mutual compassion, uplifting one another, and caring about and for each other. Finally, but not least, the church-sponsored hospital, while full *in* this world, is to make known by its practices and attitudes that it is not wholly *of* this world. Its leaders and staff members do not merely hold jobs or fill slots in organization charts, but work with zest, dedication, liveliness, vigor, and in a team spirit to convey the message that they are called by their Creator to co-creative activity and inventiveness. Imbued by this sense of vocation (which the first generation of mental health workers apparently had to a marked degree) the staff members will not only do their work cheerfully and marshal their best talents, but also invigorate the patients who have fallen into a state of lassitude or emptiness.

The qualifying conditions that I have outlined for the church-sponsored hospital are not easy to reach. It takes church-bred people who combine idealism and realism to define and implement these conditions. From my limited and spotty consultatory participation in its activities I have gained the impression that the Mennonite Mental Health Services have come close to meeting the demanding criteria I have listed—as close as any institution I know. Their history, if constantly restudied and assessed, in vigilant concern for the present, bodes well for the future.

Notes

Preface

1. Wesley Prieb was a member of the MMHS board 1972-80. He serves on the faculty of Tabor College, Hillsboro, Kansas.

2. Copies of the January 1982 *MQR* issue are available from AMS Press, Inc., 56 East 13th, New York, NY 10003.

Chapter 1

1. Harold S. Bender, "The Anabaptist Vision," *The Mennonite Quarterly Review* (April 1944), p. 5.

2. *Ibid.*, p. 14.

3. Gregory Zilboorg and George W. Henry, *A History of Medical Psychology* (New York: W. W. Norton & Co., Inc., 1941), p. 39.

4. *Ibid.*, pp. 43 ff.

5. *Ibid.*, pp. 144-74.

6. Michel Foucault, *Madness and Civilization, A History of Insanity in the Age of Reason* (New York: Random House, Inc., 1965), p. 8.

7. *Ibid.*, p. 26.

8. *Ibid.*, p. 28.

9. Zilboorg and Henry, *ibid.*, p. 561.

10. W. Earl Biddle, *Integration of Religion and Psychiatry* (New York: The Macmillan Company, 1955), p. 12.

11. *Ibid.*, p. 11.

12. Zilboorg and Henry, *ibid.*, p. 562; Biddle, *ibid.*, p. 13; Suzanne Fields, "Asylum on the Front Porch," *Innovations* (1974), pp. 15, 16; Eugeen Roosens, *Mental Patients in Town Life, Gheel—Europe's First Therapeutic Community* (Beverly Hills, London: Sage Publications, 1979), pp. 25 ff.

13. Zilboorg and Henry, *ibid.*, p. 571.

14. Richard Hunter and Ida McCalpine, *Three Hundred Years of Psychiatry* (New York: Oxford Press, 1963), p. 605.

15. *Ibid.* p. 606.

16. Zilboorg and Henry, *ibid.*, p. 572.

17. F. J. Braceland, "Psychiatry," *New Catholic Encyclopedia* (New York: McGraw Hill Book Co., 1967), vol. 11, p. 947.

18. Kim Van Atta, *An Account of the Events Surrounding the Origin of Friends Hospital, and a Brief Description of the Early Years of Friends Asylum, 1917-1820* (Philadelphia: Friends Hospital, 1976), p. 11.

19. *Ibid.*, p. 21.

20. *Ibid.*, p. 23.

21. *Ibid.*, p. 23.

22. J. Sanbourne Bockoven, *Moral Treatment in American Psychiatry* (New York: Springer Publishing Co., 1967), p. 14.

23. *Ibid.*, p. 61.

24. Zilboorg and Henry, *ibid.*, p. 583.

25. *Ibid.*, pp. 583-84.

26. Bockoven, *ibid.*, p. 39.

27. Karl Menninger, "The Genius of the Jew in Psychiatry," *A Psychiatrist's World, The Selected Papers of Karl Menninger, M.D.*, ed. Bernard H. Hall (New York: The Viking Press, 1959), p. 821.

28. Biddle, *ibid.*, p. 25

29. Paul W. Pruyser, "Sigmund Freud and His Legacy," *Beyond the Classics? Essays in the Scientific Study of Religion*, ed. Charles Y. Glock and Phillip E. Hammond (New York: Harper and Row Publishers, 1973), p. 234.

30. Biddle, *ibid.*, p. 3.

31. Arthur J. Bindman and Allen D. Spiegel, eds., *Perspectives in Community Mental Health* (Chicago: Aldine Publishing Company, 1969), p. 20.

32. R. D. Hirshelwood and Nick Manning, *Therapeutic Communities: Reflections and Communities* (London: Routledge & Kegan Paul, n.d.), p.5.

33. Bernard L. Bloom, *Community Mental Health, A General Introduction* (Monterey, Ca : Brooks/Cole Publishing Co., 1975), p. 134.

34. Henry A. Foley, *Community Mental Health Legislation* (Lexington, Maine: Lexington Books, 1975), p. 19.

35. R. P. Odenwald, "Papal Pronouncements on Psychiatry," *New Catholic Encyclopedia* (New York: McGraw Hill, 1967), vol. II, p. 951.

36. Robert A. Clark and J. Russell Elkinton, *The Quaker Heritage in Medicine* (Pacific Grove, Ca.: The Boxwood Press, 1978), pp. 15-22.

37. Van Atta, *ibid.*, p. 11.

38. *Inward Light* XLII:93 (Fall 1979), p. 3.

39. Harrison Evans, letter, May 5, 1981.

40. *Mennonite Encyclopedia*, s.v. "Bethania."

41. Delmar Stahly, "Mennonite Programs for Mental Illness," *Mennonite Life* (July 1954), p. 120.

42. *Mennonite Encyclopedia*, s.v. "Bethesda."

43. Bertram D. Smucker, "Visitation Report on Bethesda Hospital, Vineland, Ontario, March 28, 1946," unpublished, p.2.

44. Vernon Neufeld, "Director's Report on Paraguay Trip," unpublished, April 16-30, 1980, p. 3.

45. C. E. Krehbiel, "Report to the Ministers' Conference at Hillsboro, Kansas, October 1937," unpublished, p. 1.

46. Krehbiel, *ibid.*, pp. 1-6.

47. William Keeney, "Civilian Public Service and Related World War II Experiences," (Hagerstown, Maryland, October 1-2, 1971), 11 pp.

48. Melvin Gingerich, *Service for Peace, A History of Mennonite Civilian Public Service* (Akron, Pa.: The Mennonite Central Committee, 1949), p. 213.

49. Albert Q. Maisel, "Bedlam 1946, Most U.S. Mental Hospitals Are a Shame and a Disgrace," *Life* (May 6, 1946), p. 102.

50. *Ibid.*, pp. 102f.

51. *Ibid.*, p. 105.

52. Gingerich, *ibid.*, p. 216.

53. William Klassen, "The Role of the Church in Community Psychiatry," *McCormick Quarterly* 28 (July 1967), pp. 25, 26.

54. *Anniversary Review* (May 1945), p. 53.

55. Frank L. Wright, *Out of Sight Out of Mind* (Philadelphia: National Mental Health Foundation, Inc., 1947), p. 156.

56. Robert Kreider, ed., "A Symposium: Should the Churches Establish and Maintain Hospitals for the Mentally Ill?" unpublished, February 1945, p. 1.

57. *Ibid.*, p. 3.

58. *Ibid.*, p. 9.

59. *Ibid.*, p. 11.

60. The Church of the Brethren had a special committee to consider the question but recommended not to develop their own institution. They did recommend cooperating with the Mennonite efforts, initiating their own mental health education program, and working with the public mental hospital system. (Undated and unsigned "Preliminary Report on the Question of a Hospital for the Mentally Ill," sponsored by the Church of the Brethren, available in the files of Mennonite Mental Health Services.)

61. Menninger, *ibid.*, p. 424.

Chapter 2

1. Henry A. Fast, "Beginnings of Mennonite Mental Health Services," unpublished address (Newton, Kansas, October 7, 1972), p. 2.

2. *Ibid.*, p. 2.

3. *Ibid.*, p. 3.

4. Report of the Mental Hospital Study Committee to the Annual Meeting of the MCC, December 28-29, 1945. "As the necessary resources become available, the conviction may later emerge that we together are prepared to establish a church mental institution and perhaps also a home for the feeble-minded."

5. Supplementary Report of the Mental Hospital Study Committee to the Mennonite Central Committee, April 8, 1946.

6. Elmer Ediger, "Papers and Responses Presented at the 25th Anniversary Program," (Hagerstown, Maryland, October 1-2, 1971), pp. 9-10.

7. Fast, *ibid.*, p. 3.

8. Elmer Ediger, "On the Beginnings of Brook Lane Psychiatric Center and the Mennonite Mental Health Program" (Hagerstown, Maryland, October 1-2, 1971), p.1.

9. Fast, *ibid.*, p. 3.

10. MMHS minutes May 27, 1954.

11. MMHS minutes May 13, 1955.

12. Delmar Stahly, interview, Akron, Pennsylvania, February 23, 1981.

13. *Ibid.*

14. H. Clair Amstutz, M.D., personal letter, February 9, 1981.

15. Stahly, *ibid.*

16. Though legally incorporated in 1951, the Kings View board nevertheless continued in an advisory role to MCC until the reorganization of 1958.

17. Currently the practice in the five MCC-founded centers is for a 50-50 representation of church and community board members.

18. This was first requested by E. P. Mininger, chairman of the Oaklawn board, on July 10, 1960, and approved by MCC in early 1961.

19. Amstutz, *ibid.*

20. Arthur Jost, interview, February 23, 1981.

21. Aldred H. Neufeldt, "Reflections on the Growth and Development of MMHS and Implications for the Future," unpublished paper (October 12, 1978), pp. 2-3.

22. Jost, *ibid.*

Chapter 3

1. Evangeline Myers, personal letter, July 1, 1981.

2. Elmer M. Ediger, "Considerations and Recommendations on Possibility of Utilizing Leitersburg, Maryland, Farm as Mental Rest Home," October 17, 1946.

3. Dallas Pratt, M.D., letter (MMHS Sourcebook), n.d.c. December 1947.

4. Mennonite Central Committee Annual Meeting Minutes, January 2-3, 1947.

5. Ediger, Report to MMHS, April 9, 1947.

6. This differential was eliminated late in 1950.

7. Delvin Kirchhofer, Report to MMHS, June 13, 1952.

8. *Ibid.*, Report to MMHS, June 6. 1949.

9. *Ibid.*, Report to Brook Lane Advisory Committee, February 2, 1950.

10. *Ibid.*, Report to Brook Lane Advisory Committee, February 2, 1950, and Report to MMHS, May 25, 1951.

11. *Ibid.*, Report to Brook Lane Advisory Committee, February 2, 1950.

12. Myers, *ibid.*

13. Jacob Goering, Report to MMHS, December 18, 1953.

14. During most of 1957, D. C. Kauffman was in Elkhart, Indiana, helping set up the East Central Area mental health program (Oaklawn) as an MCC staff member. In 1958, when serving as Brook Lane administrator, he was invited to return to Elkhart as Oaklawn administrator, but he declined, expressing satisfaction with his Brook Lane position.

Earlier, a potential administrator with links to another MCC institution was considered for Brook Lane. When Kings View Homes temporarily closed its hospital doors in 1957, Orie Miller, executive secretary of MCC, proposed transferring Arthur Jost, Kings View administrator, to Brook Lane. The local Kings View advisory committee, however, strongly resisted this, so the transfer never occurred. Kings View reopened less than six months later.

15. Brook Lane Advisory Committee Report to MMHS, October 22, 1954.

16. Gilles R. Morin, M.D., Report to MMHS, October 17-18, 1958.

17. *Ibid.*, Report to MMHS, October 13-14, 1961.

18. *Ibid.*, Report to MMHS, April 29-30, 1960.

19. *Ibid.*, Report to the Brook Lane Board, February, 1962.

20. Howard Musselman, Report to MMHS, November 4-5, 1960.

21. *Ibid.*, Report to MMHS, April 9-10, 1963.

22. Brook Lane Board Minutes, Joint Conference Committee, March 3, 1967.

23. Brook Lane Board Minutes, May 26-27, 1967.

24. Edmund Niklewski, M.D., Report to the Brook Lane Board, February 24, 1968.

25. Musselman, Report to MMHS, September 26-27, 1969.

26. Niklewski, Report to the Brook Lane Board, February 24, 1968.

27. Musselman, Report to the Brook Lane Board, August 20, 1970.

28. Report of Special Committee on Church and Community Relations, Brook Lane Board Minutes, February 24, 1968.

29. Donovan Beachley, who earlier had been appointed as a community representative, was a member of the Church of the Brethren.

30. In 1981, of eight constituency board members, three were Mennonites and five from the Church of the Brethren.

Chapter 4

1. MCC West Coast Regional *Newsletter*, January-February 1951, Reedley, Ca., vol. 1, no. 8; *Mennonite Weekly Review*, (February 22, 1951), vol. 29, no. 8.

2. MMHS Minutes, January 25, 1947.

3. West Coast Subcommittee of Homes for the Mentally Ill Planning and Advisory Committee, Reedley, Ca., March 24, 1947, Minutes.

4. Under the Civilian Public Service (CPS) program, conscientious objectors from nonhistoric peace churches served in MCC-sponsored units and camps during World War II. MCC received funds from these nonhistoric peace church sources in repayment for services rendered to conscientious objectors from their constituencies.

5. A Symposium: "Should the Churches Establish and Maintain Hospitals for the Mentally Ill?" MCC Hospital Section, February 15, 1945 (nine contributors).

6. Communication from Elmer Ediger to Homes for Mentally Ill Committee, July 15, 1947.

7. Arthur Jost, interview, February 21, 1981.

8. MMHS Minutes, October 20, 1948.

9. MMHS Minutes, June 6, 1949.

10. Memorandum to Mental Hospital Committee Members and Friends from Arthur Jost, December 22, 1949.

11. "MCC Progress," *Newsletter*, No. 2, MCC Mental Health Service, (February 1950).

12. *Mennonite Weekly Review*, (February 22, 1951), vol. 29, no. 8.

13. Reedley *Exponent*, (February 8, 1951), vol. 60, no. 28.

14. MMHS Minutes, Recommendations from the Akron Office to Kings View Homes, December 1, 1950.

15. MCC Mental Health Service, *Newsletter*, (December 1950).

16. Arthur Jost, "Kings View Homes," Spring 1952 (unpublished article).

17. "Religious Activities for Patients," *Kings View Pointer*, (May 1952), vol. 1, no. 1.

18. Arthur Jost, interview, March 1951.

19. MMHS, Report from A. Ross Hendricks, M.D., April 9, 1958.

20. The high school was at first funded by the State of California in a private institution. This was established in 1967 through the efforts of Silas Bartsch, district superintendent at that time and later chairman of the Kings View board.

21. Arthur Jost and Vernon Neufeld, "Comprehensive Community Care," *Hospitals*, (March 16, 1970), vol. 44, pp. 85-87.

22. Frank C. Peters, letter to Arthur Jost, July 6, 1957.

23. Kings View Hospital, 1980 Promotion Presentation (tape).

24. *Hospital and Community Psychiatry*, (October 1971), vol. 22, no. 10.

25. Arthur Jost, interview, February 23, 1981.

26. *Ibid*.

Chapter 5

1. *Intelligencer Journal* (Lancaster, Pa.), May 8, 1952.

2. J. Paul Graybill, "The Lancaster Conference Plans a Mental Hospital, *Mennonite Community* (April 1950), pp. 12 f.

3. Bishop Graybill is not precise in dating the sequence of events he describes. The article implies that discussion of a conference facility began prior to 1944. Some corroboration of this is found in the notes of the bishop board meetings which are preserved in the archives of the Lancaster Mennonite Historical Society. These notes are suggestive, but not definitive; there is no minute entry prior to 1944 which specifically mentions discussion of a mental hospital.

4. Lancaster Conference, Bishop Board, Minutes, January 14, 1948.

5. Abram Metzler, interview, July 29, 1980.

6. Original members of the board were:

George Zeiset	Melvin Kauffman	Ira Eby	Noah Kreider
Elvin Lefever	John Martin	Levi Brubaker	Abram Metzler
Clarence Garber	Monroe Garber	Harry Swarr	Victor Weaver

7. Melvin Kauffman, interview, November 19, 1980.

8. Interviews with Victor Weaver, Abram Metzler, and Noah Kreider.

9. Each member of the original board who was interviewed for this history cited the support of professional people in the health care disciplines as a factor contributing to the success of Philhaven.

10. Victor Weaver, interview, August 25, 1980.

11. The Hospital Study Committee of the bishop board was renamed the Religious Welfare Committee and became a nonvoting advisory committee to the board of directors. It continued to provide a direct link with the bishops.

12. Philhaven Hospital, Board of Directors Report, March 10, 1949.

13. However, several members of the original board of directors recall that this intention was implicit in their charge.

14. Report dated March 10, 1949.

15. This phrase was recorded at the time the gift was promised and was included in the transfer of property agreement. Horace Martin recalls, in private conversation with the author, that this was an oft-used expression of Graybill Landis.

16. Monroe Garber, interview.

17. Noah Kreider, interview, August 8, 1980.

18. Weaver, *ibid*.

19. Kreider, *ibid*.

20. Metzler, *ibid*.

21. Kreider, *ibid*., relates that J. Paul Graybill "brought" the name to the board of directors.

22. Elvin G. Lefever, "The Philhaven Hospital," *Mennonite Community* (March 1952), pp. 10, 11.

23. Kauffman, *ibid*.

24. "Articles of Incorporation," Lancaster Mennonite Hospitals, May 11, 1949.

25. However, the initial contact to consider this proposal seems to have been an invitation from representatives of the Community Chest (as reflected in the board minutes and reports).

26. Rowland Shank, interviews, December 4 and 21, 1981.

27. Metzler, *ibid*.

Chapter 6

1. Minutes, Central Area Planning and Advisory Committee, December 11, 1952.

2 .Minutes, Central Area Planning and Advisory Committee, December 6, 1947.

3. Minutes, Advisory Committee, May 24, 1951.

4. Minutes, Advisory Committee, October 9, 1954.

5. Thomas F. Morrow and Boyd Peak, "A Philosophy of Helping and Its Application in a Private Psychiatric Hospital"; Morrow, "The Essence of Helping"; and Harold Vogt, "Coordinating Community Resources for Mental Health"; Prairie View, 1958, unpublished papers.

6. Morrow, "Essence," p. 1.

7. Minutes, Mennonite Mental Health Services, October 17-18, 1958.

8. Elmer M. Ediger, "Crisis in an Institution: The Near Closing of Prairie View," unpublished, 1978, p. 3.

9. *Ibid.*, p. 5.

10. *Ibid.*, p. 6.

11. *Ibid.*, p. 10.

12. R. Glasscote, D. Sanders, H. M. Forstner, A. R. Foley (Washington, D.C.: American Psychiatric Association, 1964.)

13. Merrill F. Raber and Jane Hershberger in *New Directions for Mental Health Services*, Number 9 (1981), pp. 61-74.

14. This collaboration is described in a study of Prairie View by McClug and Stunden in 1970.

15. Annual Report to the Prairie View Board, 1979.

16. Executive Director's Report to the Prairie View Board, December 21, 1977.

17. Merrill F. Raber, "An Approach for Cultivating Personal and Leadership Skills in the Community," *Primary Prevention, An Idea Whose Time Has Come*, Edited by Donald C. Klein (Rockville, MD: NIMH, 1977).

18. Raymond M. Glasscote, et. al. (Washington D.C.: American Psychiatric Association, 1980).

19. "Prairie View: Making the Whole Community Therapeutic," in *The Mental Health of Rural America*, U.S. Dept. of Health, Education, and Welfare and NIMH, 1973, pp. 93-101.

Chapter 8

1. Delmar Stahly, Report to MMHS, MMHS Minutes, May 25, 1954.

2. This interest could go back as early as the MCC decision on January 3, 1947, when the first three MCC institutions were authorized (so Elmer Ediger, the first MCC mental health director, 1947-51). E. C. Bender from Elkhart was on the MMHS board and Harold Bender of Goshen was on the MCC Executive Committee, so two persons from the area were in key positions of influence. After the three MCC hospitals were established and operating by 1954, it is to be expected that the latent interest would become more open and vocal.

3. MCC Executive Committee Minutes, March 2, 1957.

4. Kauffman left in October 1957 to serve as administrator of Brook Lane. He was invited to return to Oaklawn as administrator the following year, but declined, expressing satisfaction with the Brook Lane position.

5. East Central Area Advisory Committee Minutes, October 14, 1957. The site committee recognized that there was "clear opportunity" in all three areas. At first

preference was given to the Ft. Wayne area because it "perhaps has more need for psychiatric assistance," as well as being centrally located.

6. "A counseling resource for the Christian Ministry — And a help in the Work of the Church," (Elkhart, Ind.: Oaklawn Psychiatric Center, /1962/). n.p.

7. Otto D. Klassen, interview, Elkhart, Indiana, November 6, 1981.

8. Oaklawn Minutes, October 12, 1960.

9. Klassen, Report to MMHS, MMHS Minutes, November 2-3, 1962.

10. A complicating factor was that Elkhart General Hospital, in planning a major fund drive, had engaged a consultant firm to assess the community potential. Their recommendations were quite negative toward the Oaklawn development. See E. P. Mininger, Report to MMHS, MMHS Minutes, July 16, 1960.

11. Klassen, interview.

12. Robert W. Hartzler, interview, Elkhart, Indiana, November 6, 1981.

13. Klassen, interview.

14. MMHS Minutes, April 11, 1958. The Penn Foundation, established in 1956, did not have beds but was located across the street from a general hospital where inpatients were admitted. See Chapter 7.

15. Karen Klink, "Oaklawn Home Project Gratifying," *Elkhart Truth*, November 1, 1966.

16. Klassen, interview.

17. Klassen, "The Church Creates a Mental Health Center: Oaklawn Psychiatric Center," *McCormick Quarterly*, vol. 21 (July, 1967), p. 54 ff.

18. Klassen, Report to Oaklawn Board, August 29, 1962

19. Klassen, Hartzler, interview.

20. Klassen, interview.

21. Hartzler, Report to Oaklawn Board, May 18, 1973.

22. Klassen, interview.

23. Oaklawn Minutes, March 10, 1960.

24. Oaklawn Psychiatric Center *Record Book*, 1971, p. 5.

25. Hartzler, "Evolution of the Mennonite Mental Health Centers," Papers and Responses Presented at the 25th Anniversary Program (Hagerstown, Maryland, October 1-2, 1971), p. 5.

26. "Oaklawn Psychiatric Center to Open Soon," Elkhart County Council of Churches *Visitor*, February, 1963. n.p.

27. "Oaklawn Center's Patients Range in Age Up to 80, Mostly 20 to 40,"

28. "The Comprehensive Community Mental Health Center. Concept and Challenge," (Washington, D.C.: U.S. Department of Health, Education, and Welfare, 1964).

29. Editorial, "Downtown Site Advisable for Halfway House," *Elkhart Truth*, September 18, 1972, n.p.; Editorial, "Fine Oaklawn Series," *Elkhart Truth*, October 12, 1972, n.p.

30. Editorial, "Deserved Praise for Oaklawn Center," *Elkhart Truth*, January 23, 1965, p. 4.

31. Hartzler, "Evolution," p. 5.

32. "The Oaklawn Psychiatric Center: Its Aspirations . . . Its Background . . . Its Needs . . . And Its People," (Elkhart, Ind.: Oaklawn Psychiatric Center, n.d.), n.p.

33. Klassen, interview.

34. Hartzler, Report to Oaklawn Board, May 20, 1971.

35. Hartzler, "Evolution," p. 6.

36. Klassen, interview.

Chapter 9

1. Arthur Jost, letter to W. Kevin Hegarty, November 8, 1961.

2. John C. Penner, interview, December 15, 1981.

3. H. Clair Amstutz, William T. Snyder, and Delmar Stahly, "MCC-MMHS Exploration in Bakersfield-Reedley, California" (December 5-6, 1962), pp. 2-4.

4. *Ibid.*, pp. 3-4.

5. *Ibid.*, p. 4.

6. Penner, *ibid.*

7. Delmar Stahly, "Report of Investigation of Bakersfield Mental Hospital Prospects" (December 17, 1962).

8. Roy Just, N. Meadoff, M.D., and Charles A. Davis, M.D., "Memorandum of Understanding" (based on March 20, 1963, meeting).

9. MMHS Board, "Memorandum of Understanding and Recommendation" (in response to the March 20, 1963, Memorandum of Understanding; April 10, 1963).

10. Ernest L. Boyer, "Summary of Meeting with Bakersfield Medical Staff Re: Proposed Kern View Hospital, April 24, 1963" (April 30, 1963). The delegation also included Roy Just and the executive committee of the Kings View board.

11. John C. Penner, letter to Daniel Horst and Arthur Jost, May 6, 1963.

12. Mennonite Central Committee, Executive Committee Minutes, "Resolution to Approve the Kern View Hospital Project," May 4, 1963.

13. The coordinating committee consisted of J. C. Penner, Henry Brandt, Roy Fast, and Abe S. Ediger.

14. Kings View Board of Directors and Greater Bakersfield Memorial Hospital Board of Directors, "Lease" (June 17, 1963).

15. Henry F. Brandt, interview, December 1981.

16. The first officers and board of directors of Kern View consisted of Henry F. Brandt, chairman; Abe S. Ediger, vice chairman; Roy Fast, secretary; John C. Penner, treasurer; Roy Cabe; Paul Engle; Charles Neff; and Marlin Riegsecker.

17. National Institute of Mental Health, Region IX, "Site Visit Report, March 18 and 19, 1969" (April 25, 1969), p. 10.

18. *Ibid.*, 10 pp.

19. Arthur Jost, interview, October 1, 1981.

20. Kern View Hospital Minutes, "Administrator's Report," February 17, 1970.

21. Kern View Hospital Minutes, Joint Conference Committee Reports, March 12, 1980; May 13, 1980; August 7, 1980; and November 13, 1980.

22. Patrick C. Barker, Ph.D., "Kern View Board of Directors' Retreat Summary of Proceedings, November 13-16, 1981."

Chapter 10

1. The eight conferences participating at that time were: Conference of Mennonites in Manitoba, Mennonite Brethren Conference, Evangelical Mennonite Conference, Evangelical Mennonite Mission Conference, Evangelical Mennonite Brethren Conference, Old Colony Mennonite Church, and the Sommerfelder Mennonite Church.

2. J. F. Pauls, interview, February 12, 1981.

3. Peter J. Klassen, *Mutual Aid Among Anabaptists* (Bluffton, Association of Mennonite Aid Societies, 1963).

4. P. J. B. Reimer, "Beginnings of Eden Mental Health Centre," *Red River Valley Echo* (November 21, 1969).

5. Ben Braun, interview, January 1981.

6. Pauls, *ibid*.

7. Other members of the study group were W. Enns from Winkler, Archie Penner from Steinbach, and G. G. Neufeld from Whitewater.

8. Esther R. Epp, *The Origins of Mennonite Central Committee (Canada)*, M.A. Thesis, University of Manitoba, 1980.

9. Pauls, *Ibid*.

10. Pauls, *ibid*.

11. *Ibid*.

12. Cornelia B. Johnson, *A History of Mental Health Care in Manitoba, A Local Manifestation of an International Social Movement*. M.A. Thesis, University of Manitoba, 1980, pp. 63-64.

13. John Boeckh, et al., "Property Values and Mental Health Facilities in Metropolitan Toronto," *Canadian Geographer* XXIV:3 (1980).

14. Johnson, *ibid*, p. 82.

15. Letter of Edward Johnson, Director of Psychiatric Services, Province of Manitoba, to George Johnson, Minister of Health, Province of Manitoba, April 10, 1962.

16. J. K. Klassen, interview, Spring, 1972.

17. *Ibid*.

18. MMHS Minutes, July 13, 1957.

19. MMHS Minutes, Chairman's Report, March 24-25, 1964.

20. Reimer, *ibid*.

21. The Steinbach Hospital was unavailable and the Concordia Hospital plan was rejected by the government because they wanted to decentralize their services.

22. Johnson, letter, *ibid*.

23. *Statutes of Manitoba*, Chapter 84, 1964, passed April 19, 1964.

24. Henry Guenther, M.D., interview, February 14, 1981.

25. Eden Mental Health Centre, Annual Report, 1967-68, Administrator's Report.

26. Braun, *ibid*.

27. Guenther, *ibid*.

28. J. C. Clarkson, *Mental Health and Retardation in Manitoba*, "A Report to the Minister of Health and Social Development, Province of Manitoba," 1963.

29. Braun, *ibid*.

30. Vernon Neufeld, "Report of Visit to Eden Mental Health Centre," April 22-24, 1976, 5 pp.

31. Guenther, *ibid*.

32. *Ibid*.

33. Part of Eden's South Central regional emphasis is reflected in the provision of satellite offices in Altona and Morden. These offices are staffed by Eden and provide services and follow-up treatment for its patients.

34. Community residences were first proposed by a government study published in government policy statement. These residences were to provide halfway living and treatment for people whose needs could not be met by current facilities. This program was meant to slowly reintegrate selected patients back into community life. As of 1980 none had been built.

35. Guenther, *ibid*.

Chapter 17

1. B. Pepper, M. Kirshner, H. Ryglewics, "The Young Adult Chronic Patient: Overview of a Population," *Hospital and Community Psychiatry* 32:7 (July 1981), pp. 463-69.

Selected Bibliography

Although the Notes comprise a comprehensive listing of the primary and secondary sources used in the preparation of this volume, the following list may be suggested for further reading.

Bloom, Bernard L. *Community Mental Health, A General Introduction.* Monterey, CA: Brooks/Cole Publishing Co., 1975.

Bockoven, J. Sanbourne, M.D. *Moral Treatment in American Psychiatry.* New York: Springer Publishing Co., Inc., 1963.

Foucault, Michel. *Madness and Civilization. A History of Insanity in the Age of Reason.* New York: Random House, Inc., 1965.

Gingerich, Melvin. *Service for Peace. A History of Mennonite Civilian Public Service.* Akron Pa: Mennonite Central Committee, 1949.

Glasscote, Raymond M. et. al. *The Community Mental Health Center. An Analysis of Existing Models.* Washington, D.C.: American Psychiatric Association, 1964.

Krahn, Cornelius, ed. *Mennonite Life.* October, 1966 (Vol. 21, no. 4), 147-89.

Maisel, Albert Q. "Bedlam 1946, Most U.S. Mental Hospitals Are a Shame and a Disgrace." *Life* magazine, May 6, 1946.

Stahly, Delmar; Rempel, C. J.; Schmidt, John R.; Krahn, C. "Mennonite and Mental Health." *Mennonite Life*, July, 1954.

Van Atta, Kim. *An Account of the Events Surrounding the Origin of Friends Hospital, and A Brief Description of the Early Years of Friends Asylum,* 1817-1820. Philadelphia: Friends Hospital, 1976.

Wright, Frank L., Jr. *Out of Sight, Out of Mind.* Philadelphia: National Mental Health Foundation, Inc., 1947.

Zilboorg, Gregory, M.D. and Henry, George W., M.D. *A History of Medical Psychology.* New York: W. W. Norton & Co., Inc., 1941.

For a more extensive bibliography, see *Mennonite Quarterly Review*, January, 1982. Available from AMS Press, Inc., 56 E. 13th, New York, NY 10003.

Index